To Tom Faciszewski.
With best wishes for
a successful future.

*Steven Heleman* K0
May '89

*Complex Foot Deformities
in Children*

# Complex Foot Deformities in Children

SHERMAN S. COLEMAN, M.D.

*Professor of Orthopedic Surgery*
*The University of Utah College of Medicine*
*Salt Lake City, Utah*

LEA & FEBIGER 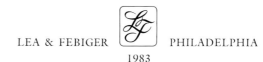 PHILADELPHIA
1983

LEA & FEBIGER
*600 Washington Square*
*Philadelphia, Pa. 19106*
*U.S.A.*

Library of Congress Cataloging in Publication Data

Coleman, Sherman S., 1922–
   Complex foot deformities in children.

   Bibliography: p.
   Includes index.
   1. Foot—Abnormalities.   2. Pediatric orthopedia.
I. Title.   [DNLM: 1. Foot—Abnormalities. WE 883 C692c]
RD781.C64        618.92′097585        82-15249
ISBN 0-8121-0857-4                        AACR2

*Printed in the United States of America*

Print Number: 3  2  1

*To Michael, Don, and Jennifer*

# Preface

Complex foot deformities in children represent a special challenge to the orthopedic surgeon. One is dealing not only with deformities of substantial proportions that may have multiple etiologic factors, but also with the element of skeletal growth. The effect of growth upon these deformities adds a special dimension that does not exist in the adult foot. Most of these deformities require some form of surgical treatment and bracing, and some form of therapy must continue throughout the entire period of the child's growth and development. As with most musculoskeletal deformities in children, the earlier the deformity can be recognized and its behavior established, the more effectively can a program of treatment be synthesized and implemented.

The implications of a child's foot deformity can often be far reaching. What initially may seem to be a simple, localized abnormality in fact may be only the outward and more obvious manifestation of a much more severe, underlying abnormality in the peripheral or central nervous system, or it may serve as an index of suspicion for the possible presence of other significant or substantial coexisting abnormalities. Thus, the potential significance and implication of a complex foot deformity will be emphasized and re-emphasized throughout the body of this text.

The components and pathologic descriptions of foot deformities require proper definition, and it is important to reduce these components to the simplest degree possible. Otherwise, one may become lost in a morass of controversial concepts, many of which trace their origin to definitions not well established or agreed upon. The terms pronation and supination, for example, have totally different meanings, depending upon whether one is referring to the forefoot, the hindfoot, or a relationship between the two. Inversion and eversion of the foot are complex positions, but adduction and abduction are much simpler descriptions, nearly always referring to the forefoot. An effort will be made to clarify descriptive definitions of the components of a foot deformity so as to establish a clearer understanding of these abnormalities.

A common-sense approach to the treatment of any musculoskeletal abnormality usually can be synthesized when one has three important sets of information: (1) a thorough knowledge of the etiology and pathogenesis of the deformity, (2) an accurate definition of the problem and its probable behavior, and (3) the options available for treatment. The intent of this text is to develop these three issues as fully and completely as possible. Parochial and self-favored methods of treatment must assume some degree of importance, but hopefully the reader will recognize that they are based upon the fundamentals mentioned earlier.

The text has been purposely restricted to the complex foot problems in children, largely because these are the deformities that provide the greatest therapeutic challenge and that require the most substantial knowledge and technical expertise in order to be appropriately treated. I hope that the narrow scope of this book will not lessen its value in the mind of the orthopedic surgeon who is genuinely interested in the problems of the child's foot.

As I reflect over the many years during which I have wrestled with these problems, it becomes impressively clear to me that we have come a long way in our understanding of these challenging conditions, and this, coupled with our improved surgical expertise, has enabled us to approach the care of these foot deformities more confidently and with greater success. This comforting and reassuring reflection must not, however, dull our awareness of the fact that future, improved knowledge, concepts, and technology may soon render obsolete some of our current therapeutic approaches. We therefore must temper any radical or rigid tendencies in our current care of these problems, and yet we must steadfastly adhere to an established and proven series of principles and concepts that will guide our hands along the way. Thus, in some areas concerning the technical aspects of treatment, some aspects of this book may be outdated at the time of its publication. Hopefully, however, the principles and concepts upon which these techniques are based will stand a reasonable test of time.

In preparing this manuscript, many individuals have been involved almost from the start. Most important and indispensable are those children whose foot problems provided the living laboratory, so to speak, that has permitted me to test and develop the concepts and approaches enunciated herein. Secondly, I have depended greatly upon my professional colleagues who have provided an endless source of information, factual and clinical, much of which I have utilized in composing these pages.

The literary research for many of the chapters has been done largely by former and current residents. Specifically, I am indebted to Drs. Lonnie Paulos, Stanley Bigos, Stanley Moss, Douglas Kehl, Bruce Blackstone, and Gary Bradley for their invaluable assistance in the preparation of several of the chapters. Many of the photographic and the radiographic studies were accomplished at the Shriners Hospital in Salt Lake City. The technicians primarily responsible were Mr. Noran Hagan and Mr. Philip Wood. I also wish to thank Mrs. Tarza Peterson, Mrs. Grace Miya, Miss Seanna Horan, and Miss Lisa Brauner for their dedicated secretarial and editorial assistance. The original drawings of the surgical procedures and other pictorial illustrations were provided by Mr. Julian Maack. Lastly, I must acknowledge the encouragement, tolerance, and understanding of my wife and family. Under the best of circumstances, it is not an easy task to write a book, even one as modest as this, but without the support of one's family, it would be impossible.

*Salt Lake City, Utah*

Sherman S. Coleman

# Contents

*Complex Foot Deformities*
*in Children*

# 1

# Evaluation and Classification

The problems posed by foot deformities in children are especially challenging because of the many factors unique to the growing foot. The complexities of the deformities resulting from many different etiologic factors further add to the challenge. In order to define the problems and to synthesize the appropriate solutions, one must be conversant with the vocabulary of foot deformities, familiar with their clinical behavior, and thoroughly knowledgeable about all therapeutic methods, both operative and nonoperative. This level of expertise requires considerable experience in the management of all types of children's foot problems.

Foot problems encountered commonly in children have been excluded from this discussion, which emphasizes rather the more uncommon, complex foot abnormalities that usually or often require surgical treatment. These particular problems are extremely diversified, not only from an etiologic point of view, but also from the standpoint of their pathomechanics and pathologic anatomy. The treatment of each of these is equally diverse and varied.

The primary goal of this text is to outline a common-sense and logical approach to these foot problems in children. In this respect, not only is definition of the problem a primary objective; the concepts of treatment and the techniques available to correct the deformities will also be presented.

Common foot problems are excluded from this discussion because these abnormalities many times are self-correcting, often have no need for complex treatment, and, in general, rarely require surgical correction. The foot deformities specifically excluded are metatarsus varus, infantile hallux varus, *physiologic* flexible flatfeet, splayfoot, infantile metatarsus primus varus, syndactyly, bunions, and other less common but rather simple problems. Also excluded are those foot deformities

*Concepts and Definitions*

associated with terminal limb deficiencies, a subject covered more appropriately in a treatise on length inequality and amputation of lower limbs.

Thus, the foot problems to be included in this text are those static or progressive deformities, both developmental (congenital) and acquired, that often require surgical intervention to achieve and maintain correction. Each one poses its own set of problems and must be approached individually.

The combination of diverse etiologic factors and complex pathologic characteristics makes a "cookbook" approach impossible. Yet, using fundamental concepts and principles, a rational and logical approach to treatment usually can be synthesized. Implicit in such a discussion is the need to agree upon the semantics and terms employed.

The term *talipes* is derived from the Latin meaning ankle (*tali-*) and foot (*pes*).[7,9,10] Thus, when used, it refers simply to a nonspecific deformity involving the ankle and foot. To some extent, this word has been misused in the past, because in many instances the ankle joint per se is not involved in the abnormality. Furthermore, the deformity is most appropriately described or implied by the suffix, e.g., equinovarus, calcaneovalgus, cavovarus. Thus, I feel that the term *talipes* is redundant and for this reason it will not be employed in this text. Far more important is the etiologic term (prefix) that identifies a more substantial issue from the diagnostic and therapeutic standpoint, e.g., paralytic equinovarus versus congenital (developmental or antenatal) equinovarus, and so forth.

Therefore, two basic terms become paramount in the definition of all foot deformities, namely, (a) the etiology of the deformity and (b) the associated or resultant descriptive, pathologic anatomy. These two determinations have great influence not only upon the diagnosis but also upon the treatment and prognosis of the particular foot deformity. Thus, from both a didactic and a practical point of view, it is important to recognize that the etiology is relatively specific but that the pathology is descriptive; therefore, it must be clearly understood that an anatomic foot deformity can result from a variety of causes.

It is essential to comprehend this simple but important concept in order to analyze the problems logically and effectively and to implement treatment of these complex foot deformities in children. Etiologically, therefore, two major categories of foot deformity can be identified: (a) congenital (developmental and antenatal) and (b) acquired. The latter can be considered further from the standpoint of whether the deformity is the result of neuromuscular, myopathic, or traumatic cause.

Specific definition or description of the components of a foot deformity requires agreement with respect to the terms employed in describing an abnormality of the foot, agreement not easily found among those who have written on foot deformities. Definitions all too frequently reflect time-honored but often inaccurate and less informed concepts of foot problems. Therefore, it becomes necessary to resort to the use of basic definitions and arbitrary interpretation when describing some of the more complex foot abnormalities. In order to appreciate the deviations from normal, however, it is essential that the normal, descriptive anatomy of the foot be understood. This means that the reader must have a thorough comprehension of the normal plantigrade foot and not simply a knowledge of the gross (surgical) anatomy of the foot. Anyone who performs surgery on a child's foot is assumed to possess this knowledge; thus, this text does not discuss the gross (surgical) anatomy of the foot.

Descriptively, the plantigrade foot enjoys considerable latitude with respect to what is considered normal. Much depends not only upon the age of the patient but also upon the normal variations that can be found from one patient to another. Despite the fact that the foot of a 1- or 2-year-old differs to some degree in appearance from that of an adolescent, however, certain basic, important similarities can be identified. During the first year or two after ambulation begins, in outward appearance, the weight-bearing foot normally exhibits no appreciable longitudinal arch. This is largely due to the normal presence of fatty tissue in the plantar aspect of the foot. Thus, what appears to be a "flatfoot" is considered more appropriately a "fat foot." This phenomenon, when coupled with the common physiologic knock-knee configuration that exists in children of this age, does indeed make the foot look even flatter. As the child grows and matures, and as the various weight-bearing and other functional stresses are placed upon the foot, the normal longitudinal arch gradually appears. It does so at different ages in different children, again reflecting the variations of normal development. Usually, during the third year of life, a distinct longitudinal arch can be identified, and this functional arch normally can be accentuated by having the child walk on his toes. During stance, the foot normally bears weight on all plantar bony prominences, but the calcaneus and the heads of the first and fifth metatarsals bear most of the weight, much as a "tripod" (see Chapter 4).

*The Anatomic and Functional Units of the Foot and Ankle*

The basic functional and anatomic segments of the foot and ankle consist of the forefoot, the midfoot, the hindfoot, and the ankle joint. From a diagnostic, biomechanical, and therapeutic standpoint, these components must be clearly understood in order that further meaningful discussion can develop regarding problem definition and appropriate treatment.[6]

It is difficult to find a specific description of the anatomic and functional components of the foot and ankle. In most writings, these have not been defined accurately. Because of the importance of such a description, from both a diagnostic and a therapeutic standpoint, it is essential that these anatomic and functional units be defined. To some extent, the separation as outlined below is arbitrary, but for the most part it is based upon an analysis of the manner in which the foot and ankle function in clinical situations.

The functional anatomy of the ankle and foot must be considered an integral structure, because the anatomy and function of both are closely inter-related. Many of the musculotendinous units that act upon the foot also cross the ankle joint and thereby indirectly affect the ankle. Because no direct muscular or tendinous attachment of any muscle of the leg to the talus exists, all active motions at the *ankle* must be achieved indirectly by motor units that act upon adjacent bones of the foot. Also, in a normally functioning ankle and foot, any motion that occurs in one component almost always affects another. It is reasonable to conclude, therefore, that from a *purely scientific* point of view, the entire ankle and foot should be treated as one unit, and that any attempt to subdivide them anatomically or functionally creates an artificial situation. Furthermore, the foot and ankle each are made up of so many bones, joints, ligaments, tendons, and muscles that it becomes impossible to define motions that occur simultaneously in all parts. In addition, it is impossible to categorize the various components of the foot and ankle so that one may define accurately what takes place between each under varying circumstances.

In view of the foregoing, if one attempts to subdivide the foot and ankle into their component parts, it is obviously not possible to do so without there being substantial overlap in their anatomy as well as in their function. By means of certain *clinical* situations, however, and from a practical point of view, it can be shown that such a subdivision is feasible. It is well known, for example, that in the presence of an ankle arthrodesis, the foot can function in a *relatively* normal fashion. Furthermore, in the presence of a triple arthrodesis, the ankle and other portions of the foot can function normally, at least from a practical standpoint. In order for this to occur, however, the adjacent articulations must alter their function somewhat because of the greater compensatory motion that is imposed on the unfused components due to the loss of motion in the adjacent, fused joints. Based upon these observations in practical, clinical situations, and recognizing the need to agree on definitions of the foot and the ankle, I believe that the following arbitrary anatomic divisions are justified on an anatomic and clinical basis.

THE ANKLE

By definition, the ankle is a *joint* composed of three bones; namely, the tibia, fibula, and talus. It moves almost exclusively around a single axis that is established and governed by the articulations between the three bones and also by the supporting ligamentous structures. The supporting structures include the deltoid ligament, the lateral collateral ligaments, and the ankle joint capsule. The medial and lateral collateral ligaments also cross the subtalar joint and, therefore, a stabilizing effect is exerted upon the foot complex as well as upon the ankle. The major motor units acting upon the ankle are the triceps surae and the anterior tibial muscle and tendon, although, as noted earlier, neither of these inserts directly onto the talus, and each moves the talus indirectly by virtue of attachments to adjacent bones. These two major motor units also exert an effect upon other components of the ankle-foot complex; however, they are considered most appropriately to be part of the ankle because their major effect is upon ankle motion.

This component of the foot is comprised of the talus, the calcaneus, the cuboid, and the navicular. From a practical point of view, the calcaneus, cuboid, and navicular bones move as a unit about the talus, not only functionally but also anatomically. The combined joint produced by these bones and their articulations with the talus has been called the peritalar (triple) joint. Any substantial motion that takes place at one portion of this joint must be accompanied by a comparable degree of motion at the other. Most of the motion of this portion of the foot occurs at the talocalcaneal and the talonavicular joints, and an integral relationship also is found between the motions that occur at the subtalar joint and those that take place at the talonavicular joint. As noted earlier, this motion can occur even if the ankle is fused or if the joints distal to the talonavicular and calcaneocuboid joints are fused.

THE HINDFOOT

The motion at the subtalar joint occurs largely around a single, oblique axis, and the motion at the talonavicular joint takes place around essentially the same axis. Some degree of dorsiflexion and plantar flexion can occur at the talonavicular joint as well as the calcaneocuboid joint. This, however, does not materially alter the concept that these joints function as a unit. It is, therefore, appropriately called the hindfoot (Fig. 1-1).

This unit is composed of the distal halves of the navicular and cuboid bones, and it extends distally to include all of the cuneiforms as well as the proximal portion of the five metatarsals and their associated joints.

THE MIDFOOT

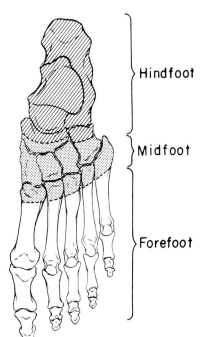

Hindfoot

Midfoot

Forefoot

FIG. 1-1. The major components of the foot. The bones and joints shaded with oblique lines represent the hindfoot. The stippled skeletal structures outline the midfoot, and the forefoot is white.

In contrast to the peritalar joint, little motion takes place in the midfoot articulations, and any motion that does occur consists mainly of dorsiflexion and plantar flexion.

A functional overlap exists between the midfoot and the hindfoot in that both are involved somewhat in dorsiflexion and plantar flexion of the foot. The function of the motor units of the foot further supports this anatomic and functional concept of the midfoot. Thus, the peroneal and anterior tibial tendons insert on the midfoot. The posterior tibial tendon inserts partially on the navicular tubercle, a defined part of the hindfoot, but it also inserts into the midfoot by means of its more distal, broad insertion into the cuneiforms and the base of the first metatarsal. This anatomic factor assumes importance when dealing with operative correction of congenital equinovarus (see Chapter 2).

The proximal metatarsals can be justifiably considered as part of the midfoot by virtue of the anatomy and function of the tarsometatarsal articulations. The first tarsometatarsal joint somewhat resembles the calcaneocuboid joint in that it is a saddle-type joint. In and of itself, this joint is capable of independent motion. The second tarsometatarsal joint is a mortise type of joint because the base of the second metatarsal articulates with, and lies within a slot created by, all three cuneiforms as well as the base of the third metatarsal. The anatomic character of this articulation, therefore, allows little functional motion. The remainder of the articulations of the tarsometatarsal joints are fairly flat and also permit only limited motion (Fig. 1-1).

THE FOREFOOT

In keeping with the anatomic and functional definitions of the various parts of the foot as previously described, the forefoot is composed of the remaining distal portions of the metatarsals and all of the phalanges (Fig. 1-1). Considerable motion takes place in all of the metatarsophalangeal joints. Although this motion is mainly dorsiflexion and plantar flexion, some degree of rotation, as well as adduction and abduction, can also occur. The motion of these joints far exceeds that of the joints of the midfoot. The long toe flexors and extensors insert into the phalanges of the toes, but in doing so, these motor units cross the other portions of the foot and ankle. Because of this, the tendons acting on the forefoot must exert an effect indirectly upon the other portions of the foot and ankle.

As will be seen in subsequent chapters that concern themselves with the surgical treatment of pathologic conditions involving various components of the ankle and foot, treatment is usually directed towards either the forefoot, the midfoot, the hindfoot, or the ankle, depending upon the identified major site of the problem. In all major instances, however, it is essential to consider the various segments of the foot and ankle as an inter-related complex, because disturbances in one portion of the foot may produce, or may be the result of, alterations in another segment of the foot and/or ankle. Clearly, the overall problem must be defined correctly before the appropriate solution can be synthesized properly. It is essential not only to identify specific deformities, but also to assess them according to whether they are supple (flexible) or rigid. This fundamental concept must be accepted so that the methods of treatment of these complex foot deformities can be properly understood and executed.

In the clinical examination at any age during growth, the *configuration* and the *flexibility* of the various components of the foot and the ankle are the two most important determinations. At birth and during the neonatal period, appraisal of the *configuration* should take into account the many intrauterine positional factors that temporarily can affect the appearance of the foot. For example, adduction or varus of the forefoot (metatarsus varus) is encountered often in the newborn just because of the fetal position that the child assumes in the few weeks or months prior to birth. The opposite configuration, ankle dorsiflexion and heel valgus, and unusual flattening of the longitudinal arch (calcaneovalgus) can also be seen commonly, likewise owing to antenatal postural or positional factors.

Except under unusual circumstances, these are considered variations from the normal, and they rarely require treatment of any kind. Extremes of these foot configurations and other aberrations at birth or any time during growth may indicate a more significant foot problem. Examples include equinus, equinovarus, cavovarus, calcaneocavus, and other such deformities. Depending upon whether they are flexible or rigid, and also depending upon the roentgenographic evaluation, they may or may not become diagnostically and therapeutically significant.

The determination of *flexibility* is an important factor in the evaluation of a child's foot, not only during the neonatal period but also throughout growth. A rigid foot usually means that an organic, structural abnormality exists, one that requires sophisticated and often extensive and prolonged treatment. Frequently, surgical intervention will be required to achieve and maintain correction. On the other hand, an unusually flexible or "floppy" foot may indicate an underlying neuromuscular or other constitutional abnormality, and these possibilities therefore mandate further investigation.

Once the influence of intrauterine positioning no longer exists or is outgrown, the normal infant's foot will exhibit a rather free range of motion. Although some variation may be apparent from one child to another, certain consistent ranges of passive motion will be evident. Giannestras lists the normal passive excursions of the foot and ankle during infancy and childhood shown in Table 1-1.[2]

It should be emphasized again that the foot and ankle nearly always must be examined together, not only because of the difficulty one can experience in separating these segments from each other, as noted previously, but also because the perceived motions may predominate in either the ankle, the foot and ankle, the hindfoot, the midfoot, or the forefoot, depending upon the examination.

*Active* ranges of motion vary substantially from *passive* ranges, largely because muscle action normally is not capable of isolating the

TABLE 1-1. *Normal Passive Motion Ranges*

| | | |
|---|---|---|
| Flexion (plantar flexion): | 50° ± 5° | (foot and ankle) |
| Extension (dorsiflexion): | | |
| Relative: | | |
| Tarsal joints unlocked: | 30° ± 5° | (combined foot and ankle) |
| True: | | |
| Tarsal joints locked: | 10° ± 5° | (almost exclusively ankle) |
| Eversion of foot: | 10° ± 5° | (forefoot and hindfoot) |
| Inversion of foot: | 10° ± 5° | (forefoot and hindfoot) |
| Adduction of forefoot: | 20° ± 5° | (forefoot) |
| Abduction of forefoot: | 15° ± 5° | (forefoot) |

different components of the foot and ankle, as just described. For example, effective forefoot adduction and abduction cannot be accomplished actively without some degree of involvement of the hindfoot, as well as ankle dorsiflexion or plantar flexion. Nor can "true" ankle motions be *actively* demonstrated. Thus, in appraising *active* foot and ankle motions, it is far more important to carefully evaluate the strength and action of the individual muscles, rather than active ranges of motion. Consequently, an accurate appraisal of muscle function, coupled with a careful study of passive motions, can adequately establish the static and dynamic functional status of the foot.

In the physical examination of the child's foot, one should establish a systematic approach that takes into account the following determinants: (a) weight-bearing or simulated weight-bearing, (b) passive flexibility, (c) muscle power, (d) sensation and reflex activity, and finally, (e) the relationships of the various bones to each other. In this final consideration, one must become familiar with certain bony prominences and depressions found in the normal foot (Fig. 1-2). Substantial deviations from these normal landmarks usually have diagnostic significance.

THE WEIGHT-BEARING FOOT

The appearance of the child's foot *in stance* varies widely from one patient to another; however, the most important determinations involve the longitudinal arch, the forefoot (whether it is plantarflexed, adducted, or abducted), the hindfoot (whether it is in the varus or valgus position), and the ankle joint, i.e., is the entire foot in equinus or is it in calcaneus? Normally, the ambulatory child appears to have a flatfoot in the first year or two of ambulation; the forefoot is slightly abducted, the heel exhibits about 5° of valgus, and there is no fixed equinus or calcaneus.

FLEXIBILITY

The importance of this determination is the significance of any *lack* of flexibility (rigidity) or, on the other hand, any degree of *excessive* flexibility (floppiness). The rigid foot usually portends a substantial problem of *therapy,* whereas the unusually flexible foot may suggest a problem in *diagnosis* (neuromuscular disturbance).

MUSCLE POWER

The method of evaluating motor power will vary greatly with the age

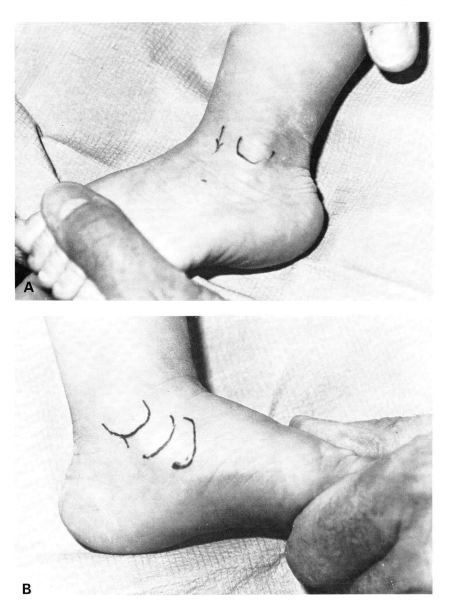

FIG. 1-2. **A,** The bony prominences and depressions present in the normal child's foot consist of a clearly defined lateral malleolus and a prominent (deep) sinus tarsus (arrow) just anterior to the lateral malleolus. **B,** On the medial side, the three easily palpable bony landmarks are the medial malleolus, the head of the talus, and the tuberosity of the navicular. These bony prominences normally lie in a direct line with each other and, when accompanied by the normal depression in the sinus tarsus on the lateral side (**A**), indicate normal relationships of the tarsal bones (**B**).

of the patient. Infants and young children rarely will be able to exhibit voluntary, selective muscle action upon command. Thus, one must resort to various indirect methods such as stroking the medial, lateral, or plantar surface of the foot in order to elicit a reflex response. By experience and intuition, the muscle power exhibited by such maneuvers can be reasonably estimated with respect to the norm. In older children, the muscle evaluations can be accomplished much more accurately once the child can respond voluntarily to commands.

SENSATION AND
REFLEX ACTIVITIY

Evaluating the sensation and reflex activity also requires a certain degree of variation in approach, largely dictated by the age of the child. In infants and young children, the evaluation of sensation requires the use of painful stimuli coupled with an evaluation of the child's reflex response, e.g., pulling away or crying. In older children, sensation can be appraised much more accurately. With experience, deep tendon reflexes are relatively easy to elicit at any age.

One must recall that certain pathologic reflexes are normally present during the first 12 months of life. In fact, Duncan observed that certain primitive tonic reflex movements of the foot in normal children can be a postural cause of deformity. He found that these reflexes could be readily elicited at birth, but that they disappear in an orderly sequence during the first year of life. Duncan preferred the term "tonic" because the reflex movements occur slowly, in contrast to the abrupt response of a tendon jerk. He identified four tonic reflexes of the foot: (1) the toe-gripping reflex, (2) the inversion reflex, (3) the eversion reflex, and (4) the dorsiflexion reflex.[1]

As noted earlier, these reflexes gradually disappear during the first year of life. On the other hand, if they persist, a foot deformity may easily result. This latter observation is well borne out by the deformities that can be seen in older children with cerebral palsy or in children in whom maturation of the central nervous system may be delayed for one reason or another. Duncan believed that these tonic reflexes may "by their occasional unopposed action, cause deformity."[1]

BONE RELATIONSHIPS

As noted previously, the physical examination of the bony prominences and the relationships of the skeletal structures in the foot are some of the most neglected yet important methods of evaluating a child's foot. The most easily palpated prominences are the medial and lateral malleoli, the calcaneus, and the head of the talus (Fig. 1-2). Less prominent are the tarsal navicular, the base of the fifth metatarsal, and the metatarsal heads. On the medial side of the foot, three prominences normally should be readily identified: the medial malleolus, the head of the talus, and the tarsal navicular (Fig. 1-2). On the lateral side, the most important topographic feature is the depression in the sinus tarsus created by the normal divergence of the talus and calcaneus. When this depression is shallow or virtually nonexistent, or when it is deep and exaggerated, one must suspect a major alteration in the talocalcaneal relationships.

A properly and carefully performed physical examination conducted in the young child (under 2 years of age) can usually give more reliable information about the true relationships of the skeletal structures than can be extracted from a roentgenographic examination. Because the skeletal structures are so largely cartilaginous during this period, the roentgenograms do not always reflect the true shape and the relationships of the bones. On the other hand, roentgenograms taken at strategic intervals can provide helpful information mostly in terms of verifying or supporting a clinical interpretation.

In evaluating a growing child's foot, it is important to recall that in the newborn and the early years of infancy a substantial portion of the skeletal structure of the foot is unossified. In this regard, it is similar to radiographic determinations in other developing skeletal structures, such as the hip and spine, in which considerable latitude of interpretation must be exercised. Consequently, all determinations must take into account both the ossified and the unossified cartilaginous structure. Therefore, unless one appreciates circumstantial radiographic considerations, the true structure of the foot may not be appropriately established. Three observations are foremost in evaluating the foot of a growing child: (1) The presence and *orderly appearance* of the ossification centers, (2) the *shape* and *size* of the visible ossification centers, and (3) the *relationships* of the centers to each other (Fig. 1-3). In order to appreciate variations from normal, it is essential to review the normal skeletal growth and development of the foot.

Standard roentgenographic studies include anteroposterior, lateral, and oblique views. These are the most well established and useful radiographic methods of evaluating the child's foot. In order to extract the most reliable and useful information, however, it is essential that the anteroposterior and lateral determinations be made with the foot in the weight-bearing or simulated weight-bearing position. If this is not done, it is impossible to attach any reliable significance to the *relationships* of the bones to each other.

Clearly, weight-bearing roentgenographic studies cannot be accomplished in young infants or in children who, for one reason or

*Radiographic Evaluation of the Foot*

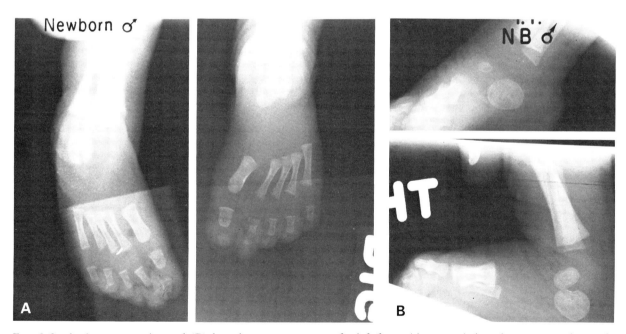

FIG. 1-3. **A,** Anteroposterior and **(B)** lateral roentgenograms of a left foot with congenital equinovarus are shown, in contrast to a normal right foot. Observe the smaller, abnormally shaped ossification centers in the left foot. The talus and calcaneus are parallel in both anteroposterior and lateral projections. The forefoot is in equinus. Compare it to the normal right foot.

another, cannot stand. In these situations, it becomes necessary that the physician or the informed x-ray technician position the foot so as to simulate weight-bearing (see Fig. 5-2). In some circumstances, various types of special positioning of the foot must be accomplished in which the physician holds the foot in specific positions at the time the film is taken. The manner in which the technician directs the x-ray beam is equally important in obtaining reliable evaluation because, if the foot is improperly positioned or the x-ray beam inappropriately directed, misleading and sometimes confusing observations will result.

Simple anteroposterior and lateral standing films are usually sufficient to evaluate the configuration of the foot and the relationships of the skeletal structures in the weight-bearing position. If one suspects a tarsal coalition, or if special positioning is needed, additional films clearly will be required (see Chapter 9). As a rule, an oblique, non-weight-bearing view of the foot is an essential, basic diagnostic study in older children.

Occasionally it is important to establish and quantitate the degree of hindfoot varus or valgus existing in a foot. The technique for such a determination has been developed by Paulos, Coleman, and Samuelson.[5] The patient stands in a full weight-bearing position on a special Plexiglas platform, and the following roentgenographic exposures are taken using a standard x-ray machine: (1) The first view is a routine anteroposterior mortise examination of the ankle, with the leg rotated inwardly about 20° so that the malleoli are equidistant from the plane of the film. (2) With the leg maintained in the same position, a second view is obtained on the same cassette, with the x-ray tube lowered and angled upward from a position 20° below the horizontal, thus providing a double exposure of the involved foot and ankle (Fig. 1-4) in two planes.

As seen in Figure 1-5, it is now possible to separate the image of the forefoot from that of the hindfoot and ankle, and thus, the relationship of the talus to the calcaneus can be measured accurately using easily recognized bony landmarks. A perpendicular line is erected, ex-

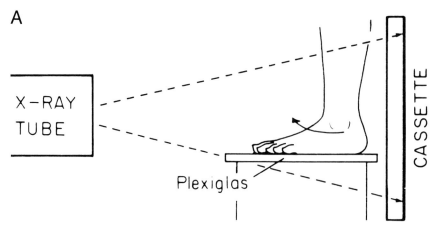

FIG. 1-4. **A,** The x-ray beam is shown as it is projected in the routine anteroposterior roentgenogram of the ankle with the malleoli held parallel to each other.

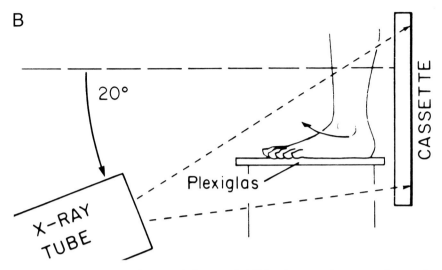

FIG. 1-4. **B,** The x-ray tube is angled upwards 20° for the second exposure (see text). (Paulos, L. E., Coleman, S. S., and Samuelson, K. M.: Pes cavovarus. Review of a surgical approach using selective soft-tissue procedures. J. Bone Joint Surg., *62A:942,* 1980.)

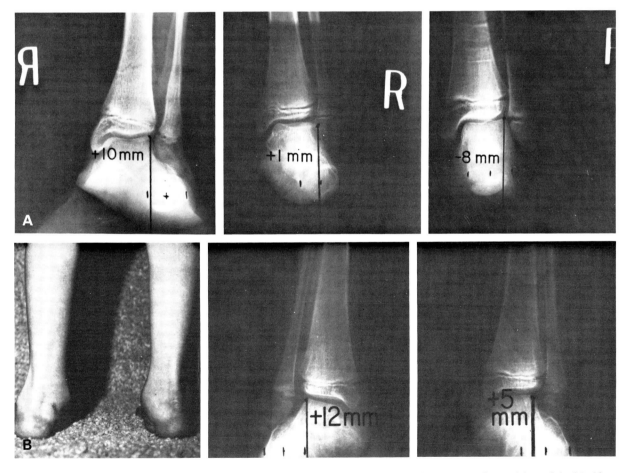

FIG. 1-5. **A,** Utilizing the technique shown in Figure 1-4, these roentgenograms demonstrate the position of the hindfoot in valgus, normal, and varus positions. (Paulos, L. E., Coleman, S. S., and Samuelson, K. M.: Pes cavovarus. Review of a surgical approach using selective soft-tissue procedures. J. Bone Joint Surg., *62A:942,* 1980.) **B,** The manner by which the hindfoot valgus is reflected by this roentgenographic technique can be readily seen.

tending from the superior lateral corner of the talar dome to the weight-bearing surface of the foot represented by the Plexiglas shadow seen at the bottom of the roentgenogram. The medial and lateral cortices of the calcaneus are marked, and the distance between these points is measured. The center mark is then struck at exactly half the measured distance. In the normal foot, the center mark falls within several millimeters on each side of the line perpendicular to the line of weight bearing. In the *varus* hindfoot, the center mark falls far medial to the perpendicular line; in the *valgus* hindfoot, it falls far lateral.

Lovell has employed arthrography in an effort to evaluate the true configuration and the relationships of the tarsal bones and the ankle joints in infants and young children, especially those with clubfeet.[4] Although this diagnostic measure is conceptually attractive, Lovell has found from a *practical* point of view that it has not provided any more information than that obtained by the routine roentgenograms mentioned previously, provided that it is coupled with a carefully performed physical examination of the foot as described earlier. I have had no personal experience with arthrography, being content with the information obtained by the roentgenographic evaluation procedures outlined previously.

Steel has explored the use of a computerized axial tomographic (CAT) scan in defining foot deformities in children.[8] He performed studies in children with equinovarus deformities, but was unable to identify any special observations that would assist in the evaluation of tarsal bone configuration or their relationships. Considering the cost and potentially increased radiation exposure of such examinations, the paucity of new or helpful information obtained by the CAT studies renders them unnecessary and inappropriate, at least at our present state of knowledge.

## The Implications of Foot Deformities in Children

When a foot deformity is encountered in a child at any age, certain specific questions should surface: Is this a positional deformity? Is it a developmental (congenital) abnormality? Is it the result of some neurologic or neuromuscular disorder? Or is it a teratologic manifestation? The obvious importance of these determinations is the bearing that they have upon treatment and prognosis. A positional deformity usually will respond effectively to a conservative nonsurgical program. A developmental anomaly will usually present all of the major therapeutic challenges that are innate and unique to all developmental abnormalities; often it may also be genetically determined. Those abnormalities that result from a neurologic problem require that the basic underlying neurologic defect be defined, and teratologic problems almost always will be accompanied by other visceral or skeletal abnormalities. Usually, treatment of these teratologic problems will be complicated and difficult, and often the result will be unsatisfactory. The implication of a developmental infantile or childhood foot deformity therefore becomes rather ominous when the far-reaching possibilities are fully appreciated.

From the foregoing, it must be clear that the exact nature of a child's foot deformity must be accurately described, defined, and documented. If the underlying cause is not readily apparent, a conscientious and thorough search must be carried out.

Many neurologic and neuromuscular abnormalities can produce foot deformities of substantial magnitude. These include arthrogryposis, myelodysplasia, spinal dysraphism, diastematomyelia, cauda equina lesions (both developmental and acquired), amyoplasia, Charcot-Marie-Tooth syndrome, Friedreich's ataxia, poliomyelitis, myelopathies, encephalopathies, and sciatic nerve palsies. In some, the foot problem will be the result of muscle imbalance due to spastic (upper-motor-neuron) paralysis, and in others the deformity will be the result of flaccid (lower-motor-neuron) paralysis. Some will be progressive lesions, and others will be static. Some may portend a poor prognosis for survival, whereas others may have no effect upon the patient's longevity.

One must weigh all of the above factors when approaching the treatment of a foot deformity resulting from or related to an underlying neuromuscular disorder. Unless one is well informed about the behavior of these conditions, proper evaluation usually requires expert assistance from those in other special disciplines such as pediatric neurology and neuroradiology. This issue is self-evident from the fact that electromyograms and selective myelograms or CAT scans of the lumbosacral spine occasionally will be necessary.

Failure to recognize that the foot deformity is the result of a much more profound and serious problem can result in both inappropriate treatment and considerable embarrassment to the physician. The frequent relationship between structural foot deformities in children and a lesion of the nervous system cannot be overemphasized (Fig. 1-6).

Structural and complex foot deformities often may coexist with other important skeletal and/or visceral developmental abnormalities. The incidence of hip disorders (dysplasia and dislocation) is substantially higher than normal in the presence of a clubfoot or some other developmental foot deformity (Fig. 1-7). Therefore, it is mandatory that the hip joints of all children who have established structural foot disorders be evaluated periodically throughout the first year of life. At 6 weeks or 3 months of age, I feel a pelvic roentgenogram should be obtained for all children with structural foot deformities in order to evaluate the hip joints more completely. Pelvic films taken at birth may appear falsely normal; it is better to wait a few weeks before taking the films. As mentioned earlier, a lower lumbosacral spine film also should be taken in order to exclude any developmental abnormality such as spinal dysraphism or diastematomyelia. One usually can rely on clinical judgment and good pediatric care to identify other coexisting musculoskeletal or visceral problems, but the important issue is to recognize that the deformed foot may be simply the tip of the iceberg.

Certain foot deformities such as tarsal coalitions (failure of segmentation), clubfeet, cavus feet, and severe planovalgus feet have strong familial tendencies and, as noted in subsequent chapters, there

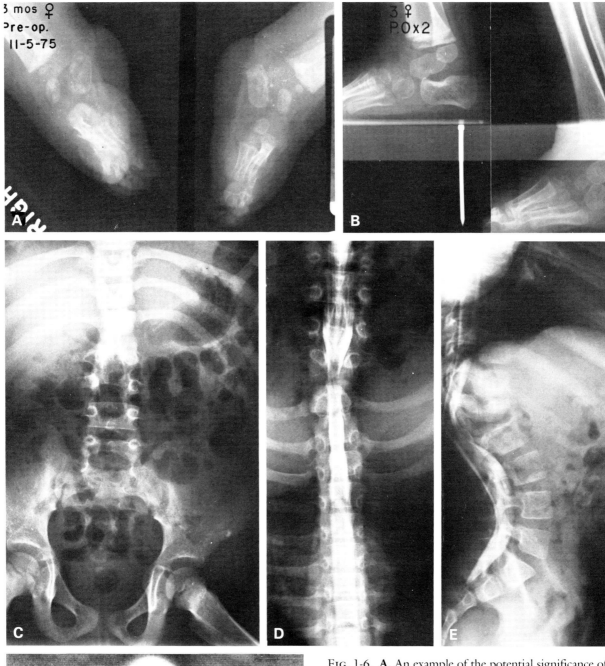

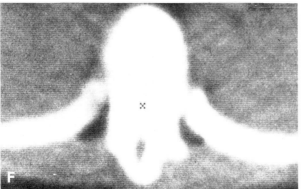

Fig. 1-6. **A,** An example of the potential significance of a structural congenital foot deformity is illustrated in the case of this 4-year-old girl born with equinovarus. After preliminary efforts with manipulation and cast correction, both feet were operated on at 1 year of age and again at 3 years (**B**). **C,** At age 4, she was evaluated for urinary problems, and a scout film was taken during cystoscopic examination. The congenital spinal abnormality is obvious. **D, E,** and **F,** Myelographic and CAT studies revealed the deformity and narrowing of the spinal canal at the level of T12. The spinal deformity and its implications should have been suspected, or the possibility eliminated, by appropriate roentgenographic studies performed when the foot deformity was discovered.

is a distinct genetic mode of transmission in certain of these foot disorders. The importance of this is simply to increase one's index of suspicion when faced with siblings and/or parents having a family history of foot abnormalities. To what extent genetic counseling is indicated naturally will depend upon the nature and severity of the deformity.

Finally, it is important to mention the implications of the different foot deformities upon treatment. To a large extent this has already been covered in earlier sections, but it seems appropriate to emphasize that the prognosis and the type and length of treatment all rest with an accurate diagnosis of the nature of the foot problem. To this end, it is axiomatic that the entire contents of this chapter must be well understood, because if a complete definition of the problem is not established, treatment of the patient's total problem may be either incomplete or inappropriate.

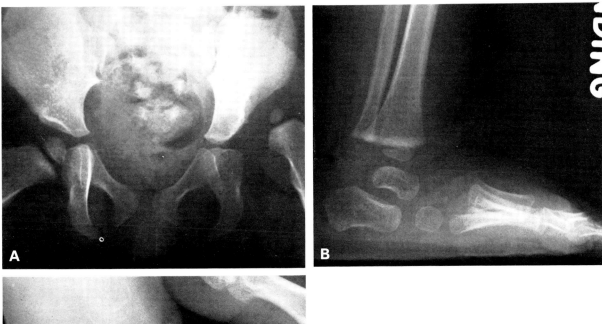

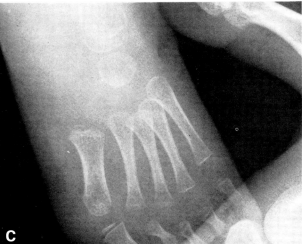

Fig. 1-7. This 2-year-old girl was born with a clubfoot. After a series of preliminary cast corrections, she underwent a posterior release at 6 months of age and a medial release at 12 months of age, both procedures done by an orthopedic surgeon. At no time was a roentgenogram taken of the pelvis or lower spine. **A,** At 2 years of age, her limp, which had been attributed to the clubfoot on that same left side, became more evident, and the first roentgenogram of her pelvis was obtained, which shows a dislocated hip of long standing. The residual stigmata of the partially corrected clubfoot can be seen in **B** and **C.** This case emphasizes the need to suspect other congenital abnormalities when a structural congenital foot deformity is present.

## Classification of Deformities

As mentioned earlier, this text is not intended to be a cyclopedic treatise on the subject of children's foot deformities. The complex abnormalities do lend themselves, however, to a logical and meaningful classification. In this regard, two broad categories can be defined: (1) developmental and/or congenital disorders and (2) acquired disorders. Developmental disorders are the result of some genetically determined or idiopathic alteration in the development of the foot that may or may not be identifiable at birth, whereas the second group consists of foot disorders acquired after birth, for which a multitude of specific and identifiable causes can usually be found.

### CONGENITAL AND DEVELOPMENTAL DISORDERS

The term "congenital" simply means that a condition exists in some form at birth. It is purely a temporal term and, in a strict sense, connotes no etiologic factor. In common usage, however, frequently it is used interchangeably with "developmental." Yet some developmental foot disorders (cavovarus, tarsal coalition, and the like) are not evident at birth, but gradually become apparent in later years of infancy or childhood. This distinction, though accurate, can be misleading; therefore, I have elected to use "congenital" whenever the deformity is present at birth or when it has a genetic cause. Examples are congenital equinovarus, congenital vertical talus, and congenital cavovarus. As noted earlier, some of these are definitely genetically determined, and as each deformity is discussed, the genetic characteristics will be appropriately described. Congenital and developmental disorders that qualify as complex deformities include the following: congenital equinovarus (Chapter 2), congenital vertical talus (Chapter 3), severe flexible and rigid valgoplanus (Chapter 6), teratologic equinovarus (Chapter 8), and tarsal coalition and serpentine foot (Chapter 9).

### ACQUIRED FOOT DISORDERS

These occur most often after birth, but in reality, some can also be the result of intrauterine positioning. Since those postural deformities due to intrauterine positioning are not included in this text, however, I refer only to postnatal conditions as having been acquired. There are many etiologic factors; most of them are related to some disturbance of the neuromuscular system, but some are the result of local causes, either traumatic or iatrogenic. Acquired disorders include paralytic and "idiopathic" cavovarus (Chapter 4), paralytic calcaneocavus (Chapter 5), paralytic planovalgus and equinovarus (Chapter 7) and a small group of acquired deformities secondary to iatrogenic sciatic nerve lesions (Chapter 9).

Based upon the preceding broad, etiologic classification, it is relatively easy to develop a discussion that centers around etiology because it is the true, underlying cause of the deformity that determines the type of treatment to be rendered, as well as the ultimate prognosis. The fact that the deformity may be similar and may even have the same descriptive name is relatively unimportant, as contrasted with the importance of the etiology. Thus, congenital equinovarus (clubfoot), even though it is superficially similar to acquired paralytic equinovarus, presents a totally different therapeutic problem.

Basically, each of these disorders is discussed separately, again with the emphasis on the importance of the etiologic and pathomechanical factors. As will become evident throughout the text, however, this classification contains some overlap, because in some deformities such as cavovarus, the cause cannot always be accurately established. Nevertheless, the principles of treatment remain the same.

An important issue in the classification and evaluation of a child's foot has to do with the patterns of inheritance of these abnormalities, specifically in relation to the congenital and developmental deformities. In each chapter, when applicable, the heritable patterns of the specific foot abnormality are discussed in detail.

## Heritable Patterns in Foot Deformities

TABLE 1-2. *Ossification Centers of the Foot: Postnatal Order of Appearance*[3]

| Primary Centers | Year | Secondary | Year |
|---|---|---|---|
| Calcaneus | Birth | Apophysis | 10 |
| Talus | Birth | | |
| Navicular | 4 | | |
| Cuboid | Birth (or shortly thereafter) | | |
| First (Medial) Cuneiform | 3 | | |
| Second Cuneiform | 4 | | |
| Third (Lateral) Cuneiform | 1 | | |
| All Metatarsals | Birth | Epiphyses | 3 |
| Phalanges | Birth | | |
| | | Epiphyses | 2–6 |

## References

1. Duncan, W. R.: Tonic reflexes of the foot. J. Bone Joint Surg., *42A*:859, 1960.
2. Giannestras, N. J.: *Foot Disorders—Medical and Surgical Management.* 1st Edition. Philadelphia, Lea & Febiger, 1967, p. 78.
3. *The Gray's Anatomy.* 36th ed. Edited by R. Warwick and P. L. Williams. Philadelphia, W. B. Saunders, 1980.
4. Lovell, W. W.: Personal communication, 1981.
5. Paulos, L. E., Coleman, S. S., and Samuelson, K. M.: Pes cavovarus. Review of a surgical approach using selective soft-tissue procedures. J. Bone Joint Surg., *62A*:942, 1980.
6. Samuelson, K. M.: Personal communication, 1980.
7. *Stedman's Medical Dictionary.* 23rd Edition. Baltimore, Williams & Wilkins, 1976.
8. Steel, H. H.: Personal communication, 1981.
9. Tachdjian, M. O.: *Pediatric Orthopedics.* Philadelphia, W. B. Saunders, 1972, p. 1264.
10. *Webster's New World Dictionary.* New York, The World Publishing Co., 1964, p. 1486.

# 2

# Equinovarus Congenita

In spite of the large number of publications concerning the causes, natural history, diagnostic features, therapeutic considerations, and results of various forms of treatment of equinovarus congenita, this foot deformity continues to pose many unanswered questions and remains a substantial therapeutic challenge to the orthopedic surgeon. Lloyd-Roberts, in 1964, emphasized the lack of progress that had been made in our understanding and in the methods of treatment of equinovarus congenita.[45] To a large extent, the same can be said today.

If one reads the published literature and attends continuing education courses on the management of equinovarus congenita, it is apparent that considerable controversy and difference of opinion continue to surface. The varying degrees of severity and as yet unknown pathologic factors make it impossible for anyone to be dogmatic about a specific method or technique of treating equinovarus congenita. The major goals of this chapter are to attempt to minimize the controversies, to emphasize the therapeutic principles, and to propose those technical solutions that, in my hands, have proven most effective. Because my own techniques are constantly changing, and because more than one method of solving the varied, manifold problems that exist in clubfoot treatment may be recognized and accepted, any dogmatic or pedantic presentation is unacceptable.

The condition has been given a variety of names, including clubfoot, congenital idiopathic clubfoot, talipes equinovarus, and equinovarus congenita. As noted in Chapter 1, when referring to the true congenital idiopathic deformity, the name equinovarus congenita is preferred because of its greater specificity in describing the etiology and pathology. The more general term clubfoot is not appropriate because it connotes no etiologic factor. Also as mentioned in Chapter 1, "equinovarus congenita" also avoids the redundancy involved in using the rather nonspecific word "talipes."

*Etiology*     The true cause of equinovarus congenita is presently unknown. With major deformities existing in both the cartilage and bony structures as well as in the soft tissues, the major question with respect to etiology centers around which of these is primary and which is secondary. Two major hypotheses have been proposed. The first contends that the equinovarus deformity is due to extrinsic or external pressures, including such factors as intrauterine postural abnormalities or oligohydramnios. The second hypothesis proposes intrinsic or endogenous factors as primary causes of abnormal development. These include such causative factors as developmental arrest, abnormal tendon and ligament attachments, neurologic defects with secondary muscle dysfunction, and primary germ plasm defects.

EXTRINSIC
HYPOTHESES

POSTURAL CAUSES. The initial hypothesis suggesting a postural etiology was proposed by Hippocrates.[32] Denis Browne also felt that intrauterine compression against the uterine wall or fetal membranes upon the developing foot could produce abnormalities of the bones and soft tissues of the foot.[10]

OLIGOHYDRAMNIOS. The concept that decreased fluid within the amniotic sac could result in increased pressure on the developing foot was proposed as a result of veterinary studies. For example, Roberts noted that an equinovarus deformity could occur in lambs born to sheep with oligohydramnios.[64] Similar findings were noted by Whittem, who studied foot deformities in calves born to oligohydramniotic cows.[88] None of these findings, however, have been confirmed in humans. Also, most of these extrinsic concepts do not hold up to critical analysis when one attempts to explain the pathology of true congenital clubfoot. On the other hand, these extrinsic factors can easily account for the postural clubfoot that responds so well and so completely to nonsurgical, conservative cast treatment, in which a short period of manipulation and cast application usually solve the problem.

INTRINSIC
HYPOTHESES

ARRESTED DEVELOPMENT. The concept that equinovarus congenita is simply the consequence of an arrested development in the early formation of the foot was proposed by Böhm.[8] He examined six fetal specimens from the fifth week (14-mm stage) through the fourth month (90-mm stage) of gestation. He noted four definite stages in the maturation of the normal, developing foot. Stage I begins at 5 weeks of gestation and is characterized by marked equinus of the ankle, with adduction of the forefoot. At this age, the navicular and cuboid are in slight medial deviation with respect to the talus and calcaneus. At 6 weeks, the talus, through continued growth, causes the navicular and the remaining tarsus to shift further in the lateral direction.

By the eighth week of gestation, Stage II is entered. At this time, the tarsal bones are in proper alignment, but the entire foot remains supinated, with the calcaneus located directly below the talus. Adduction of the forefoot also continues, along with 90° of equinus of the ankle. Stage III is entered at 10 weeks of gestation, at which time the degree of equinus begins to decrease. By 12 weeks, Stage IV of development has been reached, during which the equinus continues to decrease. During this stage, the previously supinated foot now assumes a pronated position, but slight residual metatarsal adduction persists.

Böhm felt that the deformity of equinovarus congenita was close to, if not indistinguishable from, the normal fetal foot at 5 weeks of gestation. He therefore postulated an arrest in the development of the normal foot at an early age as the possible cause of equinovarus congenita. He was unable, however, to document any significant abnormalities in the talar head or neck, with its associated medial deviation of the navicular, in any of his specimens. As will be seen in the section on pathologic anatomy, this abnormality is one of the most salient features of true congenital clubfoot.

ABNORMAL TENDON AND LIGAMENT ATTACHMENTS. Bissell postulated that abnormal tendon insertions could be a possible cause of equinovarus congenita.[7] Fried examined 56 specimens with congenital equinovarus and noted that, in all instances, the posterior tibial tendon was hypertrophic at its insertion, and also noted multiple plantar ramifications of the insertion.[23] He therefore postulated that abnormalities in the insertion of the posterior tibial tendon were the principal cause of equinovarus congenita.

Stewart and Flinchum both noted that in congenital clubfoot the Achilles tendon was inserted more medially on the calcaneus than on the normal foot.[21,73] They also encountered an abnormal insertion of the peroneus longus, and they believed that in congenital clubfoot these tendons undergo an abnormal differentiation at or near their attachments at the time of their development. The anterior tibial and triceps surae were considered to act as deforming forces, and because the peroneals were unable to counteract the combined action of these tendons, it was postulated that the foot was held in an abnormal position during development. The bony changes, therefore, were considered to be adaptive in nature, secondary to muscle imbalance. Hirsch proposed that the hindfoot deformities in congenital clubfoot were due to a tight and contracted deltoid ligament, the presumed result of a developmental defect.[33]

DEFECT IN NEUROLOGIC AND MUSCLE FUNCTION. Mau and Wiley noted abnormal histologic changes in the calf musculature in cases of equinovarus congenita.[53,89] Loss of normal striations and variations in muscle fiber size were found. Isaacs examined 111 muscle biopsy specimens of the posteromedial calf and peroneal muscle groups and found evidence to suggest early denervation.[37] Histologically, all but 19 of the specimens showed varying fiber size suggesting early denervation. Fifty-three of the specimens were examined through an electron microscope, and all showed an abnormal increase in collagen content, again suggesting denervation. These findings were present in both muscle groups studied, and from these observations it was postulated that the deformity in equinovarus congenita *could* be due to a muscle imbalance created by partial denervation of the muscle groups in the calf early in their development.

Fearnley, however, performed electromyographic studies on five patients with unilateral equinovarus congenita. The posterior muscle groups of the calf showed no evidence of fibrillation or polyphasic potential. He therefore felt that muscle imbalance, if it did exist, was simply due to delayed maturation and not to true denervation.[20]

Bechtol and Mossman examined two fetal specimens and concluded that congenital clubfoot could be the result of asymmetric muscle growth as compared to bone growth. They theorized that the bones grew more rapidly than the muscles, and that the resulting increased muscle tension produced muscle imbalance and thus created the deformity.[6]

GERM PLASM DEFECT. The most widely accepted theory on the cause of equinovarus congenita is that of a germ plasm defect.[36,38,70] Irani, Sherman, and Settle found a defective cartilage anlage of the talus.[36,69] All of the other associated deformities in the soft tissues, as well as the remaining bony changes, were considered to be adaptive responses to the position of the deformed talar head and neck. Shapiro and Glimcher further documented the concept of a germ plasm defect of the talus.[70] In a histologic study of the talus from a 9-day-old infant with unilateral equinovarus, the authors noted certain findings that could only be explained on the basis of an abnormal formation of the talus (see section on pathologic anatomy).

From this brief historical review of the theories of causation of congenital clubfoot, it is evident that the most consistent and convincing proposal is that of a primary defect in development of the tarsal bones, especially the talus. The cause of this basic defect, however, remains unknown. It is important to recognize and accept this concept because it explains why a well treated clubfoot never looks like a normal foot, why residual adduction deformity of the midfoot and forefoot is so common, and why all of our therapeutic efforts are aimed at producing sufficient corrective changes in the foot so as to *compensate* for a primary bony defect (the talus) that itself cannot be corrected satisfactorily. As is shown subsequently in the section on treatment, Roberts has conducted some recent operations on the neck of the talus in an effort to correct the deformity at its primary location.[63] This is done, however, only when the remainder of the foot has been fully corrected and also when there is no residual internal tibial torsion.

*Pathologic Anatomy*    The first detailed description of equinovarus congenita was written by Scarpa in 1818.[68] He described medial deviation of the navicular, cuboid, and calcaneus on the talus. He felt that the talus was normal and that the deformity was secondary to a shift of the other bones of the tarsus about the talus. Scarpa also felt that the soft-tissue changes were secondary to the disturbed bony relationships. Adams, in 1866, studied 30 cases of equinovarus, including fetal as well as adult specimens.[1] His opinion was that the principal deformity was within the talus, and that the remainder of the bony abnormalities as well as the soft-tissue changes were secondary to the talar abnormality.

Since this early description of the pathologic anatomy, many observations have appeared in the literature, based largely upon dissections of embryologic, fetal, and postnatal specimens of varying ages (Fig. 2-1).

Two major studies, already alluded to, have surfaced in recent years. The first was conducted by Irani and Sherman, who, in 1963, examined 11 abnormal limbs, the gestational age of which varied from 22 to 36 weeks. The uninvolved foot was used for comparison to the normal foot.[36] Settle, in the same year, examined 16 feet, all obtained from fetal specimens in the third trimester.[69]

Both studies revealed many similar observations, and the major abnormality was in the talus, which was found to be decreased in size to approximately three fourths that of the normal talus. The talus was held in plantar flexion, but exhibited essentially a normal body and a normal articulation within the ankle. The major deformity was found in the distal neck and head portion of the talus. The neck was foreshortened, and the head was directed medially and in the plantar direction. The average angulation between the head and neck and the body of the talus was found to be decreased. Normally 150 to 155°, this angle was reduced to 115 to 135° in the equinovarus feet. The subtalar articular facets were distorted and rotated medially.

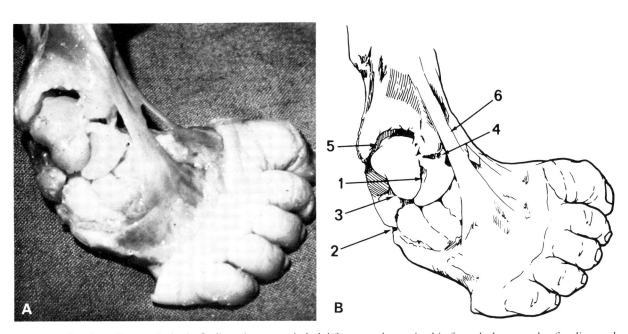

FIG. 2-1. **A**, The salient pathologic findings in congenital clubfoot are shown in this frontal photograph of a dissected specimen in a newborn. **B**, The artist's interpretation. The characteristic clubfoot deformity is apparent. 1, 2, and 3, The grossly disturbed talonavicular, calcaneocuboid, and talocalcaneal relationships are well demonstrated. 4, Note the close approximation (pseudoarticulation) that exists between the navicular and the medial malleolus. 5, The ankle mortise, however, is normal. 6, Owing to the altered relationship of the forefoot and midfoot with the hindfoot, the tendons are displaced medially. (Courtesy of I. V. Ponseti, Iowa City, Iowa.)

The navicular was decreased in size to two thirds that of normal. The navicular was medially deviated, corresponding to the direction of the distorted head and neck of the talus. Owing to this abnormal medial displacement of the navicular, an accessory joint was created between the medial malleolus and navicular.

The calcaneus likewise showed some decrease in size; furthermore, it was displaced into varus, supination, and equinus. Adaptive changes were found in the facets of the calcaneus, with the most significant alterations seen in the anterior facet, corresponding to the abnormal subtalar articulations. Because of these abnormal osseous relationships, the joints of the hindfoot, namely, the talonavicular and calcaneocuboid joints, were not only deviated medially but were also lined up one beneath the other instead of in the normal side-by-side relationship.

The remainder of the bones of the foot were essentially normal in size and configuration, but secondary positional changes were present as a result of the abnormalities just described.

The observations in both of these studies showed that the soft-tissue changes found within the capsular, ligamentous, tendinous, and muscular structures were all the result of the abnormal configuration of the skeletal elements of the foot. Gross and histologic examination of the calf muscles, spinal cord, and peripheral nerves showed no major abnormalities.

As noted earlier, Shapiro and Glimcher performed a gross and histologic study of the talus in a child who had congenital clubfoot along with multiple other congenital anomalies.[70] They confirmed the smallness of the talus, along with a medial deviation of the head and neck of the talus, which was also misshapen. In serial studies of the microscopic anatomy, the ossification center of the talus was found to be smaller than normal and was positioned eccentrically in a more lateral and anterior location. In addition, vascular abnormalities were found in the area of endochondral ossification. Shapiro and Glimcher believed that these observations supported the theory of a primary defect in the morphogenesis of the talus, producing alterations in the shape and size of the talus. They further implied that simple replacement of the navicular in front of the talus does not restore the foot to a normal appearance.

PATHOGENESIS

In a condition in which the cause is considered to be a germ plasm defect, any discussion of pathogenesis must consider the heritable factors, which have been studied in considerable detail, especially by Wynne-Davies and Idelberger.[35,91,92] Wynne-Davies showed that the incidence of equinovarus congenita is strongly influenced by race. In Caucasians, the incidence is 1.00 to 1.24 per 1000 births, approximately twice that found in the Oriental races (0.57 per 1000 births). On the other hand, Polynesians tend to have a much higher incidence (as high as 6.81 per 1000 births). In nearly all races, the male-to-female ratio is 2:1. Most studies have shown no consistent relationship between the incidence of equinovarus congenita and the patient's birth weight, birth number, or maternal age.

A definite, heritable pattern exists in equinovarus congenita. Idelberger studied the incidence of congenital clubfoot in twins as it compared to the incidence of about 0.1% in the general population. He found that the incidence in monozygous twins was elevated to 32.5% and in dizygous twins to 2.9%.[35] Wynne-Davies also noted an increased incidence among relatives of patients with equinovarus congenita, finding it to be 20 to 30 times greater in first-degree relatives and 6 times greater in second-degree relatives. The incidence in third-degree relatives was the same as that of the general population.

Proposed theories concerning the mode of inheritance of equinovarus congenita have been variable, including autosomal recessive, sex-linked recessive, and autosomal dominant patterns. The majority of current data available now suggests that the most plausible and workable pattern is that of polygenic inheritance with a threshold effect. Within this pattern, a continuum of multiple gene loci exists in which either a certain number of abnormal genes or an altered threshold is required for the abnormality to appear. According to this concept, the deformity occurs when the number of abnormal genes exceeds the threshold level. Furthermore, a more severe clinical deformity would occur if a higher load of abnormal genes were present.

The threshold appears to be sex-related, with a lower boundary level being found in males than in females. This would explain why males are affected more commonly than females. This concept can also explain the finding that the deformity tends to be less severe in males than in females because a lower number of abnormal genes is usually present in males. Correspondingly, females require a higher number of abnormal genes to manifest the deformity and therefore would tend to have a more severe or resistant deformity. This sex-linked concept can also explain why first-degree relatives of affected females are more likely to be affected than those of affected males. In a polygenic pattern of inheritance, it appears possible that the threshold for manifestation of the abnormality may also depend upon environmental as well as genetic factors.

Upon clinical examination of the clubfoot, one observes that the involved foot is, in general, smaller than the noninvolved foot (Fig. 2-2). A fixed hindfoot varus is found, with the calcaneus located beneath the talus. Forefoot adduction and supination are also seen, and the hindfoot is in fixed plantar flexion within the ankle mortise. A varying amount of forefoot plantar flexion on the hindfoot also exists, creating an associated cavus deformity in some cases (Fig. 2-3). Laterally, a palpable sinus tarsus is absent, with the head of the talus occupying most of the space. Medially, the head of the talus cannot be felt because the navicular articulates with the medial malleolus (Fig. 2-1). Associated with the foot deformities is a calf that is always decreased in

**CLINICAL APPEARANCE**

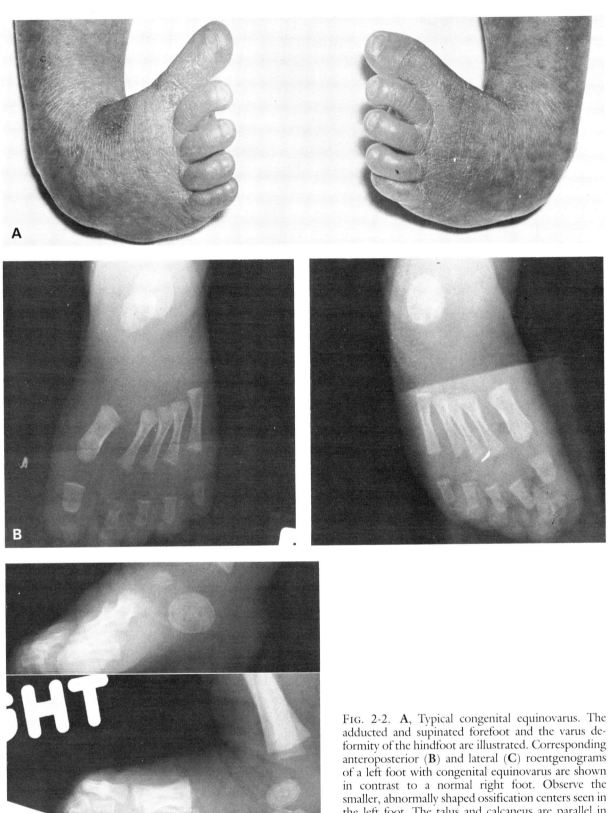

FIG. 2-2. **A**, Typical congenital equinovarus. The adducted and supinated forefoot and the varus deformity of the hindfoot are illustrated. Corresponding anteroposterior (**B**) and lateral (**C**) roentgenograms of a left foot with congenital equinovarus are shown in contrast to a normal right foot. Observe the smaller, abnormally shaped ossification centers seen in the left foot. The talus and calcaneus are parallel in both anteroposterior and lateral projections. The forefoot is in equinus. Compare it to the normal right foot.

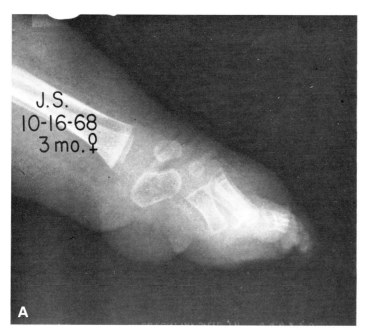 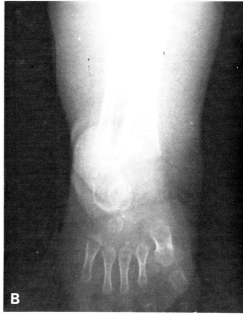

FIG. 2-3. Severe equinus of the forefoot is illustrated in this 3-month-old female with congenital equinovarus. Note the severely plantarflexed attitude of the metatarsals, especially the first metatarsal, which is projected as being foreshortened in the anteroposterior view (**B**). The angle (Meary) between the long axis of the talus and the first metatarsal approaches 90°. The severe plantar crease in the soft tissues can be seen plainly in the lateral view (**A**).

circumference on the involved side. One must also remember that a high incidence of associated, congenital hip dysplasia is found in these abnormalities.

Three broad categories of equinovarus congenita can be identified. The first is postural equinovarus, resulting most likely from extrinsic pressure exerted upon the developing foot during the late weeks of gestation. This form of equinovarus demonstrates normal configuration of the bony structures, with no disturbed talocalcaneal relationships, fixed soft-tissue contractures, or muscle imbalance. The deformity responds quickly to serial casting, resulting inevitably in a normal foot.

The second category is idiopathic congenital equinovarus (Fig. 2-2). As already discussed, it is believed to be the result of a germ plasm abnormality, in which formation of the talus is defective, along with other structural changes in the remainder of the tarsal bones, the musculature, and the soft tissues. The talocalcaneal and talonavicular joints are subluxated, and the ligamentous and capsular structures are contracted and foreshortened. This form of equinovarus congenita is the most common, and although it often appears as an isolated deformity, it is frequently associated with other congenital anomalies. Crabbe, for example, has reported the incidence of associated congenital anomalies in equinovarus congenita to be as high as 11.6%.[12]

The third category is a more severe form of equinovarus that is associated with arthrogryposis or myelodysplasia (Fig. 2-4). It is characterized by extensive and resistant soft-tissue abnormalities, as well as

*Classification*

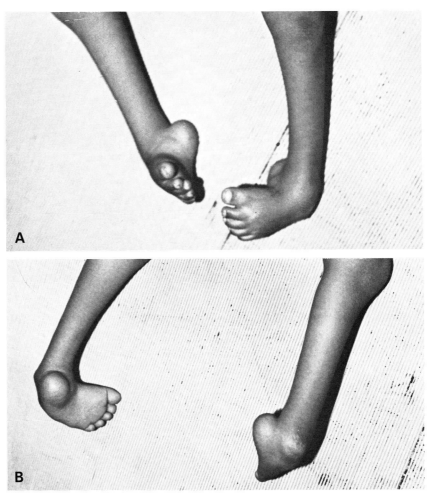

FIG. 2-4. Various views of the clubfeet typically seen in children with arthrogryposis. Note the absence of any skin creases, the flexed attitude of the toes, the atrophic calf musculature, and the "featureless" character of the limbs.

impressive resistance to conventional forms of treatment. Nearly all such feet require extensive surgical release at an early period in infancy. A convenient flowsheet depicting these types of congenital equinovarus and their clinical behavior is seen below.

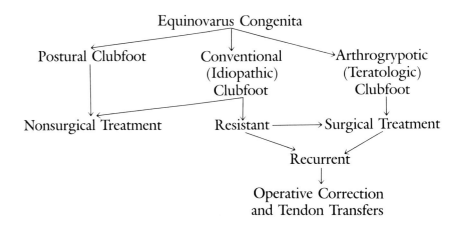

Numerous authors have advanced the radiographic criteria for diagnosis of this deformity.[31,71,81] The minimum roentgenographic views necessary are an anteroposterior and a lateral projection of the foot and ankle. The anteroposterior view should always be taken in the weight-bearing or simulated weight-bearing position because it is essential that the film demonstrate the relationships of the bones of the foot in a position of weight-bearing function. The lateral view should be taken with the foot in maximum dorsiflexion in order to evaluate hindfoot and ankle equinus (Fig. 2-5).

In the anteroposterior view, the talocalcaneal angle (angle of Kite) is the most important determinant. This angle is determined by drawing one line through the longitudinal axis of the talus and a second line through the long midaxis of the calcaneus. The first line should pass medial to the base of the first metatarsal, and the second line should pass through the base of the fifth metatarsal. The angle subtended by these two lines is the talocalcaneal angle (Fig. 2-6).

Templeton, McAlister, and Zim determined that the talocalcaneal angle varies somewhat with the child's age.[81] In infants, the normal range is from 30 to 50°, whereas in children 5 years of age or older, 20 to 35° is considered normal. Kite feels that the normal range of the talocalcaneal angle is 20 to 40°.[40] All authors agree that values less than 20° at any age are consistent with hindfoot varus.

## Radiographic Criteria

### ANTEROPOSTERIOR VIEW

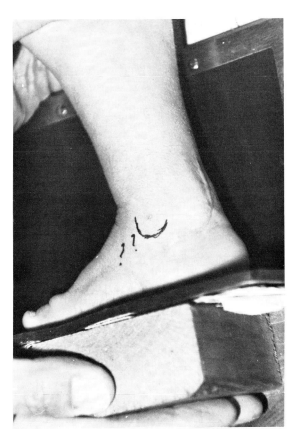

FIG. 2-5. My preferred method of performing a dorsiflexion stress test to evaluate heelcord tightness in clubfoot. The surgeon should perform the test using leaded gloves. A translucent, flat plate of Plexiglas can be held easily by means of a wooden block cemented to it. The leg is stabilized and the foot dorsiflexed firmly but gently.

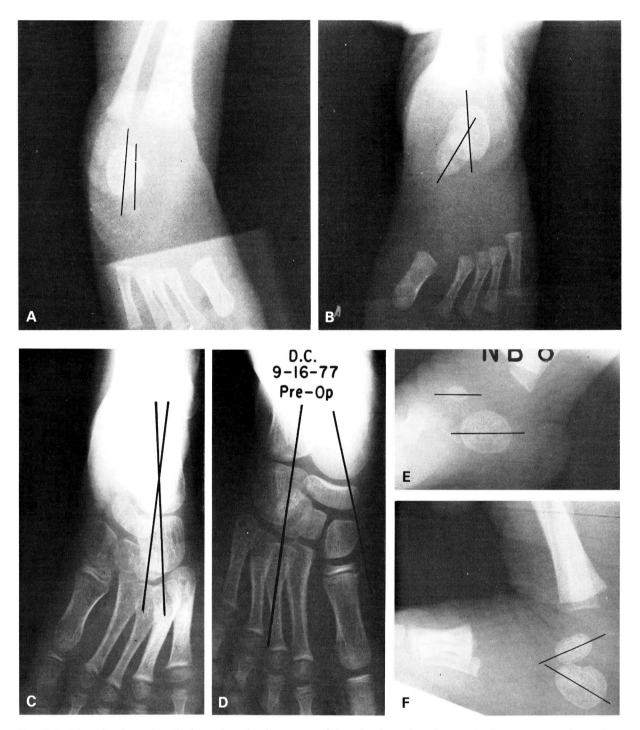

FIG. 2-6. The talocalcaneal angle determines the divergence of the talus from the calcaneus in the anteroposterior projection. Commonly known as Kite's angle, it is created by the intersection of two lines drawn through the long axis of the talus and calcaneus. **A,** In newborn and young infants, the long axis of these bones is often difficult to establish accurately compared to the normal side (**B**). This value is much less reliable than that found in older children, in whom the true shape of the ossification centers can be identified more readily. **C,** The abnormal angle is shown, as compared to the normal (**D**). The lateral talocalcaneal angle reflects to some degree the same determination as Kite's angle, i.e., it provides a relationship of the talus to the calcaneus that is similar to that seen in the lateral view. Similar lines are utilized; that is, lines drawn through the long axes of the two main tarsal bones, and similar frailties exist in the newborn examination as compared to evaluations made in older children. **E,** The lines are nearly parallel in the clubfoot. **F,** Note the convergence seen in the normal foot.

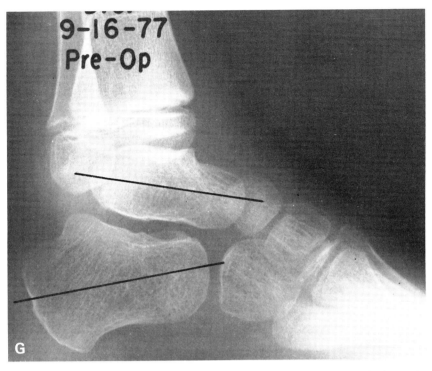

FIG. 2-6. **G,** The greater ability to assess the long axis of these bones is shown in the abnormal clubfoot.

Using the same anteroposterior view, Simons has found the talometatarsal angle to be helpful.[71] This angle is identified in the anteroposterior view by drawing one line through the center of the first metatarsal shaft and a second line through the long central axis of the talus. If the line through the talus passes medial to the line through the first metatarsal, a negative angle exists (Fig. 2-7); if the line through the talar axis extends lateral to the first metatarsal, a positive angle exists (Fig. 2-7). A normal talometatarsal angle ranges from 0 to −20°. If the talocalcaneal angle is less than 15° and the talometatarsal angle is greater than +15°, an abnormal talonavicular relationship is considered to be present.

**LATERAL VIEW**

In the lateral view, the most important determinant is the talocalcaneal angle, determined by drawing one line through the long axis of the calcaneus and a second line through the midaxis of the talus. The angle subtended by these two lines is the lateral talocalcaneal angle (Fig. 2-6). In contrast to Kite's angle, this angle is not dependent on age and normally ranges from 25 to 50°. An angle of less than 25° shows increased parallelism between the talus and calcaneus and indicates inadequate correction of the hindfoot.

In this same view, Meary has shown that a talometatarsal angle may also be determined by drawing one line through the long axis of the talus and another through the longitudinal axis of the first metatarsal shaft (Fig. 2-8).[54] In the normal configuration for a child less than 5 years of age, the talar axis passes inferior to the first metatarsal, whereas in children over 5 years of age it is parallel to the shaft of the first metatarsal. An angle greater than 15° above the shaft indicates a cavus deformity (Fig. 2-8).

**Treatment**

In general, the treatment of equinovarus congenita should begin as early as possible while the cartilaginous as well as the soft-tissue structures are able to undergo remodeling, so as to avoid or minimize permanent, abnormal, adaptive changes in the bones and soft tissues.

The objective of treatment of congenital clubfoot is to achieve as normal a foot as possible, fully recognizing, however, that a totally normal foot can never be achieved in the case of a true congenital clubfoot. The anticipated results should be a reasonably supple foot that is plantigrade, with a heel in valgus and a nearly normal medial longitudinal arch. The corrected foot should be one that facilitates gait and accepts normal shoes.

**GENERAL CONSIDERATIONS**

Over the years, it has gradually been accepted that "conservative" does not necessarily mean "nonoperative," nor that operative treatment is necessarily "radical." In many instances, it is clearly evident that a more conservative method of establishing bone and joint relationships may consist of selective, carefully performed surgical elongation of

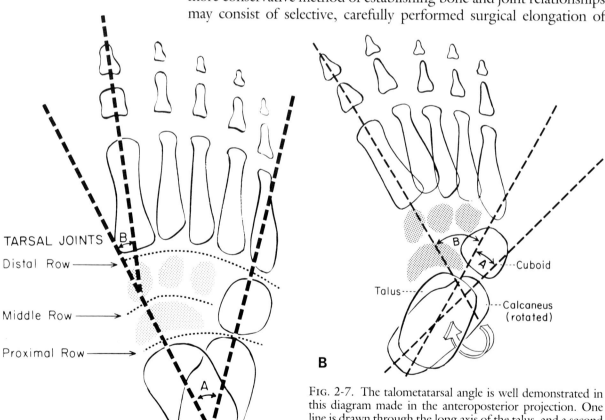

TARSAL JOINTS
Distal Row
Middle Row
Proximal Row

Talus
Cuboid
Calcaneus (rotated)

A

B

Fig. 2-7. The talometatarsal angle is well demonstrated in this diagram made in the anteroposterior projection. One line is drawn through the long axis of the talus, and a second line is drawn through the long axis of the first metatarsal shaft. **A,** The normal angle ranges from 0 to −20°, and a positive talometatarsal angle (angle B in **B**) connotes an abnormal adducted relationship between the forefoot and the hindfoot. (Simmons, G. W.: Analytical radiography of club feet. J. Bone Joint Surg., *59B*:487, 1977.)

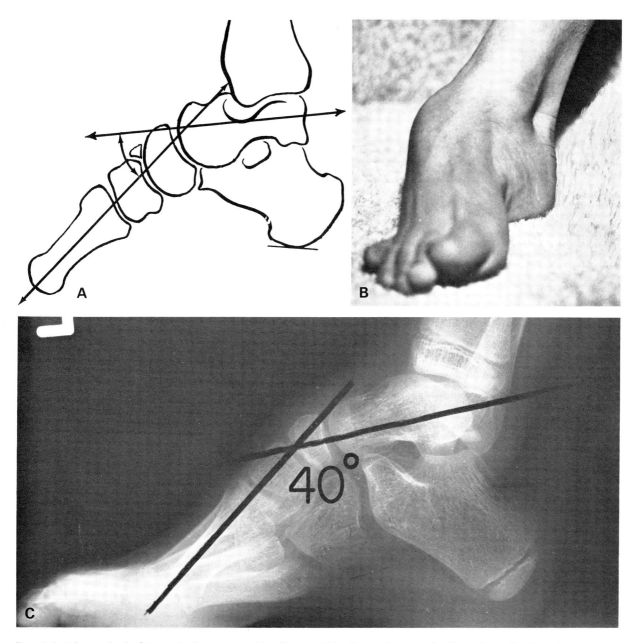

FIG. 2-8. The method of Meary is demonstrated by diagram (**A**), clinical photograph (**B**), and standing lateral roentgenogram (**C**). The talometatarsal angle as illustrated provides a relatively good representation of the degree of cavus of the forefoot on the hindfoot, but does not assist in determination of flexibility of either component (see Chapter 4).

ligaments and tendons. When confronted with a rigid, resistant, equinovarus foot, persistent manipulations and cast applications of the foot (even though gentle) actually may be a more radical method of treatment than surgical intervention.

In viewing this concept, it is attractive to use the approach of Williams and others, who have said that, in treating the child's foot, one must remember that, *relatively* speaking, the soft tissues (skin, ligaments, and tendons) may actually be "hard" and that the hard tissues (bone and articular cartilage) are, in reality, relatively soft.[90] In dealing with the tarsal bones, furthermore, one must recognize that the articular surfaces of these bones are the principal means by which these structures grow in size and develop their configuration.

Also, it is important to recall that articular cartilage is sensitive to prolonged and uninterrupted pressure, especially when denied freedom of motion, a concept that has been enunciated by Salter and Field.[66] Consequently, cartilage necrosis, growth alterations in tarsal bones, and intra-articular fibrosis and adhesions leading to rigidity are the all-too-frequent results of such excessive pressure.

MECHANISMS OF ELONGATION. It is also essential to understand the various possible mechanisms by which ligaments and capsular structures can elongate, because it is only by elongation of these particular structures, plus the tendons and their sheaths and retinacula, that the bones can be taken from their displaced or abnormal position and placed into their proper, normal position.

First, ligaments and other soft tissues can elongate by growth, as evidenced by the fact that these structures are of greater magnitude in adults than in children. This process requires months and years, and cannot be accelerated in any practical way. Second, these ligamentous structures can elongate by using their viscoelastic properties in the process known as "creep." In this situation, time and some degree of force are the two basic elements permitting or leading to lengthening by "creep." Third, the ligaments and capsules can be partially ruptured or torn by forcible manipulations of the interconnected osseous structures. The force necessary to rupture or tear these ligamentous structures must be accompanied by an equal and opposite force that must be withstood by the bones and their hyaline cartilage. As noted previously, this may lead to cartilage necrosis, bone deformation, and ultimate alterations in growth.

Finally, the ligaments and capsular structures can be lengthened surgically. Properly done with precision and care, this may be the most atraumatic and effective method of all. The major decisions one must make, however, are when, what, where, and how much to lengthen. To some extent, the answers to these difficult questions must be derived exclusively from surgical experience and intuition.

GOALS AND LIMITATIONS. Therefore, the guiding principles that govern our current treatment of the congenital clubfoot must include the need to restore to as near normal as possible the bony relationships of the talocalcaneonavicular joint, and to accomplish this by the most atraumatic method possible. It is essential then to hold this relationship (reduction) until the foot can mature. This overly simplified goal of treatment involves a multiplicity of complex considerations that will be outlined subsequently.

Treatment of the congenital clubfoot must take into account several important issues unique to this condition. These are virtually axiomatic with most individuals experienced in the treatment of this condition. First, there is a true bony deformity of the talus, as previously described in the section on pathology. Whether this deformity is primary or secondary at birth (adaptive) is still the subject of some debate, but the fact that it exists at birth makes ultimate, true, complete correction of the congenital clubfoot virtually impossible. Second, the other tarsal bones are smaller and have an abnormal configuration. For example, the calcaneus is shorter and somewhat different in shape than normal. Third, variable degrees of muscle atrophy and weakness exist in all of the leg musculature. Fourth, joint ranges of motion between the forefoot and the hindfoot and in the ankle are invariably restricted. Finally, postnatal treatment has not really been directed towards the yet unknown cause of congenital clubfoot.

When all of these considerations are accepted and contemplated, it becomes clear that treatment of the true congenital clubfoot, irrespective of how early or how skillfully administered, cannot possibly result in a foot that is indistinguishable from normal. The foot is always slightly shorter and often wider than the normal foot. The calf is usually smaller than normal. The configuration of the heel is foreshortened, and the external configuration of the heelcord where it inserts onto the calcaneus is less prominent than normal (Fig. 2-9). Many of the normal bony prominences are altered in configuration. The medial malleolus is broader than normal, the depth of the sinus tarsus is variable, and the usually clear distinction between the prominence of the talar head and the navicular tuberosity is not found. Ranges of motion are reduced, not only between the forefoot and hindfoot, but also especially in the subtalar and ankle joints. Even in the well corrected foot, the stigmata of the deformity will practically always be apparent to some degree and will persist throughout the growth of the child and into adult life. Also, as a rule, following treatment the foot will usually be either slightly over- or undercorrected.

It is advisable to recognize these rather well accepted results of congenital clubfoot treatment in order to avoid unexpected disappointment, on the part of both the surgeon and the parents. It is far better to prepare the parents early for the likely result just outlined so that they can recognize that anything better is an unexpected but welcome bonus of treatment.

SEQUENCE OF CORRECTION. The literature contains some confusion in regard to the sequence in which congenital clubfoot is corrected nonoperatively. It is often said that the forefoot is corrected first, then the hindfoot, and then the ankle. When one considers the description of the components of the foot (see Chapter 1), it becomes obvious that the forefoot cannot possibly be corrected without some aspects of the hindfoot deformity also being corrected to some degree. For example, if the surgeon manipulates the forefoot and midfoot into abduction and at the same time gently exerts pressure over the lateral aspect of the talar head, almost surely the forefoot and midfoot will not be corrected unless some change in the peritalar (hindfoot) relationships also occurs. Furthermore, the cuboid must move laterally if the navicular moves in this direction, and this automatically will dis-

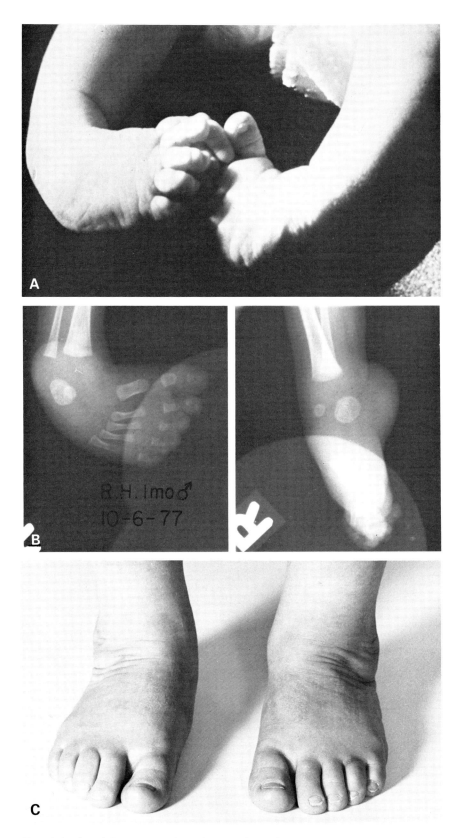

FIG. 2-9. **A** and **B**, Precorrection photographs and roentgenograms of the feet of a 5-year-old male who was treated nonoperatively by serial cast applications. **C, D,** and

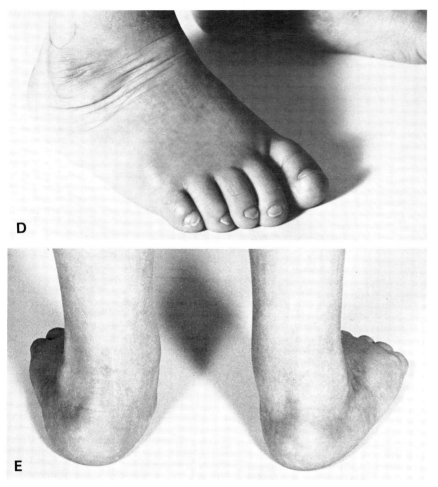

**E,** Although satisfactory clinical corrections were achieved, the feet show the mild residual stigmata of congenital equinovarus. Note the absence of the prominence of the heel and Achilles tendon.

place the calcaneus laterally to some degree from under the talus. Therefore, in most instances, the foot is corrected as a unit, and one component cannot be corrected without having some corrective influence on the other. This gives further credence to Tachdjian's statement that the primary goal in clubfoot treatment is the reduction of the subluxated talocalcaneonavicular joint.[79]

**NONOPERATIVE TREATMENT**

The history of the nonoperative treatment of equinovarus congenita can be traced to the time of Hippocrates (400 BC). As stated earlier, he believed that the deformity was created by a positional abnormality of the foot during fetal development. He felt that if the foot could be placed into a more normal position and held with bandages, the deformity would be corrected.[32] In 1836, Guerin proposed a program of forceful manipulation of the deformity into a more normal position, followed by plaster-of-Paris casts designed to hold the correction.[29] Later, in 1886, Hugh Owen Thomas also believed in forceful manipulation and developed a wrench to be used as a manipulative device in order to correct the foot more easily.[82]

In 1920, Elmslie recommended forceful correction of both the hindfoot and the ankle deformities; however, he felt that the deformities should be corrected sequentially.[18] He recommended initial, manipulative correction of the varus and adduction deformities, accompanied by a holding cast for 6 weeks. Following this, the foot was manipulated out of the equinus deformity into dorsiflexion, and a holding cast was applied for 6 weeks. Denis Browne, in 1937, proposed that the deformity of the hindfoot should be forcefully corrected into a calcaneovalgus position, and then the foot should be splinted on a holding bar in the corrected position until ambulation was begun (see section on Denis Browne technique).[10]

In 1932, Kite cited the harmful effects of forceful manipulation, recognizing that forceful correction caused joint stiffness and a resultant decrease in the cartilage joint space between tarsal bones as seen by roentgenographic examination. Kite also saw these forceful corrective efforts to be the causes of damage to the cartilage growth centers, the joint surfaces, and the soft tissues, resulting in intra-articular adhesions and joint incongruity.

Kite therefore recommended gentle, repeated efforts at correction through serial casts, using slow, continued pressure in line with the planes of tarsal joint motions. He believed that this method would gradually elongate the contracted medial capsular, ligamentous, and tendinous structures about the tarsal bones and joints; at the same time, the structures on the lateral side would gradually contract and ultimately adapt to their corrected position. Kite emphasized that this method required slow, patient efforts at correction and believed that correction of hindfoot varus required a minimum of 8 weeks, followed by a similar period of stretching the posterior ankle structures, and then the application of retention casts for several weeks.[40]

Much later, in 1963, Ponseti and Smoley agreed with Kite's principles of gentle correction by means of serial plaster casts, but they added the procedure of percutaneous tenotomy of the heelcord at age 3 months if the ankle equinus persisted.[60] More recently, Lovell, Price, and Meehan have proposed gentle, serial manipulation of the various deformities, again in line with their planes of joint motion, and with application of well molded, below-knee casts used to hold the correction that is achieved through manipulation (see following section).[49]

CAST TREATMENT. As noted previously, the general principles of gentle reduction through serial cast applications have been thoroughly described by Kite and reinforced by Lovell, Price, and Meehan, who also emphasized the need for gentle, passive manipulation in the process of correcting the congenital clubfoot. Lovell believed that the deformities of equinovarus are most appropriately corrected through slow and gentle manipulation of the foot into a normal position along the lines of joint motion; a cast is then applied to hold the foot in the improved position thus gained. Lovell also believed that well molded, below-knee plaster casts are sufficient to control the correction achieved after manipulation; however, above-knee casts are recommended in small infants.[49]

Ponseti also agreed with the concept of correction through repeated, gentle manipulation and cast applications, but felt that above-knee plaster casts are required routinely to control rotation of the talus within the ankle mortise.[60] In principle, Ponseti is correct; however, with a *well molded cast,* I have found, along with Lovell, that a below-knee plaster cast is often adequate (Fig. 2-10).

Kite proposed the following sequence of correction of the deformities in congenital equinovarus: First, the forefoot adduction and hindfoot varus should be corrected; this should be confirmed by anteroposterior radiographs showing restitution of a normal talocalcaneal angle.[40] This must be corrected before any attempts to dorsiflex the foot and ankle, because the equinus of the foot and ankle cannot possibly be corrected effectively if the heel varus has not been corrected adequately. Dorsiflexion attempted prior to correction of the hindfoot varus will create either a rocker-bottom deformity of the foot or flattening of the talotibial joint surfaces or both.

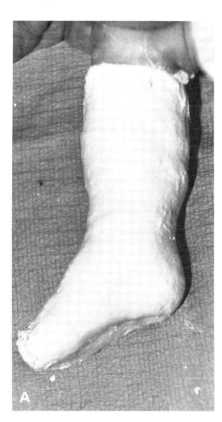 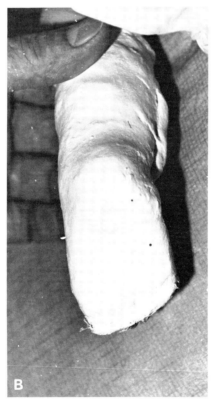

FIG. 2-10. **A,** In a properly applied below-knee cast, the posterior aspect of the heel at the point of insertion of the Achilles tendon must be well molded, and the cast should have a slight concavity over the longitudinal arch. The cast should look like a foot. **B,** The plantar aspect of the cast shows straight lateral and medial borders, and the cast should extend out to the end of the toes so that the long toe flexors will be put on stretch. In most instances of *nonoperative* casts, the parent soaks off the cast the morning that the new cast is applied. The folds of plaster on the lateral side (**B**) assist in this maneuver. If an above-knee cast is desired, it is simple to extend it upwards.

One must also remember, when attempting to correct the ankle equinus, that the heel should be pulled downward rather than the forefoot pushed upward (Fig. 2-11). Lovell and associates found that, through appropriate and patient, gentle, serial manipulation and cast applications, they were able to correct between 40 and 60% of all nonteratologic congenital equinovarus deformities.[49]

Some of the controversy surrounding the nonoperative correctability of true congenital clubfoot centers around the problem of an exact definition of the deformity. The controversy diminishes if one agrees that all feet that can be corrected without surgical treatment represent "positional" clubfeet, and that only those requiring surgical treatment are true congenital clubfeet. This, however, is an artificial "preselection" concept. As noted previously, it is well established that some congenital clubfeet, though they have all of the roentgenographic and physical signs of true clubfoot, can be successfully corrected without an operation. It is important to recognize this concept, otherwise many relatively mild, yet *true* clubfeet may be subjected unnecessarily to surgical treatment. Nearly all experienced orthopedic surgeons have satisfactorily corrected a modest number of true congenital clubfeet without any operative intervention. In my experience, the deformities most likely to respond to nonoperative measures are unilateral deformities in males who have no family history of the disorder (see later section on indications for surgical treatment).

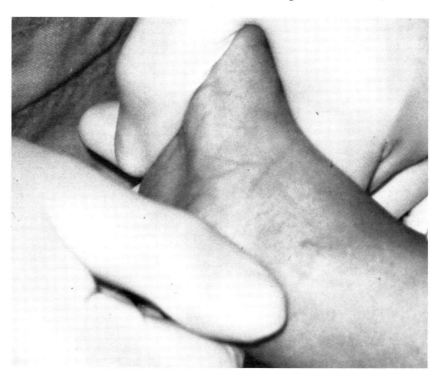

FIG. 2-11. Method of manipulating the foot at the ankle joint. The forefoot is grasped in one hand and a gentle dorsiflexion force is exerted, while the thumb and index finger of the opposite hand grasp the heel and Achilles tendon and pull downward on the heel. This is the only safe and effective way to achieve dorsiflexion of the ankle without creating a potential "break" in the midfoot (see also Fig. 2-22**A**).

DENIS BROWNE (NONCAST) TECHNIQUE. Denis Browne proposed a method of correcting the equinovarus deformity by forcibly placing the foot into the corrected (calcaneovalgus) position, which was then maintained by strapping the foot to a transverse holding bar until the child could ambulate.[10] In Thomson's modification of this technique, the foot is initially strapped or taped to foot plates attached to a crossbar.[84] Then, by progressively abducting and dorsiflexing the foot on the bar, the active physiologic motions of the infant's foot are employed to assist in correction of the clubfoot through a dynamic mechanism.

A prerequisite for this form of treatment is that the infant has good hip and knee motion on the involved side. In addition, the bar should be no wider than the infant's pelvis. A snug fit between the foot and the footplate should be maintained by retaping the foot at weekly intervals. It is essential that the treatment be started early, preferably no later than 2 to 3 weeks of age.

The program involves three phases. Phase I requires at least 5 to 6 weeks and consists of slightly overcorrecting the foot deformity through progressive external rotation and abduction of the foot as described previously. The foot is then maintained in this overcorrected position for about 5 months. Phase II consists of placing the foot in an open-toed shoe on the bar in the corrected position for an additional 6 months, or until ambulation begins.

Phase III consists of a brace and splint program. The shoe is attached to the crossbar and is used only at night. A below-knee brace with a 90° plantar flexion stop and a spring dorsiflexion assist is worn during the day. This is continued for as long as necessary and usually for a minimum of 2 to 3 years. Thomson reports that the major complication in this form of treatment is flattening of the longitudinal arch of the uninvolved foot.[83] To prevent this, he suggests applying a universal joint to the underside of the footplate beneath the normal shoe.

Paterson has adopted a slight variation of this program.[58] He prefers to gain some degree of correction by means of gentle manipulation and cast applications and then institutes the adhesive strapping program detailed in Figure 2-12. Following correction, the foot must be supported for a period of time with protective braces and splints. Observation of the foot must also continue throughout bony maturation to identify and/or prevent recurrence of the deformity.

MANIPULATION AND RETENTION OF CORRECTION BY CASTS. Tachdjian has called our attention appropriately to the need for early reduction of the subluxated talocalcaneonavicular joint, preferably by gentle and careful manipulation and the use of some appropriate retaining device, as emphasized by Lovell. The retaining device used following the manipulation may be a properly applied cast, as preferred by Kite and Lovell, or a method of adhesive strapping as favored by Paterson and others. To some extent, the choice of one over the other is principally a matter of practice, experience, and convenience. Basically, if one uses casts, it is important to change them frequently and to apply them

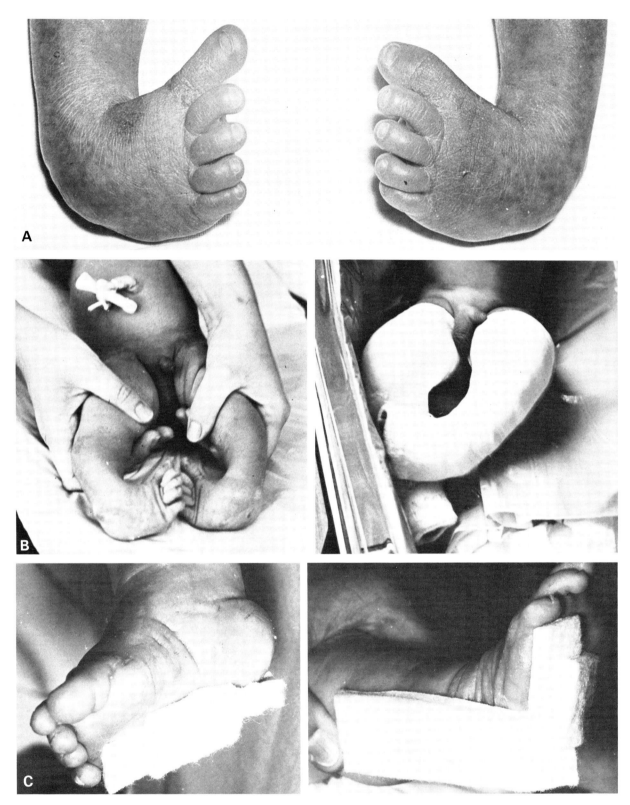

FIG. 2-12. Technique of correction of congenital clubfoot by means of Denis Browne splints. **A,** A typical congenital equinovarus deformity. **B,** The initial correction is achieved by serial manipulation and cast application. Usually 2 weeks of cast treatment are necessary before Denis Browne splints can be applied to the feet. **C,** The first step is the application of adhesive felt to the outer side of the foot and heel and to the outer side of the leg.

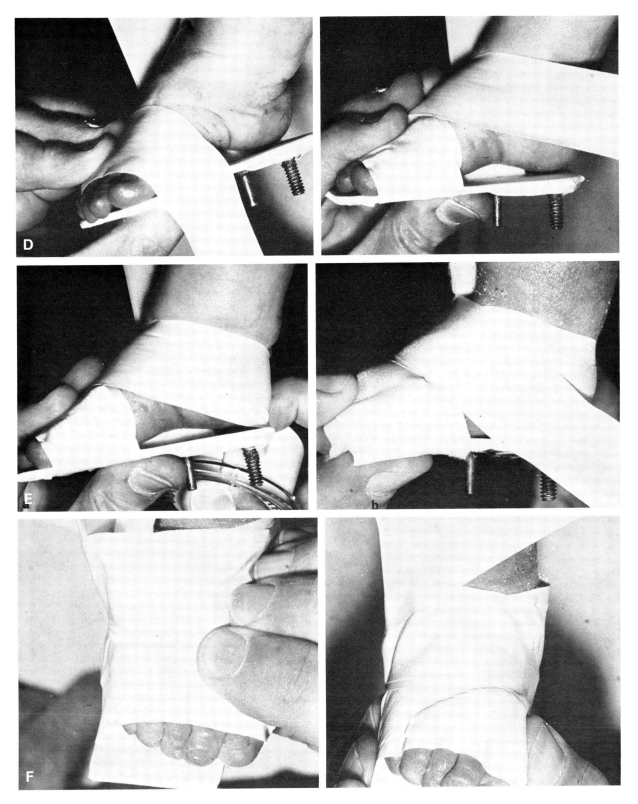

FIG. 2-12. **D**, With the padded foot held firmly on the foot plate, adhesive strapping is begun from the lateral side of the foot, fixing the forefoot and the medial aspect of the heel. (Avoid the foot plate on the turn about the heel.) **E**, Once the forefoot and hindfoot are firmly held by the tape, the foot is then fixed to the foot plate. **F**, The side plate (arrow) is then brought against the outer aspect of the leg and fixed with the strapping.

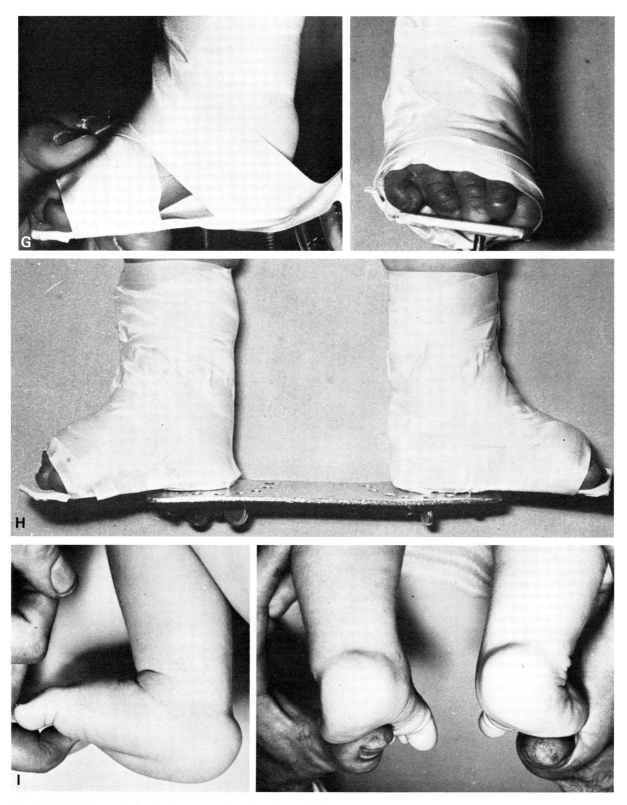

FIG. 2-12. **G,** The entire leg is then strapped to the splint, and then both feet are strapped and attached to a crossbar, which holds the legs in outward rotation (**H**). This technique may correct all components of the clubfoot deformity, but when a convexity of the sole results upon dorsiflexion of the foot, and/or when there is a deep crease or indentation just above the calcaneus (**I**), radical posterior release is then necessary.

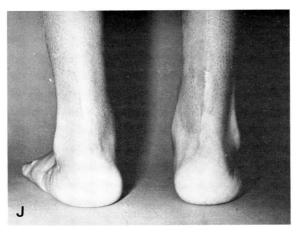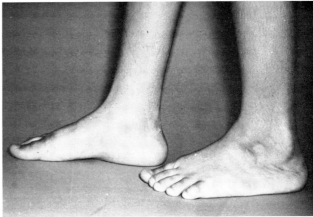

FIG. 2-12. **J,** The result of this form of treatment as shown in (**A**) is illustrated at age 14. (Courtesy of Sir Dennis Paterson, Adelaide, Australia.)

gently and skillfully. These are purely *retaining* devices and should *not* be viewed as *corrective* mechanisms. The correction should be achieved by the manipulation, which is a gentle, passive maneuver, described as follows and illustrated in Figure 2-13.

*Technique of Cast Application.* The left hand gently grasps the hindfoot (heel) of the right foot, and the thumb is placed over the prominence of the talus, which is usually palpated prominently over the lateral aspect of the foot. The right hand then grasps the forefoot. The thumb and index finger hold the metatarsophalangeal joint of the great toe, and longitudinal traction is gently exerted on the forefoot. At the same time, gentle pressure is exerted over the head of the talus.

After one or two minutes, the foot will be felt to elongate, and the prominence of the talus will usually be felt to decrease as the forefoot and other tarsal bones gently move laterally under and around the talus. The foot is held in this corrected position while a cast composed of fast-setting plaster is applied by a qualified assistant over one or two thin layers of sheet cotton. Molding of the cast is important to ensure that the cast will serve as a true retaining device. Whether one places a cast only on the foot (plaster slipper) and then connects it to the leg part separately or whether the entire below-knee cast is applied at one time is a matter of personal preference and experience. In infants with fat feet, it sometimes may be difficult to hold the below-knee cast on the limb without placing some form of adhesive substance on the skin.

Controversy exists about whether an above-knee cast is necessary or whether a below-knee cast is equally effective. In principle, the cast should extend above the knee to control rotation of the foot above the talus. From a practical standpoint, however, if one molds the cast well about all bony prominences, in most instances it is possible to leave the knee free. This has two advantages. First, the muscle action of the knee is uninhibited, thus reducing the degree of muscle atrophy that inevitably occurs during treatment. Second, the below-knee cast is much more acceptable and convenient from the parents' standpoint when it comes to such activities as changing diapers.

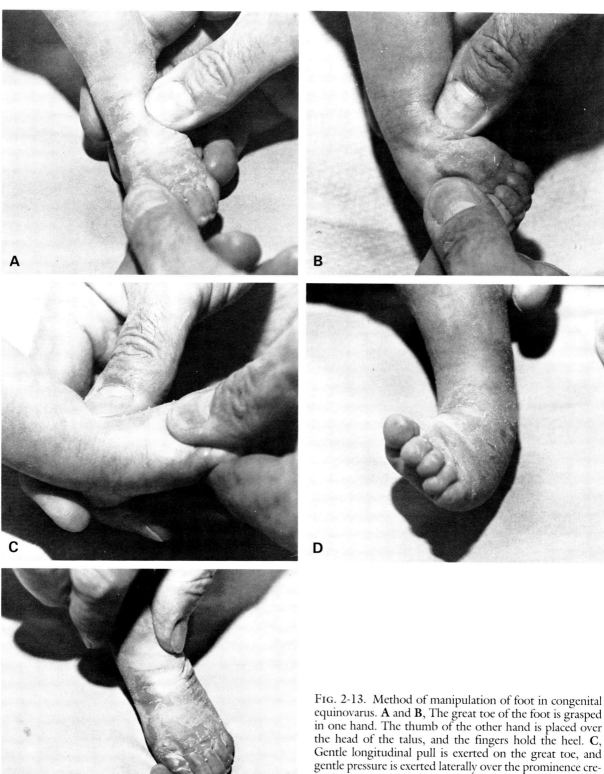

FIG. 2-13. Method of manipulation of foot in congenital equinovarus. **A** and **B**, The great toe of the foot is grasped in one hand. The thumb of the other hand is placed over the head of the talus, and the fingers hold the heel. **C**, Gentle longitudinal pull is exerted on the great toe, and gentle pressure is exerted laterally over the prominence created by the head of the talus. Often the prominence will decrease gradually as the foot rotates beneath and around the talus. **D**, The initial appearance of the foot. **E**, The degree of *clinical* correction following one manipulation. With the foot held carefully in this position, a snug cast is applied to maintain correction.

*Casting Frequency.* Casts or adhesive strapping ideally should be changed as often as is practically possible. Factors that determine the frequency of cast or adhesive application include the age of the child, the prior history of treatment, the response to treatment, and geographic and other logistic issues. Some believe that these retaining devices should be applied as soon after birth as physically possible, and that they should be changed daily when treating clubfoot in the young infant. This is considered to be the "golden" period for correction, since the ligaments at this age are more flexible and distensible, and thus correction can be achieved more rapidly and effectively. It is difficult to argue with this principle. It is not always possible to execute such a program, however, because of extenuating factors such as travel problems, convenience, and frequency of clinic or office visits.

If treatment is delayed such that the child is several weeks or months old before it is begun, casts and adhesive plaster changes need not be so frequent because the ligaments and other soft-tissue structures take longer to adapt to a new, more correct position. Also, if one is dealing with a rigid foot, the cast changes may even be more infrequent because these feet usually respond more slowly to corrective treatment. All of these factors must be taken into account when planning a nonoperative therapy regimen. The principal thing to remember is that the therapy of congenital clubfoot is a highly individualized process, and that not all feet are treated, nor do they respond to treatment, in the same way. At each cast change, the response of the foot to correction should be appraised. This is best done regularly by means of a careful physical examination.

*Casts Versus Surgical Treatment.* I feel that nonoperative techniques are indicated initially in all nonteratogenic or "typical" congenital equinovarus feet. With careful attention to the details of manipulation and the application of casts or adhesive strapping, a substantial number of these feet can be satisfactorily corrected and held by the nonoperative methods just described. By no means will all feet require some form of surgical correction; on the other hand, there is no question that many will require some form of surgical release in the early weeks or months of infancy.

How long the surgeon should persist in a nonoperative approach before realizing that he has encountered a resistant clubfoot that will require surgical methods depends upon his interpretation of the *clinical* response of the foot to nonoperative manipulative treatment. This must be based upon two important determinations, physical examination and radiologic evaluation of the foot during the process of treatment, both of which have pitfalls and limitations. Our inability to standardize and quantify these two factors is responsible for much of the uncertainty that exists regarding the need for surgical correction of a clubfoot.

The point at which improvement no longer appears to be taking place is not always a clear one, and considerable judgment and experience are necessary to make an accurate determination. I have adopted the general principle that if I am in doubt about the correction of the *foot,* then it is probably *not* corrected adequately. The decision must then be made as to whether further cast treatment is justified, or whether it is appropriate to cease nonoperative correction and proceed with surgical correction. This is a highly judgmental decision that the surgeon must make on an individual basis.

*Ankle Equinus.* On the other hand, if the *foot* has been satisfactorily corrected, as determined by clinical and roentgenographic criteria, then one may concentrate on efforts to correct equinus of the *ankle.* This is accomplished by the same basic technique, that is, the hindfoot is manipulated gently into dorsiflexion, and a retaining cast is then applied. This is usually accomplished by applying the *foot* part of the cast first (a plaster slipper) so that the sole of the foot and all of the tarsal relationships are molded as accurately as possible, and then, with the plaster-encased foot held in gentle dorsiflexion, the leg portion is applied. Whether an above- or below-knee cast is required must be determined by the skill and experience of the surgeon.

Just as with correction of the foot, these casts are usually changed at weekly intervals. After one or two efforts to dorsiflex the foot at the ankle joint, I obtain a lateral roentgenogram of the foot and ankle, with the foot held (by the treating surgeon) at the ankle joint in maximum dorsiflexion (Fig. 2-5). If the foot demonstrates satisfactory dorsiflexion, then further efforts at correction of *ankle equinus* are continued, hopefully until it is fully or acceptably corrected.

More often than not, however, in my experience the foot does not respond satisfactorily to dorsiflexion correction at the ankle, and a posterior surgical release of the ankle joint must be done (see Fig. 2-17). The decision to perform a posterior release alone at the ankle must be predicated upon the demonstration of satisfactory correction of the *forefoot, midfoot,* and *hindfoot.* If these components of the deformity are *not* corrected, then the posterior release will surely fail.

POSTCAST CARE. If one is successful in satisfactorily reducing the subluxated talocalcaneonavicular and ankle joints nonoperatively, it then becomes necessary to hold the foot and ankle in the corrected position. Also, if one accepts the fact that the bones of these feet are basically abnormal, not only in their relationships to each other, but also with respect to their size and configuration, it becomes abundantly clear that long-term splintage will be necessary. Conceptually, if one can hold the correction until growth and adaptive changes can take place effectively in the bones and soft tissues, then at some time the external holding devices can be gradually discontinued.

The specific type of splint or brace used is unimportant as long as it has the following features, namely, it can be employed both day and night, exerts both abducting and outwardly rotating forces on the forefoot and midfoot at their junction to the hindfoot, and also produces a dorsiflexion force at the ankle. The device should permit and encourage foot and ankle motions and must also permit ambulation in the older infant and young child. Several methods are available, but the techniques I have found successful are outlined as follows.

*Nonambulatory Devices.* In the young nonambulatory infant with a *unilateral* deformity, a clubfoot shoe is prescribed and is attached to a crossbar with the shoes being outwardly rotated at least 30°. The crossbar may be bent upwards in order to exert both an everting and a dorsiflexing force on the foot (Fig. 2-14). When the deformity is unilateral, the dorsiflexion function of the opposite normal foot can serve as the dynamic force producing passive dorsiflexion.

If the problem is *bilateral,* the same device may serve satisfactorily in the young nonambulatory infant. In older infants, however, I believe that a below-knee, spring-loaded dorsiflexion-assist brace is necessary to provide the necessary dynamic dorsiflexion. It must be attached to the same crossbar in order to control rotation. The brace is worn both day and night except for bathing and periods of exercise during the day.

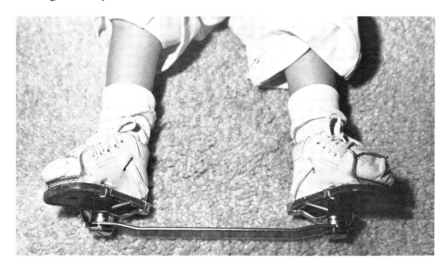

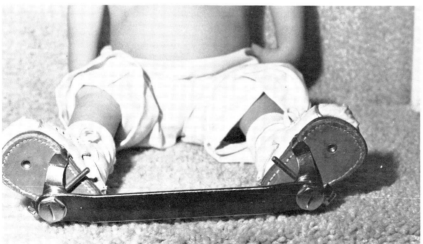

FIG. 2-14. A patient wearing clubfoot shoes attached to a Fillauer splint. In unilateral deformities, the opposite normal foot and ankle serve as the dorsiflexing force. In the case of bilateral clubfoot, spring-loaded dorsiflexion-assist braces are used, and the shoes, being attached to the crossbar, provide the outward rotation force. This combination of devices provides the dorsiflexion-everting forces necessary to maintain correction.

*Ambulatory Devices.* In the ambulatory child, a bar fixed to the shoes is not feasible. I have found that a twister cable attached to a pelvic band provides the best control of abduction or outward rotation of the foot; this device permits ambulation and can be worn day and night. In this situation, however, in order to provide passive-assistive dorsiflexion, a spring-loaded below-knee brace must also be employed in the affected limb, irrespective of whether the deformity is unilateral or bilateral. This device provides all of the external forces necessary to maintain correction (Fig. 2-15).

How long the splintage or bracing must be continued and how rapidly the patient is weaned from the device are highly individual issues. I have always contended that simple correction of the foot deformity does not guarantee that the *cause* (unknown) of the deformity has been solved, nor that whatever correction has been achieved will be maintained. Thus, I believe that some form of postcorrection splintage is mandatory until sufficient adaptive changes in the bones and soft tissues can occur. Whether this external device is used for

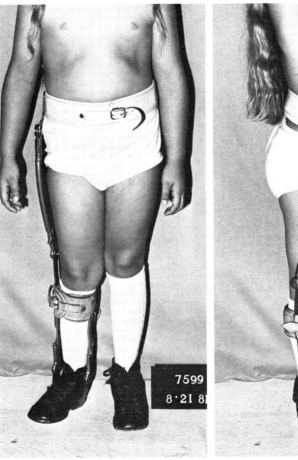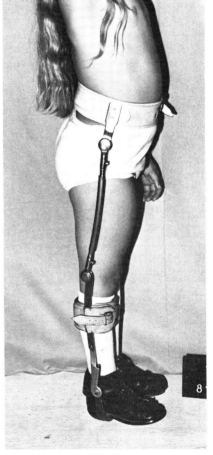

FIG. 2-15. My preferred method of retaining correction of a congenital clubfoot in a child of walking age. The same device is used whether correction is achieved operatively or nonoperatively. A pelvic band controls rotation of the foot upon the leg. The spring-loaded dorsiflexion-assist brace prevents equinus. Because the feet are free, the device can be worn day and night, and the method is well accepted by patients.

several months (as in severe clubfeet and arthrogrypotic feet) is a highly individualized matter. Unfortunately, there are no well recognized control studies to support or refute this concept. Thus, my approach must be considered largely intuitive. Nevertheless, the concept seems valid, and until further information develops refuting this practice, I plan to continue to emphasize this postcorrection splinting program.

In 1784, Lorenz of Frankfort described tenotomy of the heelcord for correction of clubfoot.[48] Stromeyer, in 1835, and subsequently Little, in 1839, both agreed that tenotomy of the Achilles tendon was beneficial in correction of the clubfoot deformity.[44,76] The concept of capsular and ligamentous soft-tissue release in surgical treatment of clubfoot was initiated in 1867 with Streckeisen, who recommended a limited medial release procedure.[75] In 1890, Phelps also recommended correction of the varus through release of the soft tissues on the medial side of the foot.[59]

OPERATIVE
TREATMENT

It was not until 1917 that Zadek and Barnett identified the need for additional release of the posterior ankle capsule, including the ligamentous structures of the posterior ankle and the Achilles tendon.[93] Shortly later, in 1920, Ober emphasized the importance of releasing the deltoid ligament in order to fully correct the hindfoot.[56] Brockman, in 1930, recommended a medial release procedure, with special emphasis upon release of the structures about the talonavicular capsule.[9] In 1940, Storen recognized the importance of both the medial structures and the posterior structures in the deformity and therefore recommended a staged medial release, followed by a posterior release about 4 weeks later.[74]

More recently in 1959, McCauley felt that if initial cast applications failed to correct the deformity, a release of the medial talonavicular calcaneal complex was necessary.[51] A second-stage posterior release for persistent equinus deformity of the ankle was employed, if needed. In 1966, Attenborough felt that posterior release was nearly always necessary to bring the talus out of equinus.[2] In 1971, Turco also recognized the need for both medial foot and posterior ankle release, and he was the first to popularize the concept of releasing both the medial and the posterior structures in one operation.[86]

The use of tarsal osteotomy and bone resection to correct the clubfoot deformity began in the middle and late nineteenth century. For example, in 1857, Solly recommended resection of the cuboid.[72] In 1875, Lund advised astragalectomy.[50] In 1875, Colley proposed removal of wedge-shaped segments of bone from the lateral side of the foot in order to achieve better correction.[11] Pugh, 8 years later, advised removing the head of the talus in the surgical treatment of clubfoot.[61] In 1912, Hoke employed serial wedging casts, but he also recommended multiple lateral-wedge resections of bone to achieve additional correction if necessary.[34] In 1934, Curtis and Muro devised a "decancellation" procedure, which consisted of removing the cancellous bone from the talus, calcaneus, and cuboid.[13] This resulted in a softening of these bones and rendered them more malleable. Forceful manipulation of the foot then produced a spurious correction of the deformity.

Evans, in 1961, believed that one of the major deformities resisting correction in equinovarus congenita was relative elongation of the lateral column of the foot.[19] He therefore recommended wedge resection of the calcaneocuboid joint as a means of shortening the lateral column. This permitted more complete correction of the foot around the talus and accomplished a purposeful fusion of the calcaneocuboid joint, which was felt to be necessary in order to maintain the reduction. Later, in 1973, Lichtblau agreed with Evans' concept concerning the need for lateral-column shortening; however, he avoided calcaneocuboid fusion by resecting only the distal portion of the calcaneus.[43] In 1963, Dwyer proposed calcaneal osteotomy as a means of correcting persistent hindfoot varus.[17]

Goldner proposes a laterally based wedge resection of the cuboid as a means of shortening the lateral column.[27] He believes that the calcaneocuboid joint should not be violated and that correction can be achieved just as well by avoiding the joint. This has a good conceptual basis, provided that there is no true deformity of the calcaneocuboid joint, which sometimes exists in the older, more resistant clubfeet. If a deformity does reside in the joint, then cuboid resection may provide a spurious clinical correction, but not anatomic correction.

GENERAL CONSIDERATIONS. Most surgeons in the past have felt that operative treatment should be performed at a time when the structures of the infantile foot have grown large enough to be safely operated upon. In most instances, this is approximately age 3 months or later. Reimann and Becker-Andersen have shown that, with proper indications and careful technique, surgical release of the infant resistant clubfoot at 3 months of age can produce satisfactory results.[62] They reported 86.4% acceptable results in a follow-up study of 140 surgical cases that were operated on at age 3 months. Westin, however, feels that the congenital clubfoot should not be operated on until the child is at least 12 months old.[87]

Both Brockman and McCauley recognized the importance of releasing the tight medial structures about the talonavicular joint when correcting equinovarus congenita surgically.[9,51] They also recognized that the major offending structures preventing correction were the contracted anterior portion of the deltoid ligament, the anterior talonavicular ligament and capsule, and the calcaneonavicular ligament. They recommended operative release of these structures through a medial approach to correct the talonavicular subluxation as well as the relationships of the calcaneus to the talus. They also employed tenotomy of the posterior tibial tendon as needed. McCauley felt that lengthening of the tendons of the toe flexors usually was not necessary because these structures stretch spontaneously with time.[9,51]

Both Stewart and Attenborough outlined the indications and technique for posterior release. They advised the importance of capsulotomy and ligamentous release at both the ankle and subtalar joints, along with lengthening of the Achilles tendon. They recommended releasing the Achilles tendon at its medial attachment to the calcaneus.[2,73] Barenfeld, Weseley, Paterson, and also DeLangh noted that if release of the ankle ligaments and Achilles tendon did not achieve sufficient dorsiflexion, release of the posterior tibiofibular ligament could also be employed.[3,15,57] Conceptually, this allows the ankle mortise to spread so as to accommodate the wider anterior portion of the talus during dorsiflexion.

When Turco popularized the one-stage posteromedial release, he described a procedure that sectioned or lengthened the medial, subtalar, and posterior ligamentous structures at one operation. He felt that this was necessary in order to gain complete correction, which he found to be impossible through sequential releases.[86] In 1979, Turco reviewed his cases 2 to 15 years postoperatively and reported good to excellent results in 85% of 140 feet.[85] He concluded that the poor results were mainly related to (a) the age of the patient at the time of surgical release, (b) any prior operation on the foot, and (c) an overcorrected foot created through surgical overcorrection of the hindfoot and subtalar structures. He believed that a more selective approach, releasing only those structures necessary for correction, could avoid overcorrection.

Turco also felt that the most appropriate time for surgical release of equinovarus deformity was between 1 and 2 years of age, thus agreeing to some extent with Westin. Turco noted poor results for releases performed before or after this age. He also felt that posteromedial release in children over 6 years of age was rarely of substantial benefit.

INDICATIONS. In anticipation of the need for surgical correction in many cases of congenital clubfoot, I have developed guidelines that have helped me in establishing indications for surgical intervention. Broadly speaking, it is essential to distinguish clearly between the teratologic (atypical) clubfoot and the true clubfoot. In the former, as noted earlier, one is dealing with a severe degree of deformity in which there may be a longstanding antenatal defect associated with or resulting from growth abnormalities in muscle function, abnormalities in joint formation, or major changes in joint structure and configuration. These feet represent a specific category of congenital equinovarus and are discussed in greater detail in Chapter 8.

The true clubfoot, on the other hand, represents a broad spectrum of deformity with respect to the degree of severity. Wide variation exists in the response to both nonoperative and surgical management. Although it is difficult to provide any rigid guidelines covering the need for surgical therapy, some patterns of clubfoot behavior have influenced my judgment and decisions with respect to the indications for surgery.

In general, I have found that the unilateral congenital clubfoot in a male, without a family history of foot deformity, will respond most consistently and successfully to nonoperative or operative management (when necessary). This clinical observation corresponds with the conclusions expressed earlier regarding the different manifestations of clubfoot in males and females. At the other end of the scale, the foot that is most resistant to correction (excluding arthrogrypotic clubfeet) is a bilateral deformity in the female infant who has a family history of clubfoot. In this foot, the likelihood that some form of surgical correction will be necessary approaches 100%. Between these two extremes is a spectrum of clubfoot deformities, in which the major factors influencing treatment are: the sex of the patient, whether the deformity is unilateral or bilateral, and whether or not the family has a history of clubfoot. These observations are summarized in the following list, which arranges the deformities in order of *increasing* resistance to correction:

Unilateral clubfoot in male

↓

Unilateral clubfoot in female

↓

Bilateral clubfoot in male

↓

Bilateral clubfoot in female

When a family history shows that a close member of the family has had congenital clubfoot, the degree of resistance and complexity of the foot deformity usually is enhanced considerably (see section on pathogenesis). Clearly, there will be many exceptions to the general rule just outlined. Nevertheless, awareness of this pattern of behavior has helped me, not only in determining the likelihood of surgical correction, but also in predicting for the family what they may expect in the way of future problems and the need for prolonged and complex treatment.

Although demographic and behavioral patterns are important, the physical and roentgenographic criteria are ultimately the critical determinants that govern the decision to proceed with surgical correction. This means that the surgeon must evaluate accurately all aspects of the problem and come to the decision for surgical treatment after having performed a careful physical examination and a critical review of the roentgenograms, and after having placed all factors into appropriate perspective.

Physical examination should include the following: general inspection of the foot, careful palpation of bony prominences and depressions, and assessment of the flexibility or rigidity of the foot.

Inspection of the foot should compare the length of the first ray of the foot to that of the other rays and should assess the relationship of the forefoot and midfoot to the hindfoot (adducted or not), the position of the calcaneus (whether in varus or valgus), and the degree of flexibility of the ankle joint. If the first ray is unusually short, this probably means that the navicular and remainder of the forefoot have not been reduced appropriately. If the forefoot and midfoot remain adducted (in varus), this usually means that the hindfoot (calcaneus) is also uncorrected. This can be verified by assessing the degree of varus (or valgus) in the heel.

Flexibility of the ankle is difficult to determine accurately because it is difficult to separate the dorsiflexion motions of the forefoot and ankle. I usually rely upon lateral dorsiflexion-stress roentgenograms for this determination (see previous section on roentgenographic criteria).

The two most important determinations in palpation of the foot are (1) the depth of the sinus tarsus on the lateral aspect of the hindfoot and (2) the relationships of the three major bony prominences on the medial side; i.e., the medial malleolus, the head of the talus, and the tarsal navicular (Fig. 2-16). When the head of the talus is not palpable on the medial side of the foot, one can conclude that the relationship of the forefoot and midfoot to the *hindfoot* has been incompletely corrected. Further efforts at correction, either nonoperative or operative, therefore will be necessary.

On the other hand, correction of the *foot* deformity may be established. Correction of *ankle equinus* must then be considered, based upon the ability of the *corrected foot* to be passively dorsiflexed at the ankle joint. As noted previously, this requires a lateral roentgenogram, with the foot held in maximum dorsiflexion. This should be done after at least 2 weeks of attempts at dorsiflexion as described previously. If gradual correction is observed and if acceptable dorsiflexion *at the ankle* can be ultimately accomplished (at least 5 to 10° above a right angle), no release will be necessary. On the other hand, if no dorsiflexion is possible or, even more importantly, if apparent dorsiflexion tends to occur at the midtarsal joints, thus leaving the hindfoot in equinus (rocker-bottom foot), then posterior ankle release is indicated (Fig. 2-17).

I have found it convenient to categorize congenital clubfeet that do not respond to nonoperative, "conservative" treatment as either *resistant* or *recurrent* (relapsing). The resistant clubfoot either does not respond or has not responded favorably to nonoperative methods of correction; as a consequence, surgical release of some form is necessary. On the other hand, if the foot was acceptably corrected at one time, as demonstrated by the aforementioned clinical and radiographic determinations, but over a period of time the deformity has recurred, it is defined as a *recurrent* (relapsed) clubfoot. This latter foot problem usually implies one of two things: either correction has been inadequately maintained, or a poorly defined muscle imbalance exists that may ultimately require tendon transfers to satisfactorily maintain correction.

In addition to recurrence of the deformity, problems in the treatment of congenital equinovarus include: fixed forefoot equinus that has a substantial cavus component (equinocavovarus), and delayed treatment (neglected clubfoot). (Teratologic (arthrogrypotic) equinovarus deformities and the presence of associated visceral and skeletal

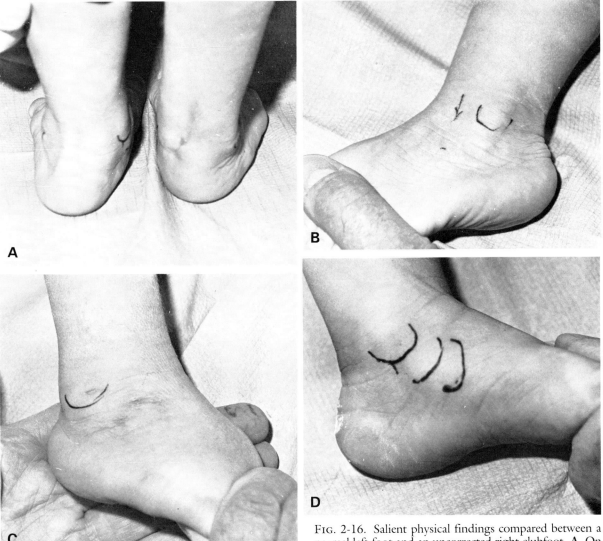

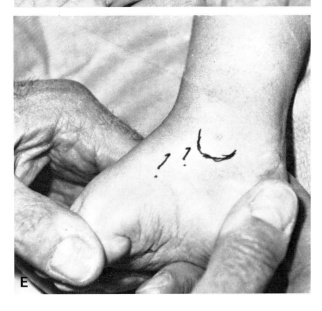

FIG. 2-16. Salient physical findings compared between a normal left foot and an uncorrected right clubfoot. **A,** On the normal left side, the heel is in slight valgus, and a clearly defined shadow is created by the Achilles tendon. On the right side, the heel is in the neutral position. The heel is widened and the Achilles tendon poorly defined. (This patient had undergone a previous heelcord lengthening; hence the scar.) **B,** On the lateral side of the normal foot, the fibula is sharply outlined and the sinus tarsus (arrow) is usually deep, representing the recess created by divergence of the talus and calcaneus. **C,** On the lateral side of the clubfoot, the fibula is less well defined, and a prominence is found in the usual location of the sinus tarsus representing the talar head. **D,** Over the medial side of the normal foot, three bony prominences are clearly defined and easily palpable: from proximal to distal, the medial malleolus, the head of the talus, and the navicular. **E,** On the medial side of the clubfoot, the medial malleolus is broader and less distinct than normal but usually can be readily identified; however, it is usually difficult to palpate the head of the talus, and the navicular may actually be found to articulate with the medial malleolus. Efforts to identify these landmarks often can be just as helpful and reliable as a roentgenogram in evaluation of a clubfoot.

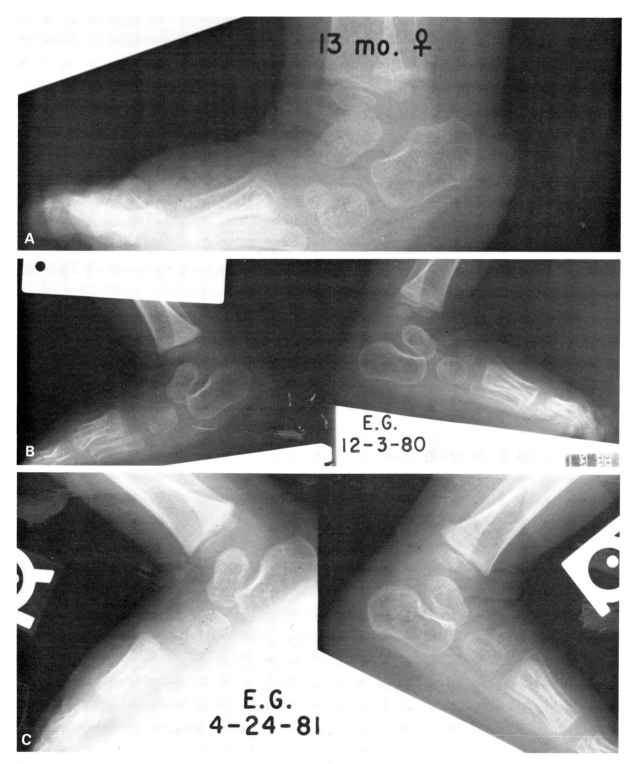

FIG. 2-17. **A,** The spurious correction of equinus is well demonstrated in this lateral roentgenogram of the foot of a 13-month-old girl who exhibited *clinical* correction, but whose roentgenograms showed equinus of the hindfoot and dorsiflexion of the forefoot and midfoot. The need for posterior release of the ankle by means of heelcord lengthening and ankle capsulotomy is evident. In this case, a selective posteromedial release was accomplished. **B,** On the other hand, a patient was expected to require a posterior release on the right foot due to possible midfoot break. **C,** After the employment of a dorsiflexion-assist brace such as that illustrated in Figure 2-15 for 5 months, however, posterior release was not considered to be necessary.

congenital abnormalities, because of their singular complications, are discussed in Chapter 8.) These situations are usually self-evident at the time of initial examination or manifest themselves sometimes early in the course of the treatment program.

THE RESISTANT CLUBFOOT. The following sections discuss two operative procedures used to correct the resistant clubfoot: the posterior release and the posterior-medial release.

*Posterior Release.* If the *foot* has been corrected, but *ankle* equinus resists nonoperative correction, then a full, complete posterior release must be delicately performed. The surgical procedure is illustrated in Figure 2-18 and described as follows.

Through a posteromedially placed curvilinear incision of appropriate length (depending upon the size of the foot), the heelcord tendon is exposed. I prefer that the convexity of the curve of the incision fall anteriorly, so that when the incision straightens out upon dorsiflexion of the foot on the ankle, it will not overlie the Achilles tendon. The incision must expose the insertion of the tendon to the calcaneus.

The Achilles tendon is lengthened in a "Z" fashion, preferably with the portion of the tendon that inserts on the medial aspect of the calcaneus being sectioned distally. Reflection of the tendon exposes a layer of fat that overlies the fascia of the deep compartment. This fat is gently rubbed away, and the deep compartment is entered with sharp dissection. Entrance into the deep compartment is easily determined because the fat of that compartment will promptly extrude through this incision in the deep fascia. This latter fascial incision is extended upwards and downwards, and the muscle and tendon of the flexor hallucis longus are identified and retracted medially. Visualization of these structures is facilitated by gently wiping away the fatty tissue of the deep compartment. This exposes the posterior aspect of the ankle joint, including all posterior ligamentous structures and the tibiofibular syndesmosis.

The ankle joint capsule and ligaments are sectioned transversely, exposing the talotibial joint. Care must be taken to cut all posterior ankle joint structures as they attach to the posterior aspects of the medial and lateral malleoli, while at the same time protecting the tendons of the flexor hallucis longus and the peroneus longus and brevis. Considerable dorsiflexion of the foot on the ankle usually will be possible when the posterior ankle ligaments are appropriately freed.

For the past several years, I have routinely performed a release of the syndesmosis between the tibia and fibula to gain greater dorsiflexion. This is done *after* the ankle joint has been released as just described. Paterson initially suggested this procedure; he concluded that in order for the wider portion of the anterior body of the talus to be placed into dorsiflexion, the ankle mortise must be allowed to spread.[57] I think this is a valid concept, and in some instances I have gained as much as 15° of increased dorsiflexion by using this procedure; to date, no identifiable complications or sequelae in the ankle joint have become evident following its accomplishment.

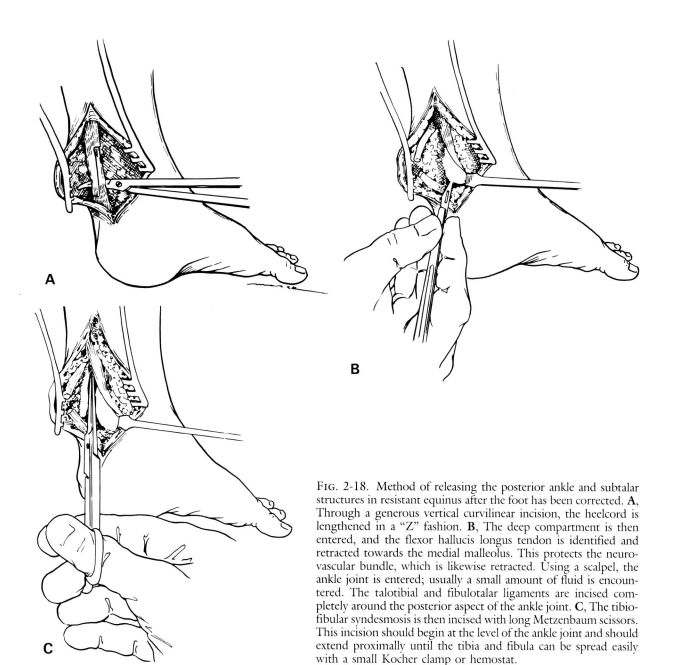

FIG. 2-18. Method of releasing the posterior ankle and subtalar structures in resistant equinus after the foot has been corrected. **A,** Through a generous vertical curvilinear incision, the heelcord is lengthened in a "Z" fashion. **B,** The deep compartment is then entered, and the flexor hallucis longus tendon is identified and retracted towards the medial malleolus. This protects the neurovascular bundle, which is likewise retracted. Using a scalpel, the ankle joint is entered; usually a small amount of fluid is encountered. The talotibial and fibulotalar ligaments are incised completely around the posterior aspect of the ankle joint. **C,** The tibiofibular syndesmosis is then incised with long Metzenbaum scissors. This incision should begin at the level of the ankle joint and should extend proximally until the tibia and fibula can be spread easily with a small Kocher clamp or hemostat.

Sectioning of the posterior aspect of the subtalar joint is purely optional; I have not found it necessary *if* the *foot* was satisfactorily corrected prior to posterior release. If any doubt exists about subtalar correction at this juncture, then the posterior aspect of the talocalcaneal joint capsule can easily be sectioned.

Postoperatively, the foot and ankle are placed in an above-knee cast. Seven days later, I routinely change the foot and ankle portion to inspect the wound and to attempt further gentle correction in the event that full or acceptable correction could not be achieved at the time of the operation. This weekly sequence continues until maximum acceptable correction of ankle equinus has been achieved. Then, in the unilateral cases, I have placed the foot in a clubfoot shoe and attached the shoe to a bar, such as a Denis Browne or Fillauer bar, with the foot held in maximum outward rotation in a similar fashion as was outlined in the section on nonoperative techniques (Fig. 2-14). A variable degree of dorsiflexion can be accomplished by bending the bar. The opposite normal foot and leg can assist in maintaining this correction in addition to providing dynamic correction.

In bilateral cases, the same program may be equally effective, but as often as not, I have found it necessary to apply a spring-loaded dorsiflexion-assist brace in which the shoes are also attached to the bar in outward rotation (Fig. 2-17). This bracing program is maintained for several months, day and night. Thereafter, the patient is slowly weaned from these devices according to the response of the foot to correction and other factors that the surgeon must weigh individually.

*Posterior-Medial Release.* In a substantial number of congenital equinovarus deformities, the foot will not respond appropriately to nonoperative cast treatment. In other words, the forefoot cannot be placed into the proper position, and the hindfoot still remains in some degree of varus, with the calcaneus remaining in its "locked" position under the talus. When this situation obtains, a *posterior-medial* release will be required.

I have experienced a substantial number of overcorrections in performing the "complete" posterior-medial release (the Turco procedure) in children with resistant clubfeet. This distressing situation is a result of performing the same routine operation on feet that vary widely in degree of deformity. Consequently, I have adopted a more selective surgical approach, in which I section or lengthen the contracted ligaments and tendinous structures only as required to achieve correction. This concept is being increasingly reinforced by many surgeons who hold that congenital equinovarus is extremely variable in its pathologic manifestations, and that the treatment thus should be individualized according to these variations. I refer to this as the "selective" posterior-medial release, whereas Tachdjian, for the same reasons, has termed it the "à la carte" approach.[78] In any case, the principle is the same, namely, that only those structures preventing correction (reduction) of the deformity are surgically sectioned or lengthened.

The following structures are most commonly responsible for holding the components of the foot in their unreduced, deformed relationships: the tibionavicular portion of the deltoid ligament, the capsule of the talonavicular joint, the posterior tibial tendon, the plantar calcaneonavicular (spring) ligament, the thickened and contracted sheaths of the posterior tibial tendon and the tendons of the long toe flexors, the talocalcaneal joint capsule, and the talocalcaneal interosseous ligament.

Which and how many of these structures need to be sectioned or lengthened can be accurately determined only during the operation and not preoperatively. The order of structures just listed is the sequence I usually follow in the medial portion of the posterior-medial release.

The structures responsible for holding the ankle in equinus are the Achilles (and plantaris) tendon and its sheath, the contracted posterior deep fascia of the calf, the ankle joint capsule, the posterior talofibular and talotibial ligaments and the tibiofibular ligaments (syndesmosis), along with the distal portion of the coextensive interosseous membrane between the tibia and fibula. In addition to lengthening the Achilles tendon, when performing the posterior release, I routinely section all of the ligaments just mentioned, almost always in the order listed here. The entire posterior-medial release is described as follows (Fig. 2-19).

A generous incision is made, centering over the prominence of the medial malleolus. It extends gently upward in a curvilinear fashion from the medial cuneiform to the Achilles tendon. Using scalpel dissection, with binocular magnification as necessary, the deep fascia overlying the anterior tibial tendon, the tibionavicular ligament and its subjacent posterior tibial tendon, the posterior tibial neurovascular bundle, and the Achilles tendon are exposed. The skin flaps are undermined, and the saphenous vein is retracted with the anterior skin flap. The first structure sectioned is the tibionavicular portion of the deltoid ligament. This is usually a strong, thick ligament and blends intimately into the sheath and part of the insertion of the posterior tibial tendon. This tendon is then freed up, but it is *not* sectioned at the talonavicular level; rather, it is lengthened in the following fashion, modified somewhat from the technique described by Barnett.[4,5]

The distal insertion of the posterior tibial tendon is identified at its attachment to the navicular. Using scalpel dissection, the tendon and its anterior and plantar extensions are freed up as far distally as the base of the first metatarsal. The tendon is sectioned at this point and allowed to retract proximally as the foot is placed into its corrected position. This avoids unnecessary scarring within the proximal sheath of the posterior tibial tendon and preserves it as a functional muscle after it is sutured back to the navicular.

Above all, the tendon should not be simply cut without repair. Except in arthrogrypotic feet and other salvage situations, in which it is often excised, the posterior tibial tendon should not be sectioned over the medial aspect of the ankle or talonavicular joint. It will nearly always become adherent and nonfunctional at this location or, even worse, a tenodesis effect may occur that would tend to increase the likelihood of forefoot adduction recurring. Also, just as in normal feet, clubfeet deserve to have a functional posterior tibial muscle, with an excursion across the talonavicular joint, and the action of this musculotendinous unit should be preserved if possible.

The talonavicular capsule is then sectioned completely, and this requires dissection over the dorsum of the foot. A small, sharp rake placed into the substance of the navicular can exert gentle, distal traction on the capsule of the talonavicular joint. This facilitates identification and release of the capsule dorsally. In the process of doing the plantar release, the plantar calcaneonavicular ligament is sectioned.

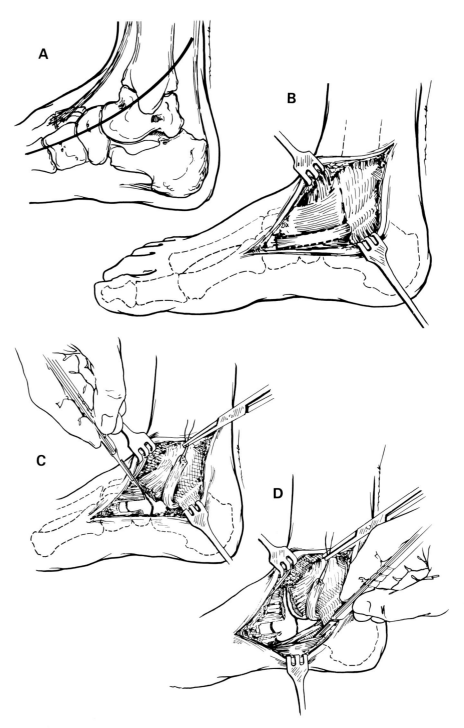

FIG. 2-19. My preferred method of performing a posteromedial release. **A,** Incision. **B,** The skin flaps are retracted to expose the laciniate ligament and the tibionavicular portion of the deltoid ligament. **C,** The distal portion of the laciniate ligament over the course of the posterior tibial tendon is incised, and the distal insertion of this tendon is exposed as far as the medial cuneiform, where it is sectioned. This requires a careful dissection of portions of the capsule of the naviculocuneiform joint and tendinous expansion of the tibialis posterior. **D,** The tendon is reflected, thus exposing the tibionavicular ligament and the underlying and coextensive talonavicular joint capsule. These are both incised near the medial malleolus, thereby leaving a generous portion of the deltoid ligament attached to the navicular.

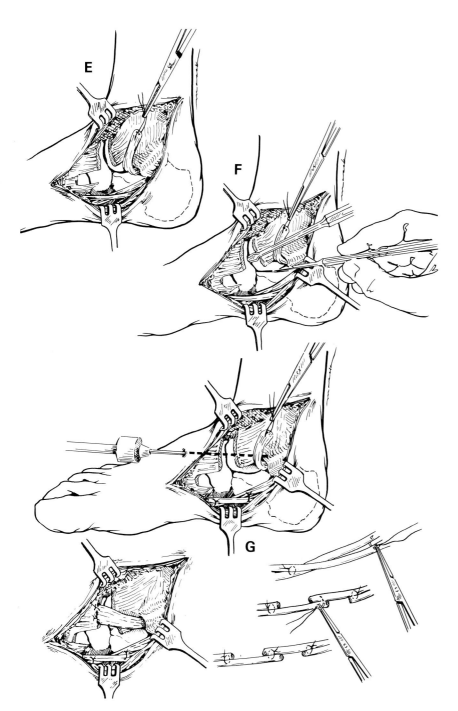

FIG. 2-19. **E,** Utilizing a small, sharp rake retractor, the navicular is gently pulled distally over the head of the talus, and the talonavicular joint capsule is further released. **F,** If necessary, the subtalar joint is then exposed and the ligaments are incised, including the talocalcaneal interosseous ligament. This amount of soft-tissue release is usually adequate to correct the triple joint. Lengthening of the long toe flexors and resection of portions of the laciniate ligament may be required. **G,** My preferred method of lengthening the flexors. If a limited plantar release is deemed necessary, it can be done through this incision (**D**). Reduction of the talonavicular relationship is maintained by a smooth Kirschner wire (**G**). A posterior release is then accomplished through a proximal extension of the incision as illustrated in Figure 2-18. The posterior tibial tendon is then sutured to the flap of tibionavicular ligament distally (left insert).

Using a curved, sharp elevator, the lateral portion of the talonavicular capsule is gently cut blindly. If necessary, a small, lateral incision, as described by Goldner, may be employed to section this important structure.[28] Care must be taken at all times to avoid damage to the delicate articular surfaces of the talonavicular joint, because in the foot these are the functional growth equivalents to the epiphyseal plates of the long bones. At this point, the correctability of the foot is assessed. In some unusual circumstances, this amount of surgical treatment is all that is required for satisfactory correction.

Recently, in unpublished data, both Roberts and McKay emphasized the value of releasing the lateral calcaneofibular ligament during the medial release procedure.[52,63] The purpose of this operation is to allow the posterior aspect of the calcaneus to be displaced medially as the anterior aspect of the calcaneus, the cuboid, and the navicular are rotated laterally under the talus. The procedure is a simple one, accomplished through a small vertical incision just lateral to the Achilles tendon, and the ligaments connecting the calcaneus to the fibula are severed. I have had no experience with this operation, although conceptually it appears that it may have merit in the severe, resistant equinovarus foot. It is technically feasible that the same release can be accomplished when the posterior portion of the posteromedial release is done, when the entire ankle, subtalar joint, fibula, and calcaneus usually can be readily exposed, as described subsequently.

If full correction cannot be achieved after these structures have been sectioned or lengthened, the sheaths of the posterior tibial tendon and the long toe flexors (laciniate ligament) may require sectioning, or preferably, they should be simply separated from their attachments to the subtalar joint by sharp dissection. In this situation, the talocalcaneal (subtalar) joint capsule, and even the talocalcaneal interosseous ligament, may also need to be sectioned. This, of course, represents accomplishment of the complete medial release, except for the lengthening of the long toe flexors.

The decision of whether or not to lengthen these tendons must await the results of the posterior ankle joint release. Tightness of these tendons, however, ordinarily will not prevent correction of the forefoot and midfoot on the hindfoot. A *smooth* Kirschner wire of appropriate size is then placed across the talonavicular joint, with the foot held in the corrected position. The posterior tibial tendon is subsequently resutured back to the soft tissues (tibionavicular ligament) of the navicular bone in its lengthened state, as described earlier.

Attention is then directed to the Achilles tendon, which is exposed by sharp scalpel dissection. The posterior aspect of the operation is then performed exactly as described earlier (see section on posterior release). After this release has been accomplished and the foot and ankle have been satisfactorily corrected, the surgeon can knowledgeably decide whether or not to lengthen the long toe flexors. Lengthening is indicated if the toes tend to flex acutely when the ankle is dorsiflexed, and if these digits cannot be passively extended in this position. I prefer to accomplish this in the sole of the foot, where these tendons are readily accessible and where peritendinous fat is ample and thus reduces the likelihood of adhesions between the tenorrhaphy and the surrounding soft tissues. At this point, the maximum possible correction of the ankle should be achieved. The Achilles tendon is then repaired with the foot held in slight dorsiflexion, and the wound is closed.

At this point it must be decided how much correction should be attempted and how much the tissues of the foot will tolerate. This requires judgment and experience, and there is no sure "cookbook" way to make such a decision. If in doubt at all, the tourniquet should be released, and the color of the skin on both sides of the incision should be assessed. Clearly, correction should never reach the point at which skin vascularity is jeopardized.

We are indebted to Turco and others for demonstrating that in most cases both the foot and ankle deformities can be safely treated in the same operative procedure, *provided that* meticulous and conscientious attention is paid to the details of the procedures and that sound judgment is exercised concerning the amount of correction achieved at the time of operation.[86]

The statement just made deserves further explanation. Although the concept of achieving full correction at the time of the operation is attractive, and in some situations can be done safely, some circumstances may prevent this. Severe, rigid foot deformities in young infants and children may not tolerate abrupt, full correction because of the threat to operative wound healing as well as to the viability of the skin and subcutaneous tissues over the medial aspect of the foot. One of the worst disasters that can befall a foot undergoing surgical correction is major full-thickness skin slough on the medial side. This is discussed in the section on complications.

In the rigid, difficult foot just alluded to, one must regard the surgical elongation of the corrected structures (posterior-medial release) as a means of permitting *subsequent* correction rather than of achieving *immediate* total correction. Lloyd-Roberts has referred to these surgical procedures as simply "incidents" in the continued non-operative management of clubfoot.[46,47] If one accepts this thesis, namely, that the surgical releases are designed simply to *assist* correction, this mandates that the operative and postoperative casts be changed at periodic intervals postoperatively to take full advantage of the releasing procedure.

Also, judgment and experience are crucial in determining how much correction can safely be achieved at the time of operation. As noted earlier, in some situations it may be necessary to release the tourniquet and inspect the skin color and appearance prior to applying the holding operative cast. As a matter of fact, many surgeons routinely deflate the tourniquet at the time of operation in order to check for any major bleeding and to inspect the viability of the skin edges. If in doubt, I follow the same policy, especially if I am concerned about the amount of correction that can be accomplished safely.

At the first cast change, usually done between 7 and 14 days postoperatively, the wound can be inspected and a well molded, snug cast applied, with the foot and ankle being placed in a position of greater correction, provided that the wound and skin appearance render it safe. Thereafter, the judgment of the surgeon must dictate the frequency of cast changes.

*Postoperative Care.* Depending upon the age of the child, the foot remains in its corrected cast for a minimum of 6 weeks and a maximum of 3 months. The pin is removed at 2 to 4 weeks, and in children under 9 months, often the foot can be placed into a clubfoot shoe and brace, as described previously (see section on posterior release). If the child is older, most often the foot is placed into a holding cast for another 6 weeks, followed by application of the shoe and brace. The brace is kept on day and night for several months, after which the child is gradually weaned from it during the day. In feet that have undergone the full posteromedial release, it is my policy to continue nighttime bracing until the foot has good mobility and good muscle control, or until age 6 years. The tendency for the foot deformity to recur up until the age of 6 years is substantial. During the entire time of bracing, an active exercise program is encouraged, using both active, active-resistive, and passive stretching exercises, as suggested by Paterson.[57]

THE RECURRENT CLUBFOOT. *Recurrent* (relapsed) clubfoot implies that the foot was satisfactorily corrected at one time, but the previous deformity has recurred. This is a difficult situation to document, because it must be based upon concrete evidence that an acceptable correction was indeed achieved at one time. Recognizing the frailties of *documenting* the physical examination of a child's foot and realizing that many factors influence and vitiate the value of radiographic interpretation, it must be apparent that such a diagnosis may be somewhat elusive. In many instances of suspected recurrent clubfoot, I have found, by critical review of the recorded physical findings and the roentgenograms, that the foot in fact had never been truly corrected, and that the problem actually represented a resistant or incompletely corrected rather than a recurrent clubfoot.

On the other hand, I have observed a substantial number of instances of congenital equinovarus that I feel have been acceptably corrected, but yet present themselves several months or a year or two later with a recurrent deformity. It is then essential that the surgeon determine the reason(s) for the recurrence. At least two major factors usually surface in this evaluation: (a) either the postcorrection bracing and splintage programs were inadequate (either through not having been prescribed or not having been carried out) or (b) a muscle imbalance has become evident, in which the strengths of the evertors and dorsiflexors have yielded to the strengths of the invertors and plantar flexors. In the former situation, one must ask whether simple recorrection will adequately solve the problem. In the latter circumstance, one that is difficult to establish or prove, the surgeon must ascertain whether or not some form of muscle-balancing procedure will be necessary in order to avoid recurrence. In either event, the surgeon must approach the foot with the understanding that the deformity must again be corrected before considering any muscle transfers. It is axiomatic that any tendon transfers must *follow* correction. Muscle transfers are designed to *maintain* correction; they are never employed to *achieve* it (see the following).

If it can be demonstrated that the recurrence is not due to inadequate treatment or dereliction in postcorrection treatment, then the surgeon must plan to correct the foot again and perform those tendon transfers that appear appropriate. In my experience, the most appropriate procedure transfers the anterior tibial tendon, either wholly or in part, to the lateral side of the foot. Whether the whole tendon is transferred or only half (split tendon transfer) must be determined on an individual basis.

The exact site of insertion of the transferred tendon must also be chosen according to the experience and judgment of the surgeon. I have found that when the entire anterior tibial tendon is transferred, the third cuneiform is the site that provides the best result in terms of the combined dorsiflexion and evertor function required to maintain correction (in contrast to Garceau and Manning's technique of placing the tendon into the fifth metatarsal base).[24] When the split anterior tendon transfer is accomplished, I usually place the lateral half of the tendon into the cuboid bone (see Fig. 7-4).

It must be emphasized again that prior to any tendon transfers, the foot and ankle *must* have been corrected adequately either nonoperatively or operatively. In the presence of a deformity, the tendon transfer cannot possibly be expected to *achieve* correction; at best it can only help *maintain* it. Failure to appreciate this important concept has resulted in many unsuccessful tendon transfers that have been done prior to correction of the foot (Fig. 2-20).

Gartland has recommended nonphasic transfers of the posterior tibial tendon to the dorsum of the foot in order to maintain correction of the clubfoot (see Fig. 7-6).[25,26] I have never found it necessary to use this procedure in a true congenital clubfoot; furthermore, I disagree with the basic concept of performing such a transfer in the case of congenital equinovarus. In my judgment, if the foot and ankle are properly corrected prior to tendon transfer, one of the anterior tibial tendon transfers described previously will be adequate. Furthermore, an intact posterior tibial tendon functioning in its normal position is an important structure in the foot of a growing child; its plantar flexion function should not be sacrificed, except in the case of a pure salvage procedure or in instances of *paralytic* equinovarus (see Chapter 7).

FIXED FOREFOOT EQUINUS. I have become more and more impressed with the importance of fixed forefoot equinus in my reviews of long-term results of past treatment. Several of my poor results can be traced to my failure to recognize this important aspect of clubfoot deformity. It is present only in a modest number of equinovarus feet, and charac-

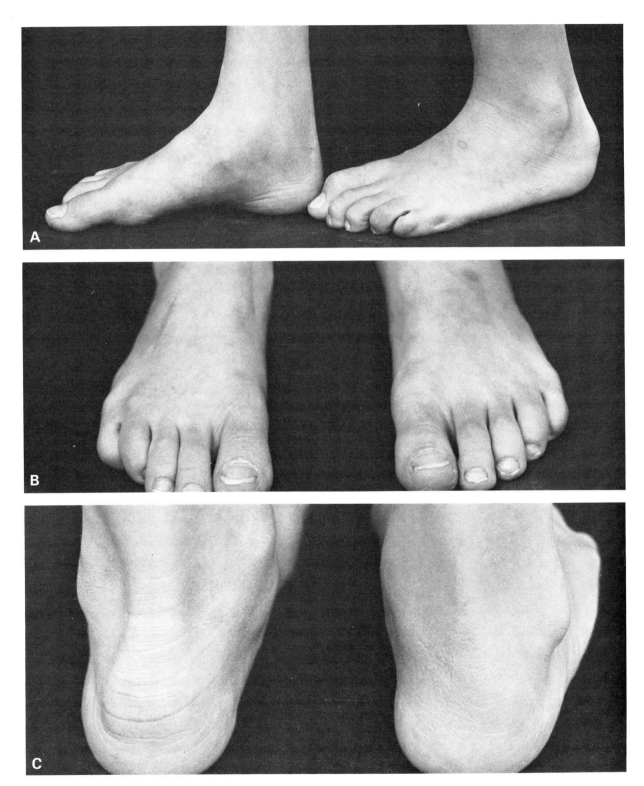

FIG. 2-20. **A, B,** and **C,** Postoperative photographs taken at age 8, 5 years after a lateral transfer of the anterior tibial tendon for "recurrent" right clubfoot deformity. The foot was corrected by manipulation and serial cast application. The ankle equinus was corrected by heelcord lengthening, posterior ankle capsulotomy, and tibiofibular syndesmotomy. Because of a tendency of the foot to develop a supination and adduction deformity of the midfoot and forefoot, a transfer of the anterior tibial tendon to the third cuneiform bone was accomplished. Note the excellent correction, but that residual stigmata of clubfoot persist.

teristically it will be found in the short, fat foot, usually in a child with bilateral deformities; it is especially likely to occur in girls. It is a substantial deformity that has not been given adequate attention in past literature. Basically, the deformity consists of marked plantar flexion of the forefoot, especially involving the first tarsometatarsal ray. In addition, the conventional equinovarus deformity is present. The combination of cavus and equinovarus justifies the term congenital *equinocavovarus*.

On clinical examination, the foot is invariably shorter than normal and is in equinus, and a prominent deep transverse crease is found in the sole of the foot. The forefoot deformity is rigid, and the plantar structures are taut and contracted. The first ray appears shorter than normal.

The *radiographic* features reflect those found on clinical examination. The striking observation separating this particular entity from the conventional congenital clubfoot is the plantarflexed forefoot, especially the first metatarsal, which in some instances may subtend an angle of 90° with respect to the long axis of the talus, as measured in the lateral view (Fig. 2-3).

This foot almost always resists nonoperative correction, and the surgeon must be prepared to operate early in nearly all such cases. Because of the extra dimension of the deformity, namely, the *forefoot* equinus, the basic surgical approach differs somewhat from that in conventional surgical treatment of clubfoot. This means that the complex foot deformity must be corrected first, and then, about 6 weeks later, the ankle. Although both the foot and ankle possibly may be corrected in one stage, I prefer a two-stage approach, based upon the principles enunciated as follows.

The principles of surgical treatment of the equinocavovarus foot are founded upon the fact that a triple abnormality of the *foot* is present, in addition to equinus deformity of the *ankle*. This triple foot deformity consists of a cavus component superimposed upon the conventional clubfoot deformity, namely the hindfoot varus and forefoot adduction. As with all general principles of foot surgery, correction of the foot should be separate from correction of any ankle deformity. Thus, to remedy the forefoot equinus (cavus), a radical plantar release is necessary; in order to correct the hindfoot varus and forefoot adduction, a medial release is required. The combination procedure, which can be done safely and effectively at one stage, is best described as a plantar-medial release. Such a procedure, combined with appropriate postsurgical corrective cast changes, can usually realign all deformed components of the foot satisfactorily. The remaining deformity is the ankle equinus, which then must be treated by the posterior release described earlier, preferably as a second stage some 6 weeks later.

Whether or not the plantar-medial release is combined with a posterior release in one stage depends upon the surgeon's ability to control the many variables involved in correcting such a complex deformity. As mentioned previously, I have found it preferable and safer to correct the deformity of the foot first, and then, 6 to 8 weeks later, to

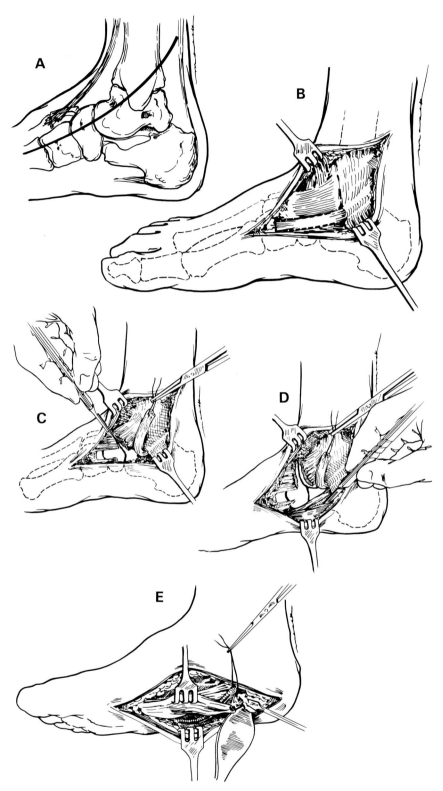

Fig. 2-21. The plantar-medial release represents a combination of the radical plantar release and the medial release. **A**, The incision represents the distal one half or two thirds of the posteromedial release incision. **B** and **C**, The medial release is accomplished first, and then the plantar portion is done (**D** and **E**). For more details of this combined procedure, refer to Figures 4-8 and 2-19.

correct the equinus of the ankle. I believe that the safety, predictability, and effectiveness of this two-stage approach outweigh any advantage of the one-stage approach in which all components of the deformity are corrected at one time. Furthermore, the two-stage approach allows adherence to the basic principle of correcting foot cavus before ankle equinus.

*Plantar-Medial Release.* An incision is made over the plantar-medial aspect of the foot, extending from the medial cuneiform to the posteromedial aspect of the foot (Fig. 2-21). The entire origin of the abductor hallucis is released from its attachments to the cuneiform, navicular, and calcaneus, thus exposing the long flexors of the digits and the neurovascular bundle as it enters the intrinsic musculature of the foot. The sheaths of the long toe flexors (Henry's knot[30]) are incised as they cover the tendons that pass distally into the sole of the foot.

The neurovascular bundle is dissected free as it enters the intrinsic musculature of the foot and divides into its medial and lateral plantar branches. Between these two branches is found a substantial origin of the abductor hallucis; this attachment must be sectioned. Next, the entire plantar musculature and plantar aponeurosis are exposed as they arise from the plantar surface of the calcaneus. These structures are sectioned completely and thoroughly from that origin and are stripped *extraperiosteally* and displaced distally as far as the calcaneocuboid joint. This completes the *plantar* aspect of the plantar-medial release.

The insertion of the anterior tibial tendon is readily identified at its attachment to the medial cuneiform bone, and, by undermining the superior skin flap, the posterior tibial tendon and the remainder of the medial aspect of the hindfoot can be readily exposed. The medial release is then performed, as described on page 65. If necessary, capsulotomies of the *plantar* surface of the naviculocuneiform, and even the tarsometatarsal joints, can be accomplished. A well padded, above-knee cast is applied, leaving the ankle in equinus yet obtaining as much forefoot and hindfoot correction as is deemed safe.

Ten days following the plantar-medial release, the cast is changed; the forefoot and midfoot are manipulated gently into abduction, dorsiflexion, and supination, and the hindfoot is carefully placed into valgus (Fig. 2-22). This tends to flatten the longitudinal arch and to place the heel into valgus. Again, it is attractive to consider this type of surgical procedure only as an "incident" in the continuing nonoperative correction of a special type of clubfoot.[46,47]

Ordinarily, a weekly cast change is necessary, attempting gradual correction but taking great care to avoid *overcorrecting* any component of this complex deformity. Four to six weeks following the operation, the pin crossing the talonavicular joint is removed and a holding cast applied. As soon as the pin tract is healed and the skin is surgically clean, a posterior release is accomplished as described previously. Six weeks later, the same postoperative care is prescribed as that used in the conventional clubfoot correction discussed previously. An exam-

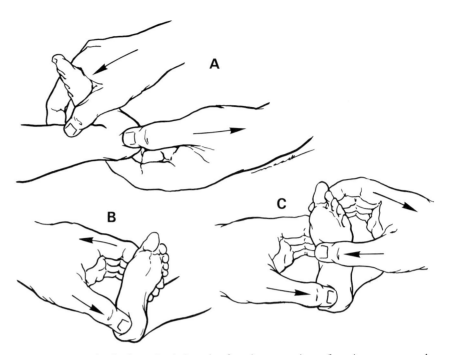

FIG. 2-22. Method of manipulating the foot in correction of equino*cavo*varus. **A**, When attempting to elongate the heelcord, the forefoot is grasped with one hand and gently dorsiflexed. At the same time, the heel is pulled distally by the thumb and index finger of the opposite hand. This combination of manipulations is essential in order to avoid a "break" of the midfoot and resulting "rocker-bottom foot." **B**, The hindfoot is gently forced into valgus by one hand, and the forefoot is supinated by the opposite hand (**C**). This, when effectively done, can elongate the medial aspect of the foot and flatten the longitudinal arch. (Redrawn from Paulos, L. E., Coleman, S. S., and Samuelson, K. M.: Pes cavovarus. Review of a surgical approach using selective soft-tissue procedures. J. Bone Joint Surg., *62A*:942, 1980.)

ple of the results of this combined, staged procedure is seen in Figure 2-23.

DELAYED TREATMENT (NEGLECTED CLUBFOOT). Delay in treatment introduces a special element in the management of congenital clubfoot. Whatever the reason for the delay, the adverse influence exerted by growth results in a more rigid deformity, usually accompanied by more advanced, adaptive changes in the bones and nearly always requiring more extensive surgical procedures to achieve correction. Thus, the neglected clubfoot represents a singular but fortunately uncommon condition that requires specialized treatment.

In many ways, and really for all practical purposes, the neglected clubfoot is equivalent and tantamount to a resistant clubfoot in an older child, namely, the foot that has never been adequately corrected. Consequently, the concepts of treatment are identical in each case, *provided that* the foot has not previously been surgically corrected.

The salient fact that separates these foot deformities from those encountered in the less resistant clubfoot in the neonate and young infant is that restoration of normal relationships of the bones often requires surgical correction of the bones themselves in addition to the conventional soft-tissue procedures outlined in earlier sections.

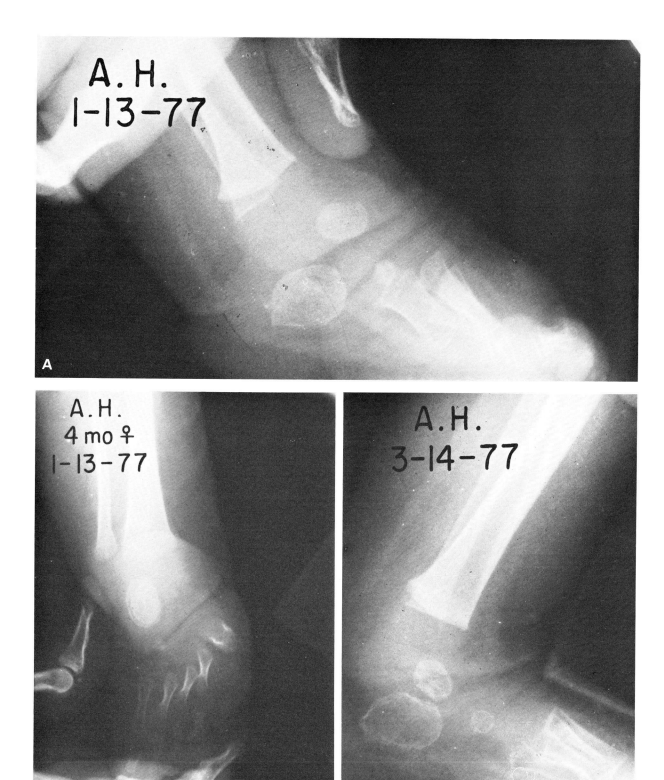

FIG. 2-23. An example of an equinocavovarus foot deformity is seen in the lateral (**A**) and anteroposterior (**B**) simulated weight-bearing views in this 4-month-old female. Note the parallelism of the talus and calcaneus and the marked plantar flexion of the first metatarsal as related to the long axis of the talus. **C**, Two months later, following a plantar-medial release, correction of the hindfoot and forefoot deformities is well shown in the lateral weight-bearing roentgenogram.

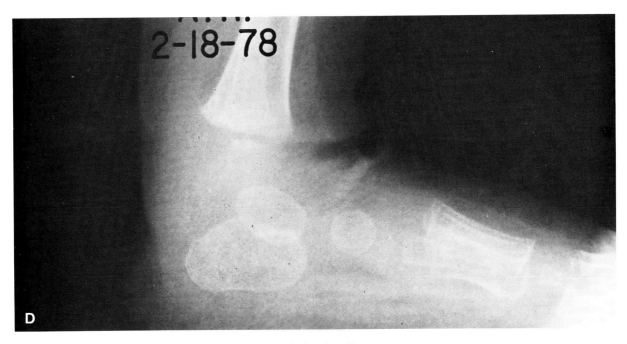

FIG. 2-23. **D,** The appearance 1 year later in the weight-bearing film.

In 1961, Evans conceived of the idea that neglected and uncorrected clubfeet in older children developed a relative "overgrowth" of the lateral column of the foot.[16] Ostensibly, this resulted from the fact that the medial column remained foreshortened owing to the lack of correction, and that function of the talonavicular articulation was also compromised. If it could be determined that substantial, adaptive, bony change had occurred, Evans felt that the lateral column had to be surgically shortened in order to restore normal relationships to the talonavicular joint.

Evans also believed not only that the lateral column should be shortened by resection of the calcaneocuboid joint, but also that the growth of that joint should be arrested by resection of the articular cartilages. Usually this led ultimately to bony fusion.

Lichtblau subscribed to the same general concept, and in a slightly different way achieved a similar goal.[43] He felt, however, that the lateral column could be shortened by resecting only the distal end of the calcaneus, thereby avoiding fusion of the joint. Recently, Goldner has recommended removing a laterally based wedge of bone from the cuboid, a technique designed to shorten the lateral column without interfering with growth in any way (see p. 269).[27]

In approaching the problem of lateral-column overgrowth, Curtis and Muro believed that the bony deformities encountered in long-standing, neglected clubfoot could be corrected only by altering the shapes of the bones.[13] They therefore recommended removing the cancellous bone tissue from the tarsal bones, especially the calcaneus and the cuboid (decancellation) and then gently manipulated the feet. This accomplished apparent but spurious correction, at least from outward appearances. The fallacy of this concept and procedure is that one creates a compensatory deformity in the tarsal bones without in fact altering the disturbed bony relationships. Thus, with growth, the deformity gradually and predictably returned, and was never lastingly corrected. In my opinion, the decancellation procedure in clubfoot is of historical interest only and should no longer be done.

My current preference for lateral-column shortening is essentially that described by Lichtblau (Fig. 2-24).[43] Even though it is anticipated that lateral-column shortening will be necessary, a modified, selective, medial release as described earlier is first accomplished. If correction is not possible, then the subtalar joint is opened and the talocalcaneal joint released.

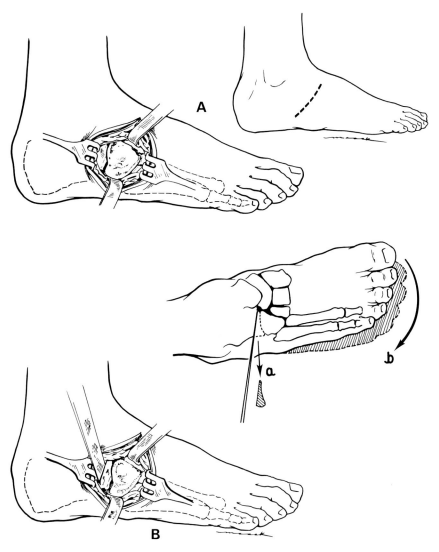

Fig. 2-24. Diagram of the lateral-column shortening procedure as described by Lichtblau. Initially a medial release is done, as illustrated in Figure 2-19; **A**, a curved incision is then made laterally over the distal end of the calcaneus, through which the calcaneocuboid joint is exposed. **B**, A wedge-shaped section of the distal end of the calcaneus is then excised with the base lateral. This resection of the calcaneus (*a*) permits further correction of the hindfoot and midfoot deformity (*b*).

If correction still cannot be achieved, the lateral side of the foot is exposed and the distal end of the calcaneus resected. This combination almost always corrects the hindfoot. In selected instances, I prefer to use percutaneous pin fixation of the resected joint in order to maintain correction. In other cases in which complete correction cannot be achieved safely at the time of the operation, however, the pin is not used, and correction is achieved gradually over the next several weeks through weekly cast changes.

This combination of medial release and calcaneal resection usually results in satisfactory correction of the neglected or resistant clubfoot in the older child between the ages of 3 and 6 years (Fig. 2-25). Again, it is important to use and emphasize the principle that soft-tissue and joint resection surgical procedures are principally methods of gaining correction when these are coupled with subsequent serial corrective cast applications. It is especially important to exercise great care in correcting these older feet so as to reduce or obviate the likelihood of skin sloughs or wound breakdown.

Shortening of the lateral column adds a distinct safety factor in this respect because it reduces the extent to which the medial structures, including the skin, must be elongated. It is my current practice to perform this method of resection of the distal calcaneus in most feet at the time of medial release in children between the ages of 3 and 6 years, especially for those feet that have been either neglected (untreated) or inadequately corrected. The age limits mentioned are not rigid figures, but do serve as fairly good guidelines.

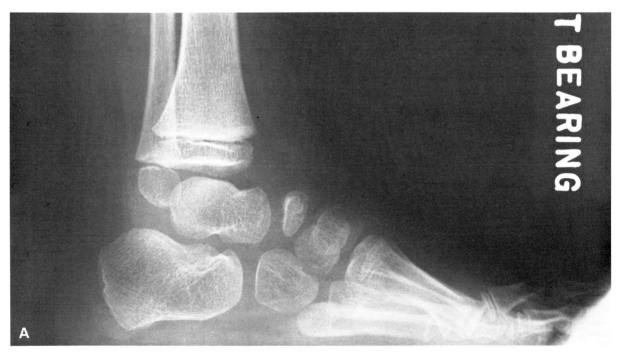

FIG. 2-25. **A** and **B**, Resistant congenital equinovarus in a 6-year-old female. Following selective medial release and lateral-column shortening (resection of the distal end of the calcaneus), the result can be seen 7 months (**C**) and 4 years later (**D** and **E**).

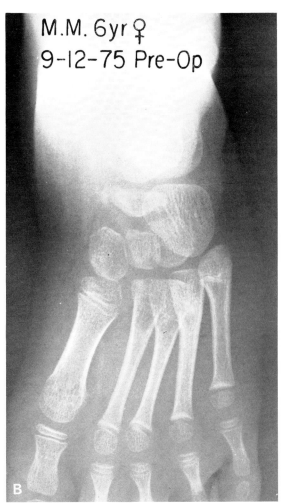

M.M. 6yr ♀
9-12-75 Pre-Op

B

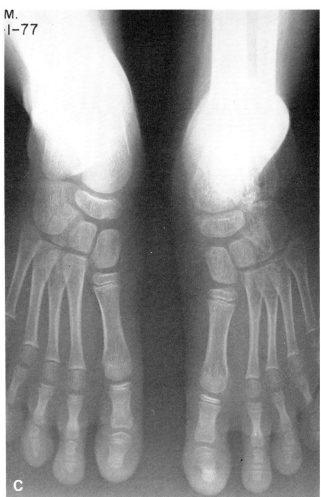

M.
-I-77

C

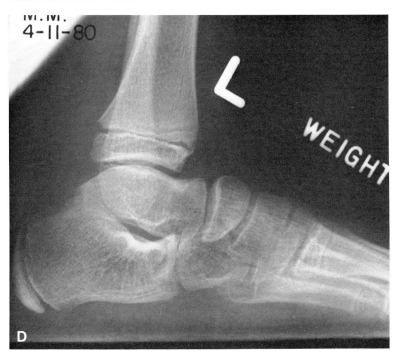

M.M.
4-11-80

WEIGHT

D

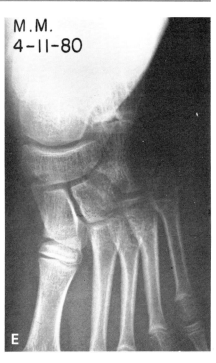

M.M.
4-11-80

E

In older children and adolescents, one is faced with a much more difficult situation because even greater adaptive bony changes will have taken place. It is possible in some instances to perform the combined medial release and lateral-column shortening in children up to 8 or 9 years of age. Beyond that age, the surgeon must consider the probable need for corrective triple arthrodesis, because soft-tissue procedures and simple bone shortening probably will not be sufficient. The age at which the more radical triple arthrodesis becomes necessary clearly will vary from one patient to another, and no rigid age limitation can be established. Triple arthrodesis is contraindicated, however, even in bilateral situations, under the skeletal age of 9 or 10 years because of the stunting effect upon growth of the foot and the potential hazard to the viability of the body of the talus.[58]

When triple arthrodesis is indicated, it is essential that the following factors be fully considered: the configuration of the foot, the character of the ankle joint, the configuration of the talar dome, the degree of ankle equinus, the probability of achieving correction exclusively by soft-tissue procedures such as posterior-ankle release, and finally, the need for *preliminary* soft-tissue releases medially. The latter are designed to reduce the amount of shortening necessary to correct the foot by bone and joint resection. This approach has been found helpful in a large series of uncorrected clubfeet that have been treated in adolescents and young adults in Iran.[65]

## Complications of Treatment

Complications are nearly always iatrogenic; they should therefore be largely preventable. Despite meticulous care and attention to detail, however, occasional untoward results are inevitable in the most conscientious treatment of some congenital clubfeet. The purpose of discussing these unattractive situations is to emphasize the potential hazards in treatment, to review the possible means of either preventing them or lessening their gravity, and to describe their treatment. It is convenient to classify these complications according to whether they result from nonoperative or operative treatment.

### NONOPERATIVE COMPLICATIONS

During the process of nonoperative treatment, the following potential complications must be watched for: distal tibial metaphyseal fracture, traumatic damage to the distal tibial epiphysis, pressure sores and skin ulcerations, rocker-bottom foot, flat-top talus, pressure necrosis of cartilage, and spurious corrections of the forefoot at the tarsometatarsal level. Some of these complications are relatively insignificant and either resolve spontaneously or respond to rather simple measures, whereas others may severely compromise the ultimate result of treatment.

DISTAL TIBIAL FRACTURE. Fracture of the distal tibia is usually the result of too forceful manipulations of the foot (Fig. 2-26). The foot and leg of the young infant that have been immobilized during cast treatment, resulting in somewhat atrophic bones, are predisposed to this complication. Rarely, the distal tibial epiphysis may actually be displaced in the hypertrophic zone of physeal cartilage; more significantly, the distal tibial epiphysis rarely may actually become damaged, producing a permanent deformity (Fig. 2-27). Recognition of this complication in the distal *metaphyses* by appropriate roentgenographic examination, followed by simple cast immobilization until the fracture is healed, usually solves this complication. I have seen no compromising sequelae from this condition, provided it was recognized early and treated appropriately.

SORES AND ULCERATIONS. Pressure sores and skin ulcerations are usually due to inept casting, in which excessive pressure has been exerted on the skin. They may also be due simply to an allergenic response to

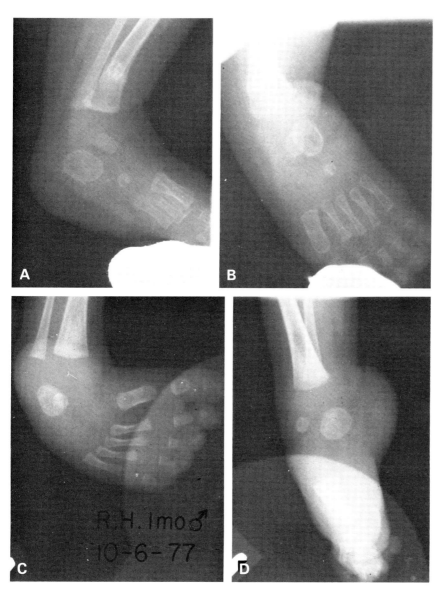

FIG. 2-26. **A** and **B**, An example of a fracture of the distal tibia resulting from manipulation and cast application of a clubfoot. This is a relatively innocuous complication as long as it is recognized. **C** and **D**, Precorrection roentgenograms.

adhesives or to the cast materials, or to skin maceration that results from wrinkling of the skin over the lateral aspect of the foot produced during the correction process. The treatment of this complication requires identification of the causative factors and application of appropriate corrective measures such as well molded casts and discontinuation of adhesives. Significant sequelae are rare.

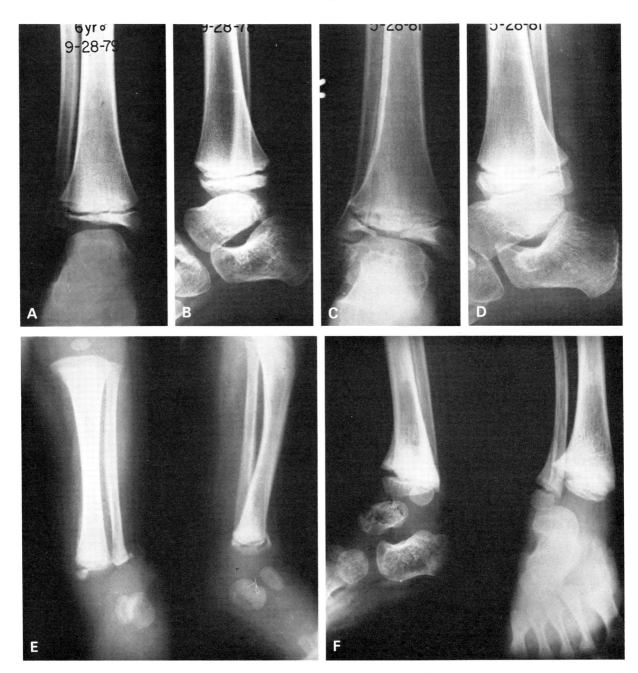

FIG. 2-27. Types of damage to the distal tibial epiphysis. **A** and **B**, Flattening and irregularity of the epiphysis are seen in these roentgenograms of a 6-year-old boy who was treated in early infancy by casts for congenital clubfoot. **C** and **D**, The dramatic change in the tibial epiphysis 2 years later is evident. **E** and **F**, More severe and complex changes in this epiphysis are seen, most surely due to the pressure manipulations and forced cast treatment. (The examples of epiphyseal damage illustrated in **E** and **F** are presented by courtesy of Mr. J. Green, Manchester, England.)

ROCKER-BOTTOM FOOT. The development of a rocker-bottom foot is one of the most distressing complications of nonoperative clubfoot treatment. Invariably this is the result of attempts to dorsiflex the foot at the ankle, either in the presence of tight posterior structures (Fig. 2-17) and/or before the hindfoot has been adequately corrected. The major difficulty lies in the fact that an iatrogenic deformity is produced, resulting in stretching or elongation of the plantar structures, with a spurious correction having occurred at the level of the foot rather than at the ankle. Unless this complication is recognized early, irreversible changes in the bones and ligamentous structures may occur, leading to a permanent flatfoot deformity.

Because of the potential for this complication in the treatment of *any* congenital clubfoot, the surgeon must exercise great care to ensure that the hindfoot has been fully or adequately corrected before *any* efforts are made to correct ankle equinus. Equally important, beginning efforts to dorsiflex the ankle must be documented by lateral, dorsiflexion-stress roentgenograms to show that dorsiflexion is occurring at the proper site (Figs. 2-5 and 2-17). Clearly, it is better to avoid this complication than to have to treat it. Once it has been produced, however, the foot again must be placed into equinus so that the bones of the foot are realigned; a posterior release then must be accomplished prior to any further nonoperative attempts to correct ankle equinus.

In some instances in which a substantial degree of rocker-bottom has been produced, I place a smooth pin across the talonavicular joint and plicate the plantar calcaneonavicular (spring) ligament and the posterior tibial tendon. This is done in an effort to restore the stability and maintain as normal an alignment of the talonavicular joint as possible. Recognized early and treated aggressively, this complication may result in minimal, if any, sequelae. A severe, persisting rocker-bottom deformity may be disabling, however, ultimately requiring a salvage procedure, such as a triple arthrodesis.

FLAT-TOP TALUS. Flat-top talus is the direct result of excessive pressure exerted on the articular surfaces of the talus and the tibia during attempts at dorsiflexion in the presence of tight posterior structures. It is the companion complication to rocker-bottom deformity and results from the same mechanism. In this particular instance, the ligaments and tendons on the plantar surface remain relatively intact, and in the presence of tight, contracted posterior structures, all dorsiflexion forces are then transmitted directly to the talotibial joint. Keim and Richie have termed this the "nutcracker" effect (Fig. 2-28).[39]

The pathomechanics of this important complication have been well described by Dunn and Samuelson.[16] The seriousness of the situation lies in the fact that a reciprocal deformity is created between the talar dome and the tibial plafond that prevents effective dorsiflexion and plantar flexion at the ankle joint. Not only is a deformity of the bones produced, but also, because of the excessive pressure of the articular surfaces, some degree of cartilage necrosis and arthrofibrosis of the ankle inevitably results.

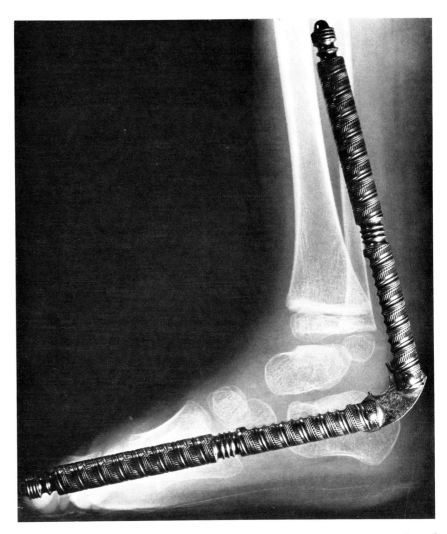

FIG. 2-28. The "nutcracker" mechanism in producing flattening or compression of the top of the talus is illustrated in this conception of the effect of dorsiflexion forces being exerted on a foot, in which the posterior ankle structures are contracted and inelastic, or the hindfoot is uncorrected, or both. (Keim, H. A. and Richie, G. W.: "Nutcracker" treatment of clubfoot. JAMA, *189*:615, 1964. Copyright 1964, American Medical Association.)

Unfortunately, unless one can prevent the condition or recognize it early enough to avoid aggravating it, no treatment is effective once bone deformity has become established. The important issue is to avoid any forceful attempts at dorsiflexion, and if the posterior structures are unduly tight and thus resist or prevent correction of ankle equinus, the ankle joint must be treated by posterior release as described previously.

In assessing the possible presence of flat-top talus, it is important to take lateral roentgenograms of the ankle in the correct projection. This pitfall has been emphasized by Larsen, and more recently by Dunn and Samuelson.[16,42] A *presumed* lateral view that suggests flattening of the talar dome in reality may be simply an oblique view of the ankle in which the talar dome *appears* flattened. In reality, the appearance is purely projectional. A hint that this situation exists is the observation that the fibular malleolus appears more posterior than normal. By viewing the ankle with the malleoli in proper relationships with each other on the roentgenogram, the true configuration of the ankle joint can be established and the possibility of a flat-top talus can be accurately assessed (Fig. 2-29).

CARTILAGE NECROSIS. Pressure necrosis of the articular cartilage of the various tarsal bones is the direct result of exerting too much force on the bones of the foot and ankle during corrective manipulation. As noted earlier, these articular cartilages are the growth centers of the tarsal bones and, therefore, nonphysiologic pressure can produce not only necrosis with resultant joint fibrosis and stiffness, but also permanent deformities of the bones. This leads to a shortened, rigid foot that may ultimately become painful as well as cosmetically unacceptable. The only effective way to deal with this complication is to prevent it. This means that one must practice gentleness in manipulation and care in cast application and must be prepared to perform early, meticulous surgical releases when nonoperative, corrective efforts have ceased to be adequate.

TARSOMETATARSAL CORRECTION. As the foot is manipulated and the holding casts are applied, correction of the forefoot and midfoot adduction will occur occasionally at the tarsometatarsal joints rather than at the talonavicular joint. This particular complication is not serious if recognized early and corrected appropriately. It is the result of continued forcing of the forefoot into abduction in the presence of the contracted and inelastic talonavicular joint capsule and ligaments. Thus, the metatarsals and/or cuneiforms are placed progressively into more abduction, whereas the hindfoot remains uncorrected. Treatment requires early surgical correction of the hindfoot by medial or posterior-medial release so that correction will occur at the proper location. If treated early, this complication rarely will have any sequelae.

Because open surgical procedures are used in the *operative* management of clubfoot, the complications are potentially greater in magnitude. They are largely related either to necrosis of skin, bone, and cartilage or to infection of the operative wound. These threatening and sometimes disastrous circumstances must be seriously considered whenever a clubfoot is operated on. It is important to emphasize that clubfeet are subjected to surgical treatment either because they have resisted nonoperative correction or have recurred following earlier correction. In both instances, these feet are usually more rigid, and the soft tissues, especially the skin, are less mobile.

Even though a foot usually can be adequately corrected at the time of operation, maintenance of this correction in the operative cast is seldom wise because of the danger to the skin and subcutaneous tissues as they are stretched over the medial side of the foot. Minor areas of skin necrosis can be tolerated reasonably well, but major degrees of

COMPLICATIONS DUE TO
OPERATIVE TREATMENT

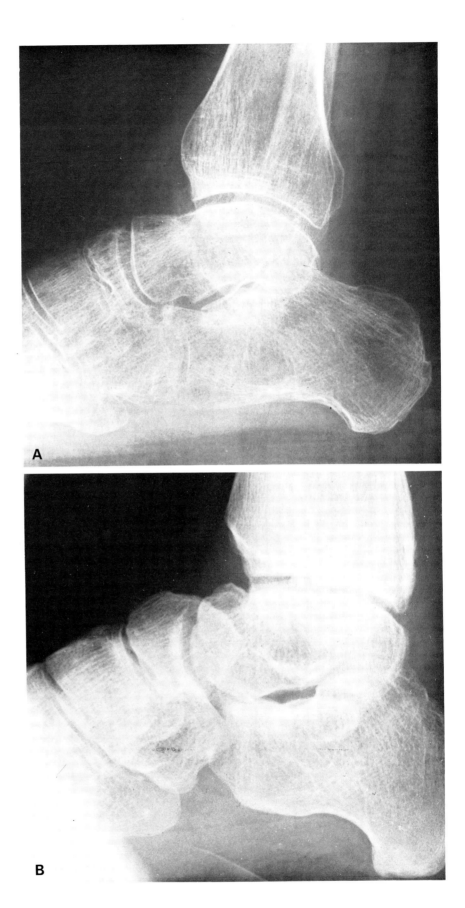

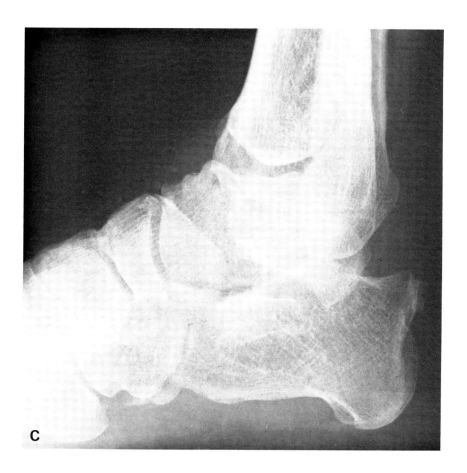

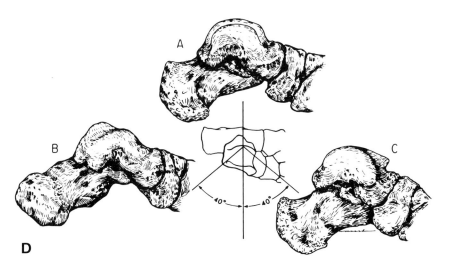

FIG. 2-29. The radiographic features of "flat-top" talus are illustrated in these roentgenograms and diagrams. **A**, Mild flat-top talus; **B**, moderate deformity; **C**, a severe degree of flattening. **D**, The importance of the radiographic projection in evaluating the true configuration of the dome of the talus is illustrated. (Dunn, H. K. and Samuelson, K. M.: Flat-top talus. A long term report of twenty club feet. J. Bone Joint Surg., *56A*:58, 1974.)

necrosis involving full-thickness skin loss can be disastrous. Goldner has solved this threat to skin viability by means of split- or full-thickness skin grafts.[28] These are applied at the time of closure when, upon release of the tourniquet, there is substantial concern regarding the health of the skin margins when full correction is attempted. I have done this on a few occasions, especially in feet that have been operated on previously, and it is an attractive option when the circumstances suggest such a need. The skin is readily available over the lateral aspect of the foot where the wrinkles usually form during correction.

If full-thickness skin loss occurs, substantial loss of correction also invariably takes place. Unyielding, often adherent scars develop, and in some instances, if the scarring is deep, it not only acts as a deforming force that prevents correction (except by major salvage procedures), but also contributes to an inexorable recurrence and accentuation of the deformity. Many times, major plastic skin surgery becomes necessary; even this may not provide healthy, distensible skin after a substantial skin slough has occurred (Fig. 2-30). The same serious situation can result from a deep wound infection that requires open debridement and packing for appropriate treatment.

Necrosis of bone may occur owing to extensive severance of soft tissues, including major portions of the blood supply to the talus and the navicular. Also, unless meticulous care is exercised during the surgical procedure, the cartilage surfaces may be irreparably damaged, leading to intra-articular fibrosis and joint stiffness.

Overcorrection is much more likely to occur following injudicious and promiscuous (nonselective) open surgical releases of ligaments and tendon sheaths than as the result of nonoperative procedures. One of the most unattractive results of surgical procedures for clubfoot is substantial overcorrection, which produces a stiff, flat foot that is a major functional and shoe-fitting problem (Fig. 2-31). On the other hand, the overcorrection may be more apparent than real, actually representing a true deformity of the calcaneus. In this situation, it is essential to take an axial view of the calcaneus to identify the deformity. If this deformity is severe enough, correction may require a medial displacement osteotomy of the calcaneus (Fig. 2-32). In rare, severe cases, ankle disarticulation may be the only means of salvage.

Hypertrophic scars may also represent a significant complication, especially if they develop in the skin directly over the Achilles tendon. Although such scars are not common, in some instances they can produce a difficult treatment problem. This emphasizes the importance of placing incisions so that they are not over bony prominences, in the areas of shoe contact, or over tendons that lie relatively close to the skin.

In reviewing the complications that can occur following open surgical correction of clubfoot, it becomes abundantly clear that their prevention is infinitely preferable to any form of treatment. The surgeon must treat the delicate tendinous, ligamentous, and cartilaginous structures of the foot with meticulous care whenever performing oper-

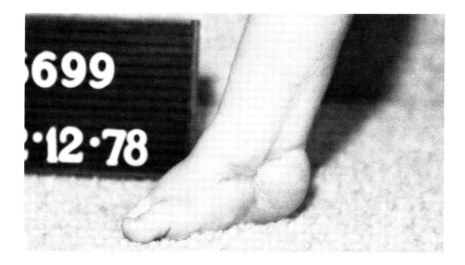

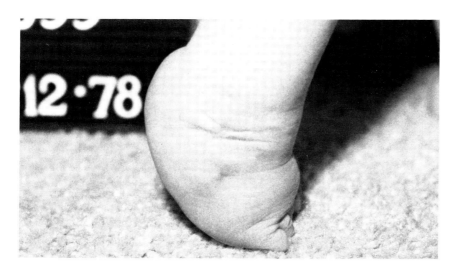

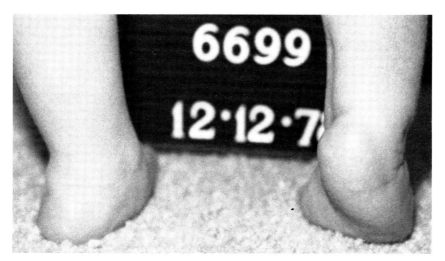

FIG. 2-30. Photographs showing extensive scarring due to skin slough following an operation for clubfoot. The scarring aggravates and accentuates the equinovarus deformity, making any procedure other than astragalectomy almost impossible.

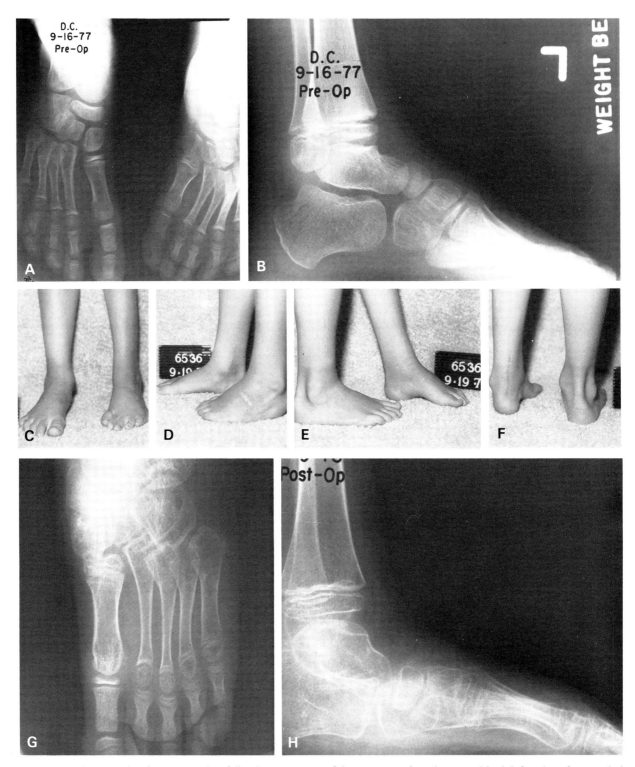

FIG. 2-31. An example of overcorrection following treatment of the cavovarus foot due to residual deformity of congenital clubfoot is illustrated in these pre- and postoperative roentgenograms. **A** and **B**, The cavovarus deformity is clearly demonstrated in standing films. **C, D, E,** and **F**, Comparison standing photographs. This deformity persisted despite previous medial and posterior releases. The normal right foot is shown for comparison. **G** and **H**, Two years later, following a plantar-medial release and multiple postoperative cast changes, overcorrection of the foot is obvious. Had a more *selective* plantar-medial release been accomplished and less aggressive postoperative correction efforts exercised, a better result might have been realized.

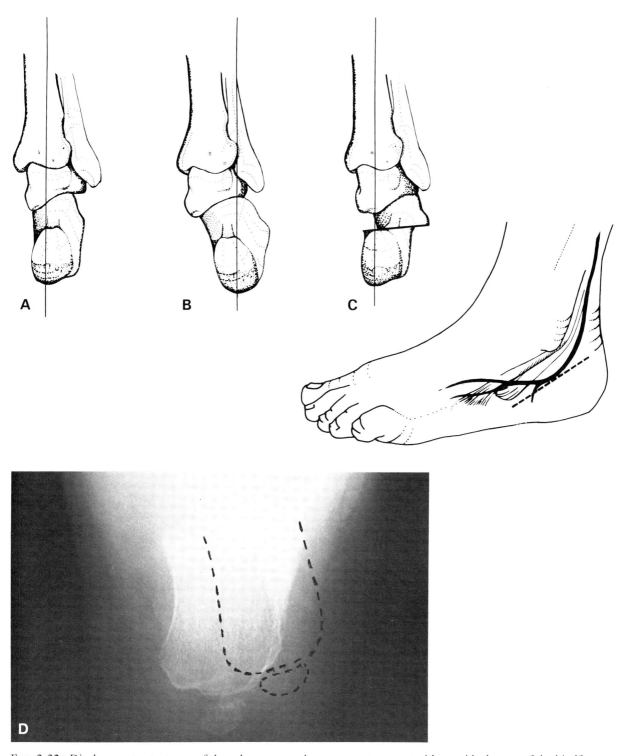

FIG. 2-32. Displacement osteotomy of the calcaneus may be necessary to correct either residual varus of the hindfoot or overcorrection (valgus) of the hindfoot. Axial radiographs of the calcaneus are essential in order to determine whether the problem is in the subtalar joint or the calcaneus. The technique of performing a medial displacement calcaneal osteotomy for excessive heel valgus is illustrated. *Insert,* The skin incision and its relationship to the sural nerve. **A,** The normal appearance of the calcaneus (posterior axial view). **B,** The valgus deformity; **C,** the correction achieved by calcaneal osteotomy. **D,** A postoperative standing roentgenogram showing the results of the osteotomy. The preoperative deformity is shown by the dotted line (the only available preoperative film was not a weight-bearing one and did not adequately illustrate the deformity). (Courtesy of Dr. John Hall, Boston Children's Hospital, Boston, Massachusetts.)

ative releases. Once the joints have been entered, the capsular and ligamentous structures severed, and the tendons lengthened, a variable degree of scarring and reparative response is inevitable. It is essential that the surgeon reduce to the absolute minimum any surgical trauma to these structures so as to avoid or lessen the degree of scarring, stiffness, and compromised function.

*Salvage and Late Reconstructive Procedures for Complications and Residual Deformities In Congenital Equinovarus*

Most congenital clubfeet, having been treated properly without substantial or meaningful complications, will become plantigrade, serviceable, and relatively symptom free. All will have some residual stigmata of the true congenital equinovarus, but few will require salvage operations. Salvage procedures are designed to achieve a plantigrade foot by means of major bone and joint operations, in which bones are sectioned or excised and functional joints are sacrificed. In the latter instance, the ultimate salvage procedure includes the complete removal of the foot, namely, an ankle disarticulation using the Syme principle.[14] Clearly, prior to consideration of these operative procedures, all conventional and more conservative methods of correcting the clubfoot shall have been exhausted.

It is convenient to divide these salvage operations into those designed to correct residual deformities of either the forefoot and midfoot, the hindfoot, or the ankle. These deformities can all be corrected effectively, provided that the plantar skin is healthy and has good sensation and that at the conclusion of the salvage procedure, the foot will be large enough and will have the appropriate shape so that shoe fitting will not be a major problem.

FOREFOOT PROCEDURES

When any salvage *forefoot* procedure is to be considered, it is axiomatic that the *hindfoot* will have already been acceptably corrected. This is extremely important, because any corrective procedure carried out on the forefoot will predictably fail if the talus and calcaneus (hindfoot) remain inadequately corrected.

Most often, the deformity requiring correction will be adduction or varus of the forefoot, either at the midtarsal (naviculocuneiform) or tarsometatarsal level. In these instances, depending upon a variety of circumstances, three procedures are best suited to achieve surgical correction. These include metatarsal osteotomy, opening-wedge osteotomy of the first cuneiform bone, and tarsometatarsal capsulotomy. Any one of these operations can correct adduction (varus) as well as equinus deformities in the forefoot. It should be emphasized again that these procedures are rarely indicated and should be used only when forefoot adduction or forefoot equinus persists, but *always* in the presence of an adequately corrected hindfoot.

METATARSAL OSTEOTOMY. Metatarsal osteotomy is best accomplished at the level of the base of the metatarsal near the metatarsocuneiform joint. The technique of metatarsal osteotomy is simple or complex, depending upon whether all of the metatarsals are sectioned or only the first. I have rarely seen the need to perform an osteotomy of all five metatarsals, and usually the forefoot can be corrected as desired with an opening-wedge or crescentic osteotomy of the first metatarsal. If all five metatarsals require osteotomy, the procedure described by Tachdjian can be used (Fig. 2-33).[80]

Because the physis of the first metatarsal is located at its proximal end, care must be taken not to damage the physis at the time of osteotomy in those children whose epiphyses are still open.

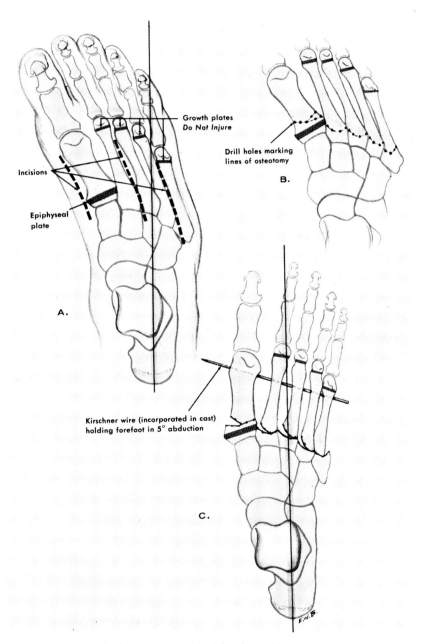

Fig. 2-33. A method of correcting residual forefoot adduction by metatarsal osteotomy. Whether all five metatarsals or only the first should be resected is a decision that must be made at the time of the operation. (Tachdjian, M. O.: *Pediatric Orthopedics*. Philadelphia, W. B. Saunders, 1972, p. 1341.)

Osteotomy of the Medial Cuneiform Bone. Fowler, Brooks, and Parrish have described an osteotomy of the medial cuneiform bone that enables one to correct two deformities of the forefoot. It consists of an opening-wedge osteotomy that can correct adduction (varus) of the forefoot and/or forefoot equinus, depending upon the direction in which the osteotomy is opened (Fig. 2-34).[22] One of the virtues of the osteotomy is that it can elongate a foreshortened medial column (thus lengthening the foot) and can correct some degree of equinus of the forefoot at the same time.

An incision is made over the medial aspect of the foot, extending from the base of the first metatarsal to just below and posterior to the medial malleolus. The incision is deepened to expose the abductor hallucis, and a formal radical plantar release is usually necessary (see p. 75). The medial cuneiform is then exposed subperiosteally, taking care to preserve the insertion of the anterior tibial tendon. Once the cuneiform is properly exposed, it is sectioned at its midpoint, and the osteotomy is opened as widely as possible using a small lamina spreader.

It is essential that the osteotomy be filled with either autogenous or homogenous bone grafts and that it be transfixed by an internal fixation device, such as a threaded pin or a small-fragment bicortical

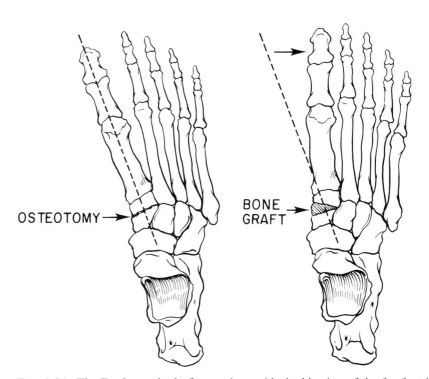

FIG. 2-34. The Fowler method of correcting residual adduction of the forefoot in either congenital equinovarus or residual deformities of a cavovarus foot. The abnormal angle of the first cuneiform metatarsal joint is corrected by the opening-wedge osteotomy. The defect is replaced by a triangle-shaped bone graft (autogenous or homogenous), and the osteotomy must be held in the corrected position by a transfixion pin.

screw. The pin must be threaded in order to prevent collapse of the osteotomy site. This device must remain in position for a minimum of 6 weeks, during which time weight-bearing should not be allowed. Once the osteotomy is healed, a graduated weight-bearing program is begun, either with or without a cast (Fig. 2-35).

TARSOMETATARSAL CAPSULOTOMY. Heyman, Herndon, and Strong described a procedure that they considered "a conservative operative procedure for the correction of residual and resistant adduction deformity of the forepart of the foot in the treatment of congenital clubfoot."[31] This consisted of mobilizing the tarsometatarsal joints by severing the tarsometatarsal and intermetatarsal ligaments and joint capsules. It is indicated most appropriately in children between the ages of 3 and 8 years in whom the hindfoot is corrected but fixed or rigid forefoot adduction persists. The operation is done through a dorsally placed transverse incision that adequately exposes all five tarsometatarsal joints. It is described as follows (Fig. 2-36).

A transverse, slightly curvilinear incision is made over the dorsum of the foot at the level of the tarsometatarsal joints. The incision extends from the base of the first to the base of the fifth metatarsal. Since it is basically a transverse incision, it may interfere to some degree with return circulation, and it is therefore important to preserve as many of

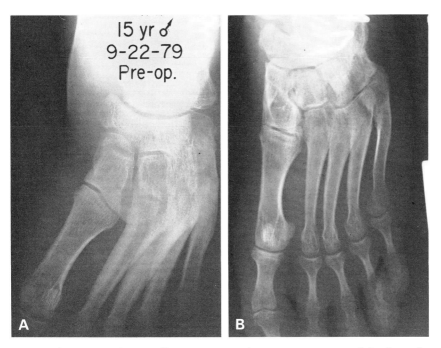

FIG. 2-35. Preoperative standing anteroposterior roentgenograms of the foot of a 15-year-old male with residual forefoot adduction; the patient underwent surgical treatment of equinovarus as a child. **A,** The abnormal angle of the first metatarsocuneiform joint is demonstrated. **B,** Sixteen months postoperatively, the angle and the adducted forefoot have been substantially improved. In this case, a triple arthrodesis was also accomplished (see Figure 2-39).

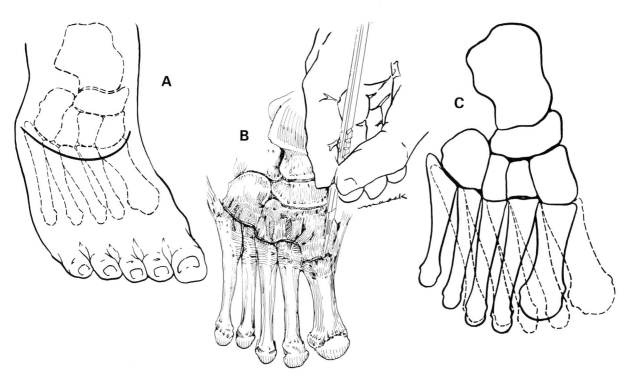

FIG. 2-36. **A**, The tarsometatarsal capsulotomy and ligament release of Heyman, Herndon, and Strong is best done through a generous curvilinear transverse incision that centers over these tarsometatarsal joints. **B**, By sharp dissection, the ligaments and capsular structures are severed completely. For satisfactory correction, these structures must be severed not only dorsally, medially, and laterally, but also on the plantar surface. Care must be taken not to damage the long flexor, anterotibial, posterotibial, and peroneal tendons. **C**, If the intermetatarsal ligaments are satisfactorily released, then the metatarsals can move and slide on each other and the forefoot can be placed effectively into abduction. (After Tachdjian, M. O.: *Pediatric Orthopedics*. Philadelphia, W. B. Saunders, 1972, pp. 1337-1339.)

the cutaneous nerves and veins as possible during this operation. Some, however, must be severed to ensure complete enough exposure to accomplish the procedure. The capsules of the joints are identified carefully and cut sharply. This must include the dorsal, plantar, and intermetatarsal ligaments of all five metatarsals. At the same time, some degree of stability must be maintained so that the metatarsals are not displaced in the dorsal direction. Care must also be taken to preserve the dorsalis pedis artery and vein. Once an adequate release has been achieved, the skin is closed and a below-knee cast applied, with the foot held as close to the corrected position as possible.

I have performed this procedure on a number of children, and it has been my experience that the surgical release should be followed by a series of below-knee corrective casts in order to achieve the greatest degree of correction. After 6 weeks, the foot is placed in an outflare or "toe-out" shoe, which is worn for several months or even a year or more.

This is a valuable procedure, but the indications and prerequisites must be adhered to assiduously; otherwise, it may fail. Specifically, the deformity must be in the forefoot and should be rigid (that is, not passively correctable); the hindfoot *must* have been corrected. The ideal age for the procedure is somewhere between 3 and 8 years.

In older children and in salvage situations, correction of the hindfoot is much more challenging than correction of the forefoot. The disturbed relationships of the talus, calcaneus, and navicular, the alterations in the shape of these bones, the stiffness of the associated joints due to intra-articular fibrosis, and the scarring of the soft tissues secondary to previous surgical procedures are the main difficulties producing the need for salvage hindfoot procedures.

If the problem is predominantly in the subtalar joint, a compensatory valgus-producing *displacement* osteotomy of the calcaneus can be done. If the hindfoot remains uncorrected in the presence of severe scarring, intra-articular stiffness and fibrosis, or bony deformity, then astragalectomy may be the only solution in the younger child between 4 and 8 years of age. This situation usually obtains in cases of severe arthrogrypotic clubfeet; on the other hand, if the patient is over 9 years of age, triple arthrodesis may be the most appropriate procedure.

Finally, and fortunately rarely, the foot may be so deformed that it is beyond salvage by these simpler procedures. In such instances, disarticulation at the ankle is an acceptable solution. Clearly, it does not salvage the foot, but does serve to salvage the limb.

DISPLACEMENT OSTEOTOMY. Displacement osteotomy of the calcaneus is a procedure I rarely have occasion to perform. It is essential to clearly define its purpose so as to avoid any confusion with the crescentic (posterior displacement) calcaneal osteotomy as described by Samilson and Mitchell or the Dwyer (valgus or varus) calcaneal osteotomy.[17,55,67] These latter procedures have completely different indications and goals, and consequently they should not be included in a discussion on clubfoot treatment. They are discussed in the sections appropriate to their use; namely, paralytic calcaneocavus and cavovarus deformities.

The calcaneal lateral displacement osteotomy is designed to correct the varus configuration of the heel (hindfoot), but without altering the bony relationships of the subtalar or talonavicular joint. Thus, one produces a compensatory deformity in order to achieve clinical valgus of the heel. The reverse (medial) displacement for correction of excessive valgus or overcorrection has already been discussed. It must be done in older children in order to be lastingly effective; furthermore, it is done primarily as an effort to avoid astragalectomy or triple arthrodesis. It is important to emphasize that growth will tend to produce recurrence of the varus deformity because the osteotomy has not changed the direction of growth of the tarsal bones that is derived from the subtalar joint cartilage.

ASTRAGALECTOMY. Astragalectomy is a rather drastic salvage procedure because it destroys, by its removal, the entire pantalar (or peritalar) articulation. It should be done only in children between 4 and 8 years of age and only when all other less radical procedures have failed to correct the hindfoot. It has several disadvantages. It decreases the height of the foot, eliminates major tarsal joints, creates a nearthrosis between the tibia and calcaneus, and renders further salvage proce-

## HINDFOOT PROCEDURES

dures nearly impossible. Its most frequent indication is in the severe arthrogrypotic foot deformity, but in rare instances of severe, rigid clubfoot in otherwise normal children, the procedure will occasionally be required (Fig. 2-37). The usual indications are: (a) a foot with excessive scarring, often with loss of soft tissues medially, (b) a rigid, deformed foot, (c) a foot in which a medial release and lateral-column shortening cannot be safely accomplished, and finally, (d) a foot with the characteristics just mentioned that is too immature (under 9 to 10 years of age) for triple arthrodesis.

I have used this operation sparingly in children who do not have arthrogryposis. The technique is rather simple, involving only severance of all ligamentous structures attached to the talus, so that the bone can be extricated from its position in the ankle joint. I prefer an anterolateral incision, centering over the ankle joint and sinus tarsus, that allows ready access to all these structures and does not enter the usually scarred medial side of the foot. The procedure is described as follows.

Even though the most direct approach to the talus is through a generous anterolateral incision as mentioned previously, one may be guided by other previously made scars that may make other incisions safer from the standpoint of viability of the skin. In any event, complete exposure of all attachments of the talus to both malleoli, the navicular, and the calcaneus is essential. The astragalus is carefully removed and the remainder of the foot displaced posteriorly so that the anterior aspect of the tibia articulates with the navicular and the plafond of the tibia articulates with the superior aspect of the calcaneus. A smooth Steinmann pin placed upward through the calcaneus into the medullary cavity of the tibia is almost essential in order to hold this position (Fig. 2-38). It is especially important to maintain the relationship between the tibia and the navicular; otherwise, the forefoot will fall into a varus and adducted position when the cast is removed. A nonweight-bearing, below-knee cast is left on for 6 weeks, at which time the pin is removed and a walking below-knee cast applied. Four weeks later, this can be removed, and a straight-last shoe is prescribed. In most instances, a serviceable foot can be produced (Fig. 2-37).

Triple Arthrodesis. Triple arthrodesis is the ultimate salvage procedure in surgical treatment for clubfoot because, if properly done, it corrects the bony relationships, produces a serviceable plantigrade foot, and retains ankle motion. Its main disadvantages are that the talocalcaneonavicular joint is destroyed by the arthrodesis and the foot is made slightly smaller. Nevertheless, one of the most time-honored and time-proven orthopedic operations is a well performed triple arthrodesis. Not only can the hindfoot be well corrected, but if fixed ankle equinus is a problem because of scarring of the posterior structures, then a Lambrinudi-type triple arthrodesis can effectively correct ankle equinus, and at the same time the hindfoot can be corrected (Fig. 2-39).[41]

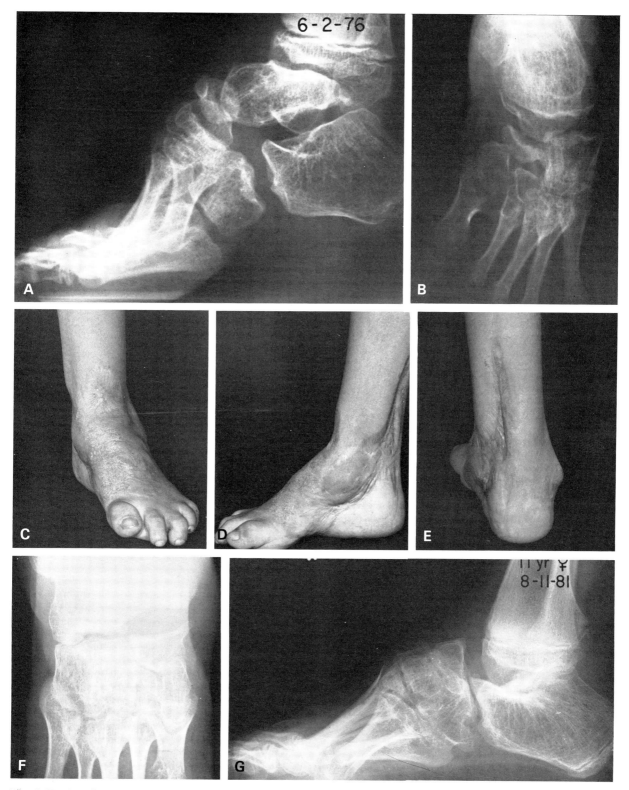

FIG. 2-37. Standing lateral (**A**) and anteroposterior (**B**) roentgenograms of the foot of a 6-year-old girl who had undergone posteromedial release 3 years earlier for congenital equinovarus. This was followed by extensive skin sloughs necessitating full-thickness skin grafts and pedicle skin flaps. Owing to the gross alteration in the configuration of the bones, efforts at reconstruction were considered contraindicated. Consequently, an astragalectomy was accomplished, producing the clinical result seen in **C** through **E**. **F** and **G**, The standing roentgenograms show a plantigrade though substantially shorter foot.

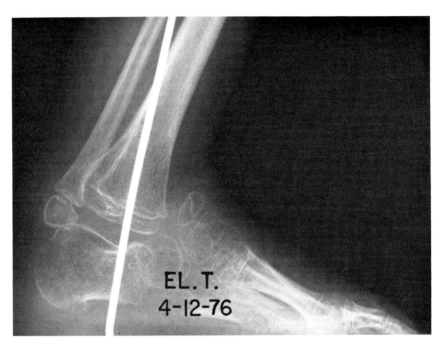

FIG. 2-38. Astragalectomy requires that a smooth Steinmann pin be placed through the calcaneus and into the tibia in order to hold the foot displaced posteriorly on the tibia and to maintain the tibia in proper relationship to the calcaneus.

The techniques for performing a corrective triple arthrodesis and a Lambrinudi triple arthrodesis are described as follows and shown diagrammatically in Figures 2-40 and 2-41.

The exposure for each is the same, but the technique of removal of the osteocartilaginous wedges is substantially different. These differences are best illustrated in the diagrams. It is essential that these remodeled bones and joints be carefully held by staples or transfixion pins in order to maintain perfect correction.

ANKLE DISARTICULATION. Ankle disarticulation fortunately is rarely indicated as salvage treatment for clubfoot. Nevertheless, in the rare instance of a recalcitrant foot that is rigid, scarred, deformed, and foreshortened, removal may be the only practical solution. If the heel skin is good and disarticulation is done properly, a serviceable amputation results. It is durable, generally free of complications, and extremely functional. This really should not be considered a salvage procedure, however; rather, it is a total capitulation in which complete failure of clubfoot treatment must be acknowledged. The operative procedure is well described in standard operative texts on amputations.

ANKLE PROCEDURES

CLOSING-WEDGE OSTEOTOMY OF THE DISTAL TIBIA. Several of the foregoing salvage operations can effectively treat residual ankle equinus, specifically, the astragalectomy and the Lambrinudi triple arthrodesis. An alternative salvage or "holding" operation can be done, however, in instances of persistent ankle equinus. This is usually done in chil-

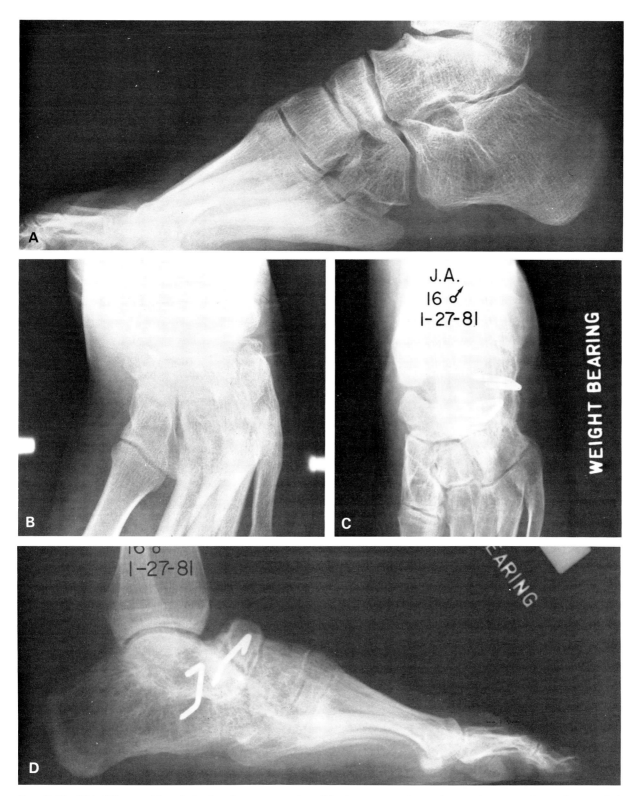

FIG. 2-39. This 15-year-old male had undergone a series of both nonoperative and operative corrections of congenital equinovarus. He continued to have major symptoms of deformity, with the development of plantar callosities under the head of his first metatarsal and the base of his fifth metatarsal. **A** and **B**, The roentgenograms demonstrate substantial adduction and equinus deformity of the forefoot and varus of the hindfoot. A Lambrinudi triple arthrodesis and an opening-wedge osteotomy of the medial cuneiform were accomplished, resulting in the satisfactory correction seen in **C** and **D**.

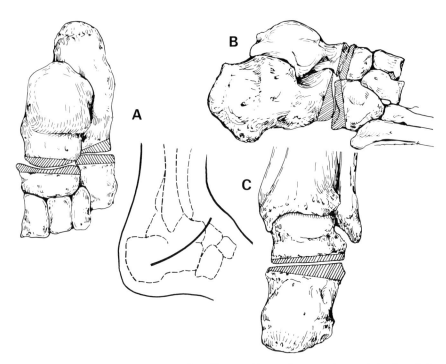

FIG. 2-40. The wedge resections of cartilage and bone that must be made in the triple joint when correcting the fixed, bony deformity in congenital equinovarus, by means of which all residual deformities of the hindfoot can be corrected.

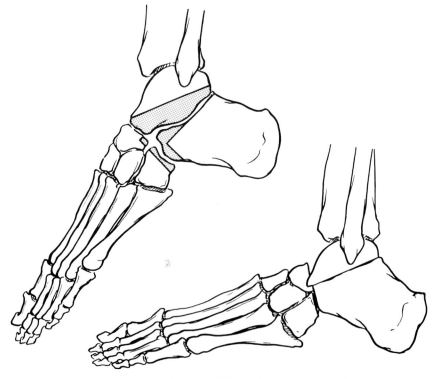

FIG. 2-41. Lambrinudi triple arthrodesis. The wedges are removed in the triple joint as seen in the stippled areas. The entire foot can then be brought out of the equinus position around the talus. Note that the equinus has been corrected while the talus has not changed its position in the ankle mortise. This procedure is helpful in treating certain types of clubfeet when the talus cannot be dorsiflexed.

dren in whom the posterior ankle structures are excessively scarred, the foot deformity is not severe enough to justify astragalectomy, and the foot has insufficient skeletal maturity to undergo the Lambrinudi triple arthrodesis.

The procedure consists of a closing-wedge osteotomy of the tibia at the supramalleolar region, just above the distal tibial physis, as described subsequently and illustrated in Figure 2-42. It can achieve spurious correction of equinus of at least 30°; unfortunately, the correction does not last long because, with growth, the equinus deformity gradually recurs.

The distal tibia is usually approached through an anterior longitudinal incision placed just above the ankle joint. Obviously, damage to the distal tibial physis must be avoided. The distal tibia is exposed subperiosteally, with care taken to leave undisturbed the periosteal attachment of the distal tibial physis. An anteriorly based wedge of bone of 30° or more is removed from the tibia just above the physis. It is nearly always necessary to perform osteotomy on the fibula in order to achieve full correction, especially in older children. Because the ankle joint does not permit dorsiflexion, simple, gentle, upward force on the sole of the foot closes the osteotomy and provides *clinical* correction. The closer to the physis the osteotomy is done, the more acceptable will be the correction.

After wound closure, an above-knee cast is applied, with the foot held in maximum dorsiflexion. The osteotomy should be healed solidly within 6 weeks. After the cast is removed, a polypropylene splint is applied to maintain correction. This splint should be used day and night for as long as the child grows to discourage or obviate recurrence of the deformity.

ROTATIONAL OSTEOTOMY OF THE TIBIA. Considerable controversy has arisen concerning the existence of internal (inward) tibial torsion in congenital equinovarus. If it does exist, it is also uncertain whether it is a secondary result or a primary part of the problem. In clubfoot, it is more difficult to diagnose increased inward tibial torsion because the medial malleolus is nearly always wider than normal, and the exact relationships between the medial and lateral malleoli are more difficult to establish. In many instances in the past, I have mistakenly attributed a residual toeing-in attitude of the forefoot following treatment of congenital equinovarus to inward tibial torsion. In most instances, however, the toeing-in was due to an inadequately corrected hindfoot. Thus, even though tibial rotational osteotomy produced an improved function and appearance, the correction was a spurious one.

Nevertheless, an occasional patient with congenital equinovarus will exhibit a substantial degree of inward tibial torsion, severe enough to justify rotational osteotomy (Fig. 2-43). Before making the diagnosis and prior to accomplishing the procedure, it must be clearly established both clinically and radiographically that the foot is corrected adequately. If not, then the foot, and not the tibial torsion, should be corrected.

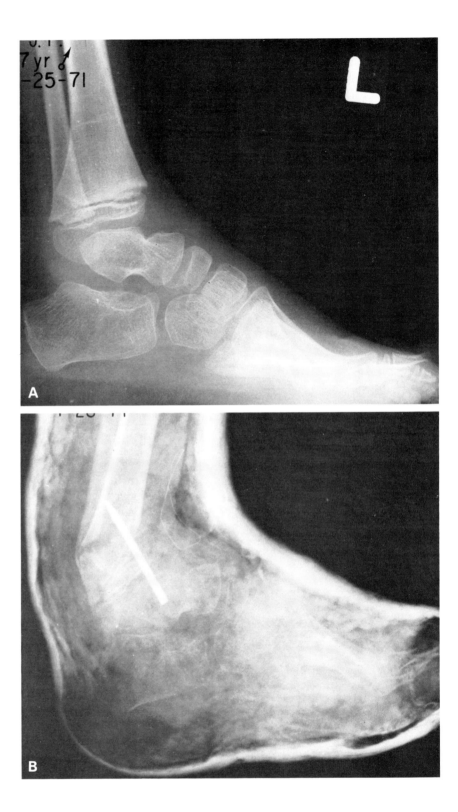

FIG. 2-42. A 7-year-old boy had persistent equinus of the foot and ankle despite two prior posterior release procedures. **A,** Note the equinus attitude and flat-top talus in the lateral weight-bearing roentgenogram. **B,** The immediate postoperative lateral roentgenograms following distal tibial closing-wedge osteotomy.

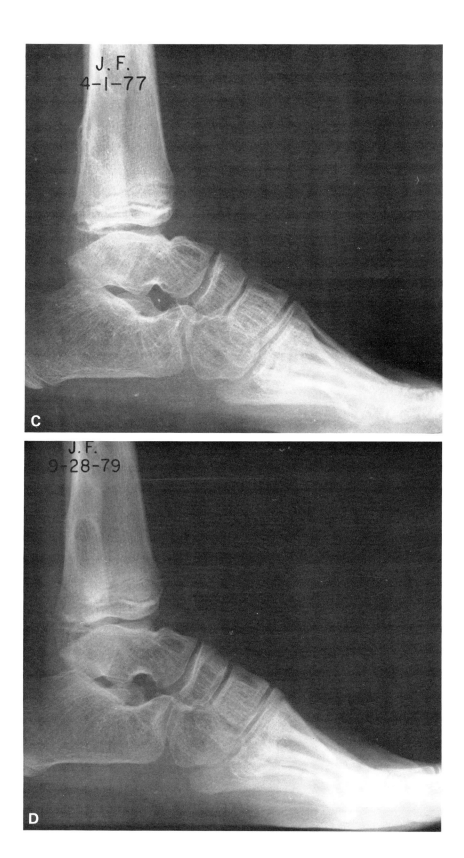

Fig. 2-42. **C,** Six and eight (**D**) years later, the distal tibia has undergone complete remodeling; however, the equinus deformity has remained satisfactorily corrected.

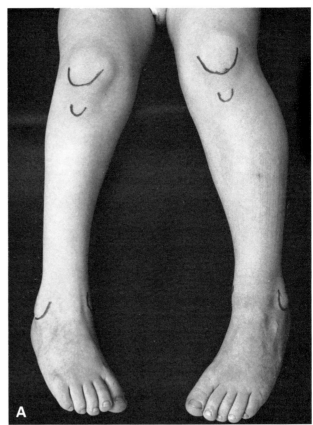

FIG. 2-43. **A,** Preoperative physical evidence of substantial inward tibial torsion. **B** and **C,** Lateral standing roentgenograms of the feet show satisfactory nonoperative correction. **D,** Postoperative roentgenograms show the supramalleolar osteotomies performed by my technique in a similar case. **E,** The postoperative roentgenograms showing the healed osteotomy; **F, G,** and **H,** clinical photos taken 6 months later. **I,** The newborn precorrection photos.

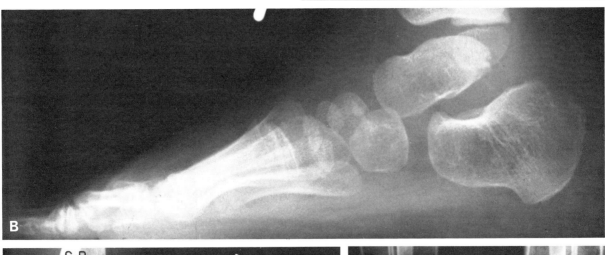

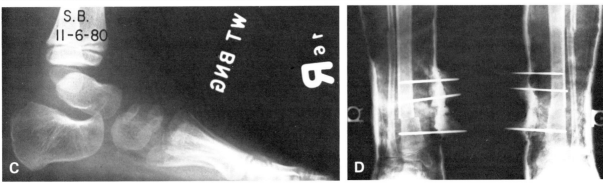

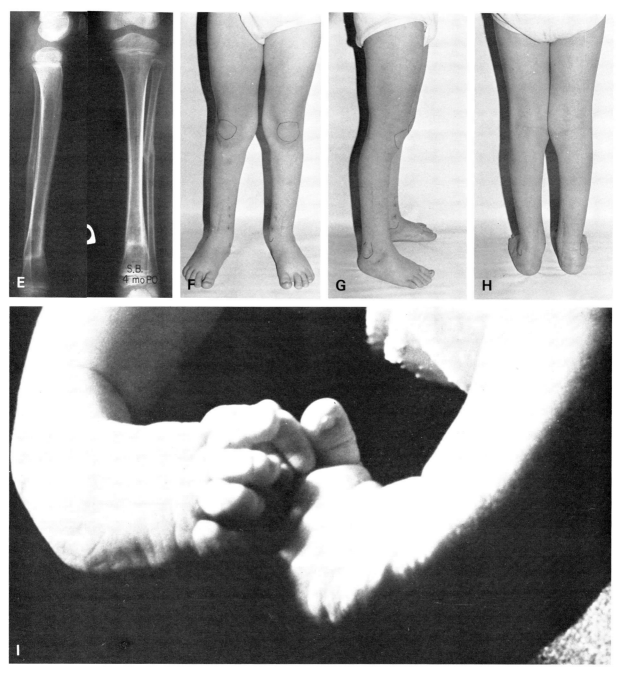

Fig. 2-43. *continued*

If rotational tibial osteotomy is done, I prefer to accomplish it at the supramalleolar level. It is much safer because it is far removed from the trifurcation of the popliteal artery proximally; it is easier and is as effective as proximal tibial osteotomy. Also, because it is done in the distal portion of the tibia, the well known complication of genu valgus resulting from proximal tibial osteotomy is avoided.

The fibula must first be sectioned obliquely at a higher level through a small, 1-inch incision. It is done at this higher level to aid in stability of the tibial osteotomy and also to reduce the likelihood of any neurovascular compromise due to excessive swelling that would result if the osteotomies were done at the same level.

After the fibular incision is closed, a 2-inch incision is made directly over the anterior aspect of the distal tibia. Just as in the angulation osteotomy described earlier, the distal tibia is exposed subperiosteally, with care taken to preserve the periosteal attachments to the distal tibial physis. Through generous stab wounds on the medial side, two ⅛-inch threaded Steinmann pins are placed through both cortices of the tibia above the proposed osteotomy site, and one pin is placed below. The amount of rotation desired can be easily established by the angle at which the pins are placed. Once the periosteum is stripped completely around the tibia, a transverse osteotomy is made with an oscillating saw. The desired rotation is achieved by rotating the distal pin outwardly. A surprising degree of stability is evident if the periosteum has not been cut posteriorly. After the wound is closed, an above-knee cast incorporating the pins is applied.

Because transfixion pins are used above and below the osteotomy in this subcutaneous area of the tibia, internal fixation is not required. The pins must be incorporated in an above-knee cast for 6 weeks, after which time sufficient healing will be evident so that the pins can be removed and a below-knee walking cast applied for an additional 4 weeks. Within the next 6 weeks, complete recovery usually will be achieved.

*References*

1. Adams, W.: *Clubfoot. Its Causes, Pathology and Treatment.* London, J. and A. Churchill, 1866.
2. Attenborough, C. G.: Severe congenital talipes equinovarus. J. Bone Joint Surg., *48B:*31, 1966.
3. Barenfeld, Ph.A., and Weseley, M. S.: Surgical treatment of congenital club foot. Clin. Orthop., *84:*79, 1972.
4. Barnett, R.: Surgical treatment of clubfeet. Read at Shriners Surgeon's Meeting, Mexico City, 1979.
5. Barnett, R.: Personal communication. Shrine Chief Surgeons Meeting, Mexico City, 1979.
6. Bechtol, C. O., and Mossman, H. W.: Club-foot. An embryological study of associated muscle abnormalities. J. Bone Joint Surg., *32A:*827, 1950.
7. Bissell, J. B.: The morbid anatomy of congenital talipes equino-varus. Arch. Pediatr., *5:*406, 1888.
8. Böhm, M.: The embryologic origin of clubfoot. J. Bone Joint Surg., *11:*229, 1929.
9. Brockman, E. P.: *Congenital Clubfoot (Talipes Equinovarus).* New York, William Wood & Co., 1930.
10. Browne, D.: Modern methods of treatment of clubfoot. Br. Med. J., *2:*512, 1937.
11. Colley (1875), cited by Kite, J. H.: The treatment of congenital clubfoot. JAMA, *99:*1156, 1932.
12. Crabbe, W.: Aetiology of congenital talipes. Br. Med. J., *2:*1060, 1960.
13. Curtis, F. E., and Muro, F.: Decancellation of os calcis, astragalus and cuboid in correction of congenital talipes equinovarus. J. Bone Joint Surg., *16:*110, 1934.
14. Davidson, W. H., and Bohne, W. H. O.: The Syme amputation in children. J. Bone Joint Surg., *57A:*905, 1975.
15. DeLangh, R.: Treatment of clubfoot by posterior capsulectomy. Clin. Orthop., *106:*248, 1975.

16. Dunn, H. K., and Samuelson, K. M.: Flat-top talus, a long-term report of twenty club feet. J. Bone Joint Surg., *56A*:57, 1974.

17. Dwyer, F. C.: The treatment of relapsed clubfoot by the insertion of a wedge into the calcaneum. J. Bone Joint Surg., *45B*:67, 1963.

18. Elmslie, R. C.: The principles of treatment of congenital talipes equinovarus. J. Orthop. Surg., *2*:669, 1920.

19. Evans, D.: Relapsed club foot. J. Bone Joint Surg., *43B*:722, 1961.

20. Fearnley, M. E., cited as personal communication by Attenborough, C. G.: Early posterior soft tissue release in severe congenital talipes equinovarus. Clin. Orthop., *84*:71, 1972.

21. Flinchum, D.: Pathological anatomy in talipes equinovarus. J. Bone Joint Surg., *35A*:111, 1953.

22. Fowler, S. B., Brooks, A. L., and Parrish, T. F.: The cavovarus foot. Proc. AAOS, J. Bone Joint Surg., *41A*:757, 1959.

23. Fried, A.: Recurrent congenital clubfoot. The role of the m. tibialis posterior in etiology and treatment. J. Bone Joint Surg., *41A*:243, 1959.

24. Garceau, G. J., and Manning, K. R.: Transposition of the anterior tibial tendon in the treatment of recurrent congenital club-foot. J. Bone Joint Surg., *29*:1044, 1947.

25. Gartland, J. J.: Posterior tibial transplant in the surgical treatment of recurrent clubfoot. A preliminary report. J. Bone Joint Surg., *46A*:1217, 1964.

26. Gartland, J. J., and Sargent, R. E.: Posterior tibial transplant in the surgical treatment of recurrent clubfoot. Clin. Orthop., *84*:66, 1972.

27. Goldner, J. L.: Personal communication, 1979.

28. Goldner, J. L.: Personal communication, St. Lukes Hospital Symposium, Houston, Texas, April 1981.

29. Guerin, M.: Division of the tendon Achilles in club foot. Lancet, *2*:648, 1935.

30. Henry, A. K.: *Extensile Exposure.* 2nd edition. New York, Churchill Livingstone, 1970, pp. 300–309.

31. Heyman, C. H., Herndon, C. H., and Strong, J. M.: Mobilization of the tarso-metatarsal and intermetatarsal joints for the correction of resistant adduction of the forepart of the foot in congenital clubfoot or congenital metatarsus varus. J. Bone Joint Surg., *40A*:299, 1958.

32. Hippocrates, Volume III. *Loeb Classical Library* (trans. E. T. Withington). London, Heinemann, 1927.

33. Hirsch, C.: Observations on early operative treatment of congenital clubfoot. Bull. Hosp. Joint Dis., *21*:173, 1960.

34. Hoke, M.: An operative plan for the correction of relapsed and untreated talipes equinovarus. Am. J. Orthop. Surg., *9*:379, 1912.

35. Idelberger, K.: Die Ergebnisse der Zwillingsforschung beim angeborenen Klumpfuss. Verh. Dtsch. Orthop. Bes., *33*:272, 1939.

36. Irani, R. N., and Sherman, M. S.: The pathological anatomy of clubfoot. J. Bone Joint Surg., *45A*:45, 1963.

37. Isaacs, H.: The muscles in club foot. J. Bone Joint Surg., *59B*:465, 1977.

38. Kaplan, E. B.: Comparative anatomy of the talus in relation to idiopathic clubfoot. Clin. Orthop., *85*:32, 1972.

39. Keim, H. A., and Richie, G. W.: "Nutcracker" treatment of clubfoot. JAMA, *189*:613, 1964.

40. Kite, J. H.: The treatment of congenital clubfoot. JAMA, *99*:1156, 1932.

41. Lambrinudi, C.: A method of correcting equinus and calcaneus deformities at the sub-astragaloid joint. Proc. R. Soc. Med., *26*:788, 1933.

42. Larsen, L.: Personal communication, San Francisco, 1972.

43. Lichtblau, S.: A medial and lateral release operation for club foot. A preliminary report. J. Bone Joint Surg., *55A*:1377, 1973.

44. Little, W. J.: *A Treatise on the Nature of Club-Foot and Analogous Distortions: Including Their Treatment Both With or Without Surgical Operation.* London, W. Jeffs, 1839.

45. Lloyd-Roberts, G. C.: Congenital club-foot. J. Bone Joint Surg., *46A:369,* 1964.
46. Lloyd-Roberts, G. C.: Personal communication, International Pediatric Orthopedics Seminar, Chicago, May, 1979.
47. Lloyd-Roberts, G. C.: Sixth Annual International Pediatric Orthopedics Seminar, San Francisco, 1978.
48. Lorenz (1784), cited by Fergusson, W. A.: A system of practical surgery. Philadelphia, Lea & Blanchard, 1843, p. 350.
49. Lovell, W. W., Price, C. T., and Meehan, P. L.: The foot. In *Pediatric Orthopaedics.* Edited by W. W. Lovell and R. B. Winter. Philadelphia, J. B. Lippincott, 1978, p. 911.
50. Lund (1875), cited by Kite, J. H.: The treatment of congenital clubfoot. JAMA, *99:*1156, 1932.
51. McCauley, J. C.: Treatment of clubfoot. In *AAOS Instructional Course Lectures.* Vol. 16. St. Louis, C. V. Mosby, 1959, p. 93.
52. McKay, D.: Personal communication, 1980.
53. Mau, C.: Muskelbefunde und ihre Bedeutung Beim Angeborenen Klumfussleiden. Arch. Orthop. Unfallchir., *28:292,* 1930.
54. Meary, R.: On the measurement of the angle between the talus and the first metatarsal. Symposium: Le Pied Creux Essentiel. Rev. Chir. Orthop., *53:389,* 1967.
55. Mitchell, G. P.: Posterior displacement osteotomy at the os calcis. J. Bone Joint Surg., *59B:233,* 1977.
56. Ober, F. R.: An operation for the relief of congenital equinovarus deformity. J. Orthop. Surg., *2:558,* 1920.
57. Paterson, D.: Personal communication, Salt Lake City, Utah, 1975.
58. Paterson, D.: Personal communication, 1981.
59. Phelps, A. M.: Congres. int des Sci. med. Copenhagen, 1884, II Sect. de Chir. 183, 1886.
60. Ponseti, I. V., and Smoley, E. M.: Congenital clubfoot: The results of treatment. J. Bone Joint Surg., *45A:261,* 1963.
61. Pugh, (1883), cited by Kite, J. H.: The treatment of congenital clubfoot. JAMA, *99:*1156, 1932.
62. Reimann, I., and Becker-Andersen, H.: Early surgical treatment of congenital club foot. Clin. Orthop., *102:200,* 1974.
63. Roberts, J. R.: Personal communication, 1980.
64. Roberts, J.: The inheritance of lethal muscle contracture in sheep. J. Genetics, *21:57,* 1929.
65. Sajadi, K.: Personal communication, Teheran, Iran, January, 1975.
66. Salter, R. B., and Field, P.: The effects of continuous compression on living articular cartilage. J. Bone Joint Surg., *42A:31,* 1960.
67. Samilson, R. L.: Crescentic osteotomy of the os calcis for calcaneocavus feet. In *Foot Science.* Edited by J. Bateman. Philadelphia, W. B. Saunders, 1976, pp. 18–25.
68. Scarpa, A.: A memoir on the congenital club foot in children. Translated from the Italian by J. W. Wishart. Edinburgh, Constable, 1818.
69. Settle, G. W.: The anatomy of congenital talipes equinovarus: Sixteen dissected specimens. J. Bone Joint Surg., *45A:*1341, 1963.
70. Shapiro, F., and Glimcher, J. J.: Gross and histological abnormalities of the talus in congenital club foot. J. Bone Joint Surg., *61A:522,* 1979.
71. Simons, G.: Analytical radiography of club foot. J. Bone Joint Surg., *59B:485,* 1977.
72. Solly (1857), cited by Kite, J. H.: The treatment of congenital clubfoot. JAMA, *99:*1156, 1932.
73. Stewart, S. F.: Club-foot: Its incidence, cause and treatment, anatomical-physiological study. J. Bone Joint Surg., *33A:577,* 1951.

74. Storen, H.: Experiences with operative treatment of clubfoot in older children and adults. Acta. Orthop. Scand., *11:*135, 1940.

75. Streckeisen (1867), cited by Baumgartner, R., and Taillard, W.: Treatment of congenital clubfoot at the Kinderspital Basel. Ann. Paediatr. Basel, *200:*363, 1963.

76. Stromeyer, L., cited by Little, W. J.: A treatise on the nature of clubfoot and analogous dissertations: Including their treatment both with and without surgical operation. London, W. Jeffs, 1939.

77. Struckman, J. S.: Triple arthrodesis in young children. Presented at the Western Orthopedic Association Meeting, 1970. (J. Bone Joint Surg., *53A:*396, 1971.)

78. Tachdjian, M. O.: Personal communication, 1980.

79. Tachdjian, M. O.: 6th Annual International Pediatric Orthopedics Seminar, San Francisco, 1978.

80. Tachdjian, M. O.: *Pediatric Orthopedics.* Philadelphia, W. B. Saunders, 1972.

81. Templeton, A. W., McAlister, W. H., and Zim, I. D.: Standardization of terminology and evaluation of osseous relationships in congenitally abnormal feet. AJR, *93:*374, 1965.

82. Thomas, H. O., cited by Preston, E. T., and Fell, T. W.: Congenital idiopathic club foot. Clin. Orthop., *122:*102, 1977.

83. Thomson, S. A.: Modified Denis Browne splint for unilateral club-foot to protect normal foot. J. Bone Joint Surg., *37:*1286, 1955.

84. Thomson, S. A.: Treatment of congenital talipes equinovarus with a modification of the Denis Browne method and splint. J. Bone Joint Surg., *24:*291, 1942.

85. Turco, V. J.: Resistant congenital club foot. One-stage posteromedial release with internal fixation. J. Bone Joint Surg., *61A:*805, 1979.

86. Turco, V. J.: Surgical correction of the resistant clubfoot. One-stage posteromedial release with internal fixation: A preliminary report. J. Bone Joint Surg., *53A:*477, 1971.

87. Westin, G. W.: Personal communication, 1980.

88. Whittem, J. H.: Congenital abnormalities in calves: Arthrogryposis and hydranencephaly. J. Pathol. Bacteriol. *73:*375, 1957.

89. Wiley, A. M.: Club foot. An anatomical and experimental study of muscle growth. J. Bone Joint Surg., *41B:*821, 1959.

90. Williams, P.: Personal communication, Melbourne, Australia, 1975.

91. Wynne-Davies, R.: Family studies and the cause of congenital clubfoot—talipes equinovarus, talipes calcaneovalgus and metatarsus varus. J. Bone Joint Surg., *46B:*445, 1964.

92. Wynne-Davies, R.: Genetic and environmental factors in the etiology of talipes equinovarus. Clin. Orthop., *84:*9, 1972.

93. Zadek, I., and Barnett, E.: The importance of the ligaments of the ankle in correction of congenital clubfoot. JAMA, *69:*1057, 1917.

# 3

# Congenital Vertical Talus (Congenital Convex Pes Valgus)

This foot deformity is uncommon, but because it is often not accurately diagnosed at birth, its true incidence is not well established. The fact that the deformity is often not diagnosed early is indeed unfortunate because, as with most complex foot deformities, the earlier specific treatment can be administered, the simpler it will be, and the more satisfactory will be the result. *Superficially,* this foot deformity simulates the more common calcaneovalgus foot, a fact largely responsible for its frequently late diagnosis. The continued inability of even pediatricians and orthopedic surgeons to make this distinction early probably reflects the rarity of the condition and results in the difficulty the physician faces in learning about its early newborn and neonatal diagnostic features (Fig. 3-1). One of the goals of this chapter is to illustrate and emphasize the diagnostic clinical and radiographic features of this deformity at various ages, not only to enhance early diagnosis and treatment, but also to reduce the severity of the problems that result from late diagnosis.

According to Lamy and Weissman, Henken produced the first complete study on the clinical and radiographic features of this deformity in 1914.[13,16] Henken was a pupil of Nove Josserand, a recognized authority on foot problems at that time. Many years later, in 1939, Lamy and Weissman described the convexity of the plantar aspect of the foot, the valgus of the heel, and the abduction of the forefoot found in this unique abnormality. Based upon these clinical observations and appropriate radiographic determinations, they called the deformity "congenital convex pes valgus." These authors further described the talonavicular dislocation, the vertical position of the talus, and the equinus attitude of the calcaneus and identified the associated musculotendinous contractures. They encountered the deformity more frequently in boys than in girls. Curiously, they preferred complete astragalectomy for treatment, but did not recommend a specific age for the procedure.

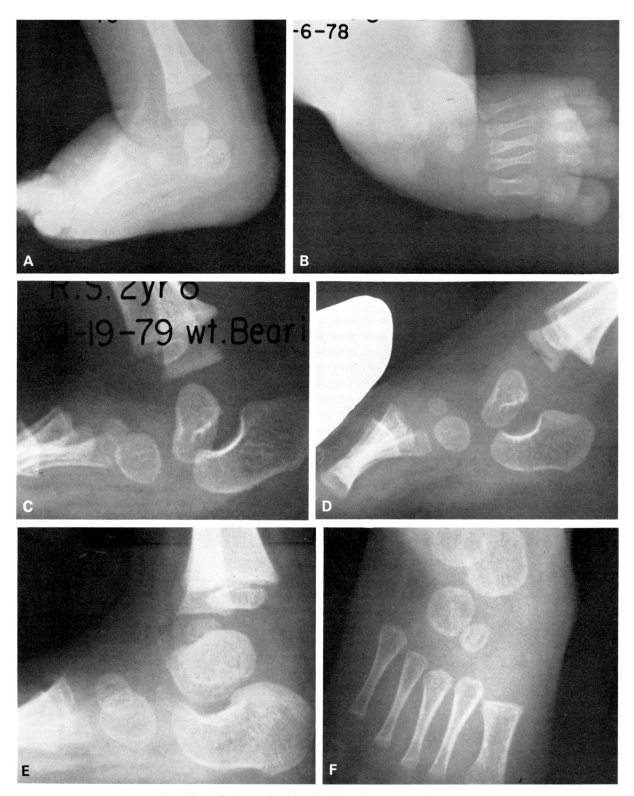

FIG. 3-1. Roentgenograms of the foot of a 2-month-old male with calcaneovalgus feet. Despite these anteroposterior and lateral roentgenograms showing a vertical talus on the left (**A** and **B**), no plantar flexion stress films were taken. Sixteen months later, the roentgenograms show a typical congenital vertical talus, demonstrated well in the plantar flexion stress films (**C** and **D**). The results of the two-stage procedures are seen radiographically and clinically 18 months later in **E**, **F**, **G**, and **H**.

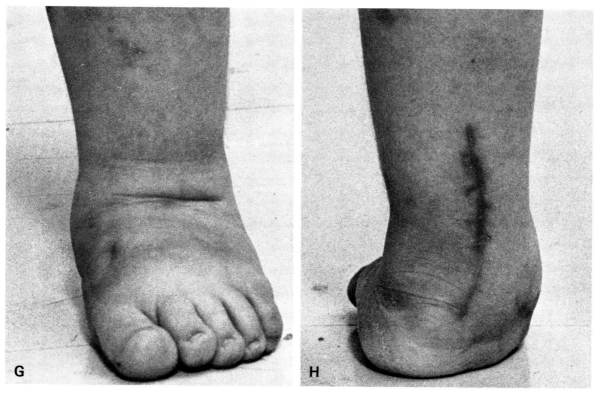

FIG. 3-1. *continued*

In 1950, Hark proposed a more sophisticated surgical approach to the problem.[11] He felt that corrective cast applications would lessen the deformity but not correct it completely. His operative approach was directed towards correcting the two most obvious abnormalities, the equinus of the hindfoot and the dorsal dislocation of the talonavicular (midtarsal) joint. In this regard, his procedure simulated that initially suggested by Rocher and Pouyanne in 1934.[22] Hark performed a posterior release at the ankle joint and pulled the calcaneus downward out of equinus, using a Steinmann pin driven into the os calcis to maintain the correction. He then lengthened the extensor tendons, reduced the talonavicular joint, and placed a pin across this joint. Except for the Steinmann pins, which were incorporated into a cast, no other stabilization procedure was performed.

Osmond-Clarke also experienced failure with nonoperative methods and therefore resorted to surgical treatment.[19] He noted that the talonavicular joint was unstable following surgical reduction and therefore believed that dynamic stabilization was necessary. Thus, he transferred the peroneus brevis into the neck of the talus in order to obviate the tendency for the talus to resume its vertical position. Unfortunately, only one case was reported, and no long-term follow-up was provided. Cowell also advocates this conceptual approach to the unstable talonavicular joint, although he uses the anterior tibial tendon instead of the peroneus brevis.[7]

Outland and Sherk's review, in 1960, of the many surgical techniques that had been used up to that time presented an imposing and confusing list of operative procedures that emphasized the tremendous technical challenge posed by this deformity.[20] They believed that osseous stabilization of the subtalar joint by means of a subtalar bone block was essential to maintain correction. Otherwise, the procedure they recommended was similar to that described by Hark. Herndon and Heyman also recognized the almost universal need for surgical correction and cautioned about the possibility of osseous necrosis of the talus, especially if the dorsal capsule of the ankle joint were damaged surgically.[14]

Eyre-Brook deserves credit for demonstrating the need for lateral stress plantar flexion roentgenograms in making or confirming the diagnosis of a fixed talonavicular dislocation.[9] He pointed out that in true congenital vertical talus, the talonavicular relationships will not change with forced plantar flexion, whereas in simple, uncomplicated, or paralytic flatfeet, these relationships revert to normal in forced plantar flexion (Fig. 3-2). He also noted that the peroneus brevis may actively assume a dorsal position over the head and neck of the talus. Eyre-Brook also popularized the therapeutic concept of "medial pillar

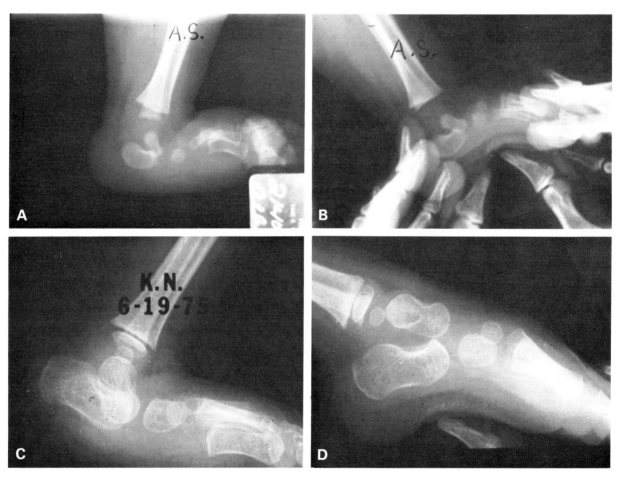

FIG. 3-2 **A,** The congenital vertical talus is shown in the lateral roentgenogram. **B,** Forced plantar flexion produces no discernible change in the relationships of the hindfoot or midfoot. **C,** In contrast, the complete restoration of normal relationships can be seen in this paralytic vertical talus following forced plantar flexion (**D**).

shortening," an idea he received from Batchelor in 1945.[3] It was first described, however, by Lange in 1912 and later by Lamy and Weissman.[17]

Harrold observed that many children with congenital vertical talus had other substantial musculoskeletal anomalies.[12] Especially common were arthrogryposis and various trisomy genetic defects. He also felt that *if* treatment was begun at birth, closed reduction by means of serial cast applications was possible in some rare cases. When surgical treatment was indicated, he preferred the technique of Heyman and Herndon.

Ellis and Scheer, in 1974, found that they could not report one successful nonoperative correction out of 17 consecutive cases of congenital vertical talus.[8] They emphasized the importance of considering age when attempting to evaluate treatment methods. They also cautioned about the substantial likelihood of aseptic necrosis of the talus and emphasized the importance of early surgical treatment for the best results.

In 1977, Clark, D'Ambrosia, and Ferguson again affirmed the importance of the "overgrown" medial column and referred to Eyre-Brook's contribution.[5] They proposed excision of the entire tarsal navicular bone, accompanied by transfixion of the cuneiform to the talus, and lengthening of the Achilles tendon. These authors felt that this simpler technique avoided any jeopardy to the talus since they reported no instances of talar osseous necrosis.

The issue of talar necrosis following treatment was further expanded by Ogata, Schoenecker, and Sheridan, who analyzed 36 patients with surgically treated congenital vertical talus.[18] In this review, they called attention to an apparent familial tendency in congenital vertical talus, a previously obscure issue.

In summary, the deformity known as congenital vertical talus has clearly challenged the imagination and technical skill of surgeons for many years. No obvious clearcut technical answer to the problem can be claimed at present. In a condition in which the etiology and pathogenesis are so poorly understood (see the following) and so many abnormalities may coexist, one must be content with making the diagnosis, identifying the pathology, and providing the most effective corrective procedures.

As one reviews the evolution of the understanding of this condition, it also becomes evident that substantial controversy has existed regarding the proper term for this foot deformity. As can be seen from the foregoing, it has been termed differently according to whether greater emphasis was given to the configuration of the foot or to the disturbed relationships between the bones. Any term used to describe the deformity will be incomplete, and for this and other reasons I prefer the simple expression "congenital vertical talus."

## Etiology

The cause of this deformity remains obscure. No obvious or consistent causal factor can be identified, although it is well accepted that congenital vertical talus, more often than not, is accompanied by some other coexisting developmental skeletal or neuromuscular abnormality (see later section on associated abnormalities).[4] These anomalies seem causally unrelated, which would suggest that the foot deformity, in most instances, is simply part of a poorly defined group of congenital anomalies.

The condition is more common in boys than in girls. The heritable pattern of this disorder is poorly defined, and no good evidence supports a consistent genetic factor. Interestingly, Aschner, Engelmann, Lamy, and Weissman reported the occurrence in a parent and child, and Armkriech encountered the deformity in identical twins.[1,2,16]

It is only infrequently (and, in my experience, rarely) that a *true* congenital vertical talus exists *without* the presence of another substantial or major musculoskeletal defect. One should therefore suspect other musculoskeletal or visceral abnormalities when a true, fixed, and rigid congenital vertical talus is identified.

## Pathology and Pathogenesis

Because its cause is unknown, it is difficult to identify or establish the pathogenesis of this deformity. A review of its pathologic features provides some insight into the pathogenesis. The heelcord and posterior ankle capsule are contracted, and the hindfoot is in equinus (Fig. 3-3). Often the posterior aspect of the heel cannot be placed on the ground. The forefoot is in fixed dorsiflexion, and the extensor tendons are contracted. Also present is a fixed talonavicular dislocation, in which the navicular lies on the anterior and dorsal aspect of the neck of the talus.

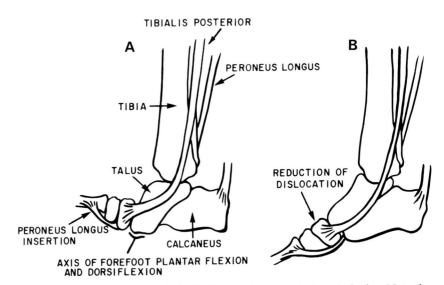

FIG. 3-3. **A,** The essential pathologic features in congenital vertical talus. Note that the calcaneus is in relative plantar flexion, the talus is almost vertical to the long axis of the foot, and the forefoot and midfoot are displaced dorsally upon the head and neck of the talus, thus making the forefoot plantar flexors actually dorsiflexors. The goal of reducing the remainder of the foot about the talus is seen in **B.** (Coleman, S. S., Stelling, F. H., and Jarrett, J.: Pathomechanics and treatment of congenital vertical talus. Clin. Orthop., *70:*65, 1970.)

The talus, as indicated in the name of the condition, has a nearly vertical relationship with the remainder of the foot. Because of this, the plantar flexors of the forefoot (the peroneals and posterior tibial tendons) are displaced *dorsal* to the talonavicular joint; consequently, these musculotendinous units, normally plantar flexors, tend to become dorsiflexors. Thus, not only are the tarsal bone and joint relationships disturbed, but a dynamic muscle imbalance is also present.

Prolonged fixed disturbance of the tarsal bone relationships, present both ante- and postnatally, gradually leads to alterations in the articulating facets, an observation borne out by Patterson, Fitz, and Smith's unique autopsy studies on a stillborn infant with congenital vertical talus.[21] Owing to these prolonged and substantial alterations in the configuration of the bones and facets and in the relationships of the bones, the deformity tends strongly to recur even after satisfactory surgical correction, especially in older children. It is less likely to recur if corrected before walking age. These observations clearly imply the need for early treatment.

At birth, the foot exhibits a convexity on its plantar aspect and is held in dorsiflexion; often the dorsum of the foot is held against the anterior aspect of the leg. The foot is rigid to a variable degree and typically cannot be substantially plantar flexed. Sometimes the tarsometatarsal joints may be sufficiently mobile that plantar flexion *seems* to occur. This spurious appearance can be readily identified and clarified, however, by appropriate roentgenograms (Fig. 3-2) (see section on roentgenographic examination).

In most instances, the involved foot is slightly smaller than its normal companion foot, and the calf is reduced in girth. In addition to the plantar convex configuration of the sole, the forefoot is abducted, and the hindfoot is in excessive valgus (Fig. 3-4). The combination of these deformities provides the basis for the term "convex (sole) pes valgus (heel)." The vertical position of the talus is responsible for the prominence in the sole of the foot, but it is much more apparent on the lateral roentgenogram (see Fig. 3-7). Thus the name "convex pes valgus" reflects the clinical appearance, and "vertical talus" more accurately, though incompletely, depicts the radiographic appearance.

Upon more detailed clinical examination, especially in older infants, one can feel a depression over the anterior aspect of the ankle joint just proximal to the navicular bone. This reflects the abnormal talonavicular relationships, in which the navicular lies on the neck of the talus rather than in its normal position directly distal to the talar head (Fig. 3-5). The most important aspect of this finding is the fact that this depression persists even with attempted maximum plantar flexion of the foot. The prominence of the head of the talus in the sole of the foot is also apparent and does not change appreciably with attempted plantar flexion. Thus, in true congenital vertical talus, a fixed or rigid talonavicular dislocation exists that passive manipulation cannot substantially alter. This can be demonstrated readily by a lateral

*Clinical Features*

roentgenogram taken with the foot held in maximum plantar flexion, as noted earlier (Fig. 3-2).

*Roentgenographic Examination*

It is important that true congenital vertical talus be distinguished from other conditions that simulate it. In most instances a careful clinical examination as just described can accomplish this. In some instances,

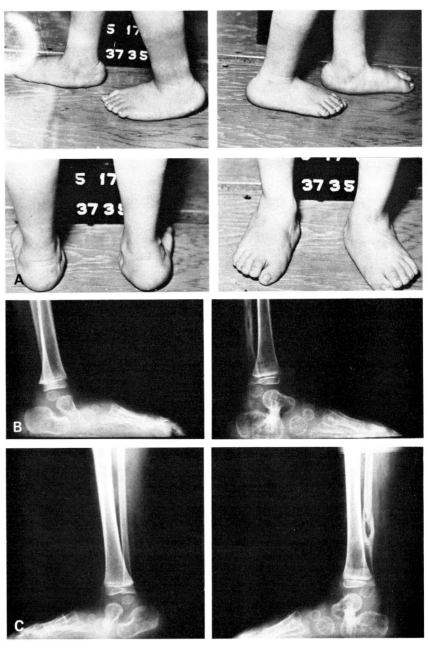

FIG. 3-4. **A**, Clinical appearance of congenital vertical talus in a 3-year-old male. Note the convexity of the sole of the foot, the valgus of the heel, which hardly touches the floor on stance, and the prominence of the talus over the plantar medial aspect of the foot. **B** and **C**, The pre- and postoperative films. (Coleman, S. S., Stelling, F. H., and Jarrett, J.: Pathomechanics and treatment of congenital vertical talus. Clin. Orthop., *70*:65, 1970.)

however, appropriate roentgenograms, especially lateral films, can best determine this difference. In order to appreciate the criteria for this distinction, it is essential to describe the distinguishing radiographic features of congenital vertical talus.

As emphasized in Chapter 1, all basic roentgenographic examinations of the child's foot should be made in the weight-bearing or simulated weight-bearing position. In instances of substantial deformity, "stress" examinations should also be performed, in which the foot is held in specific positions. These maneuvers are used primarily to assess flexibility (reducibility) or rigidity. It is especially important to perform a thorough roentgenographic study on any foot suspected of having congenital vertical talus. If the foot is truly abnormal, the roentgenograms confirm the suspicion (Fig. 3-5) and help the physician considerably in providing early diagnosis and, correspondingly, earlier and more effective treatment.

In a true congenital vertical talus, the ossification centers of the foot are smaller than normal, their configurations abnormal, and their relationships to each other clearly disturbed (Fig. 3-6), as demonstrated by Storen.[24] Thus, the diagnosis of congenital vertical talus is easily established in a properly performed and accurately interpreted roentgenogram. The abnormal size and configuration of the ossification centers are readily apparent in a comparison to roentgenograms of the opposite normal foot or of the foot of a normal newborn or neonate (Fig. 3-6). The radiographic stigmata of these abnormalities persist to some degree throughout the growth and development of the foot.

The disturbed relationships between the tarsal ossification centers are important, but the parameters used to detect them vary with the

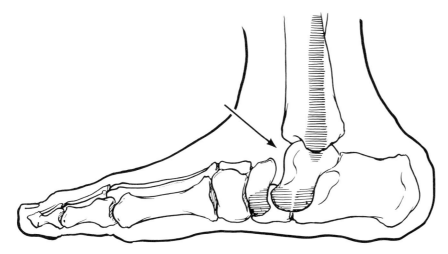

FIG. 3-5. Area of palpable depression created by the displaced navicular on the dorsal (anterior) aspect of the talus in congenital vertical talus. This depression is not present in normal feet. Also, the abnormal relationships of the navicular on the superior neck of the talus explain the presence of the concavity as well as the line of increased density seen radiographically on the talar neck that is produced by this abnormal articulation (see Figure 3-7).

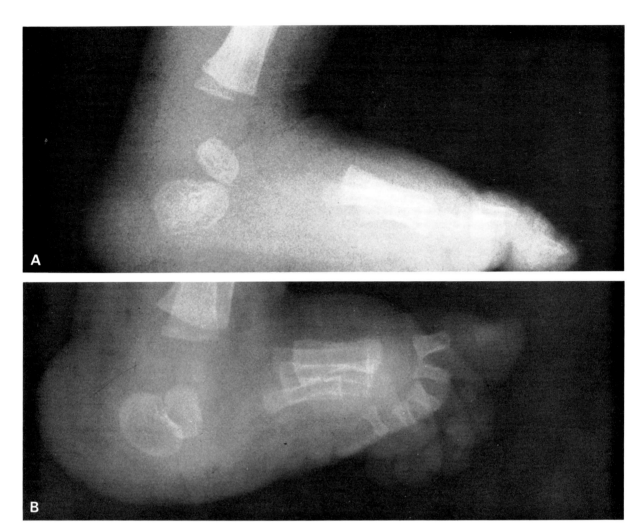

FIG. 3-6. Lateral simulated weight-bearing roentgenograms of the feet of a 2-month-old child. **A,** The normal shapes and relationships of the tarsal bones as well as the normal configuration of the entire foot. **B,** Contrast these observations with the opposite foot having a typical congenital vertical talus. Not only are the tarsal bones of a different shape, but their relationships are disturbed. The configuration of the foot is likewise distorted. Lateral radiography is a valuable diagnostic aid in the early diagnosis of congenital vertical talus.

child's age and the degree of ossification. Early in infancy, and even through age 2 or 3 years, the tarsal navicular is not yet ossified, and its abnormal position on the superior surface of the neck of the talus can only be suspected. Evidence that the unossified navicular *does* reside in this location is relatively easy to determine, however, because a depression is nearly always found in the anterior aspect of the neck of the talus, and a localized increase in thickness of the cortical bone is often seen in this same area, suggesting that the navicular has been articulating there (Fig. 3-7). Also, the cuneiform and cuboid ossification centers nearly always are displaced more dorsally than normal; this is especially evident in the lateral roentgenogram taken in forced plantar flexion (Fig. 3-2). Later, in early childhood, these abnormal relationships are more readily apparent because the tarsal bones have ossified further. In older children in whom adaptive skeletal changes have occurred, the typical severe, advanced deformity is diagnostic (Fig. 3-8).

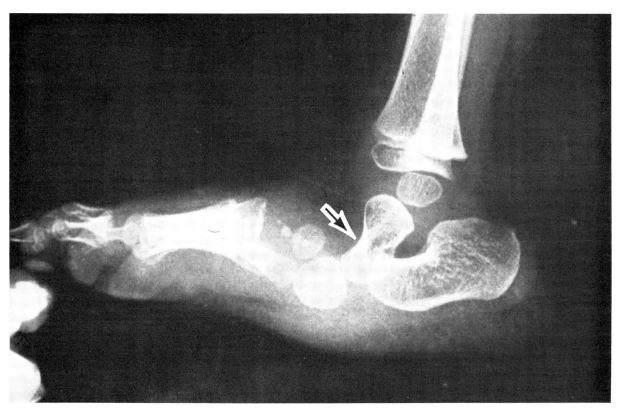

FIG. 3-7. Standing lateral roentgenogram of a 3-year-old male with typical congenital vertical talus. Note the concave configuration over the anterior aspect of the neck of the talus (arrow). This is the location of the navicular bone as yet unossified. The concavity and the increased cortical thickening are diagnostic signs of the abnormal talonavicular relationships. This film demonstrates well the vertical attitude of the talus.

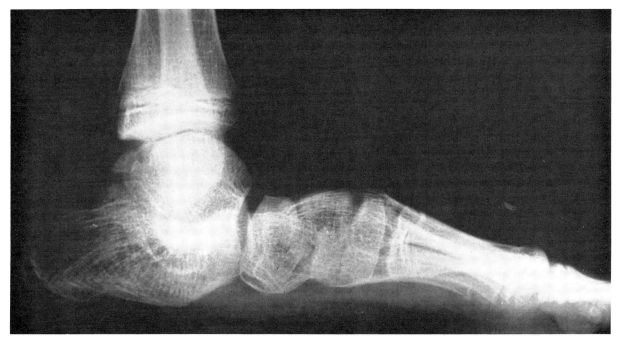

FIG. 3-8. Lateral standing film of a patient with congenital vertical talus that was *not treated* surgically. Note the completely vertical position of the talus and the navicular situated anteriorly on the neck of the talus.

In analyzing our patients with congenital vertical talus, two distinct categories become evident. In the simpler group, the major abnormality is seen as a disturbance of the talonavicular and talocalcaneal relationships. The calcaneocuboid articulations are preserved. The calcaneus is in less absolute equinus or none, and the talocalcaneal subluxation is accentuated. This group is called Type I (Fig. 3-9). In Type II, not only is a talonavicular dislocation seen, but also a disturbed relationship at the calcaneocuboid joint; in addition, the calcaneus is in a greater degree of absolute equinus. In essence, in the second case, a varying degree of subluxation or dislocation of the entire forefoot on the hindfoot is found (Fig. 3-9).[6] This categorization has important implications for treatment. When the calcaneocuboid joint is involved (Type II), it must be reduced and stabilized, in addition to the corrective procedures performed on the talonavicular and talocalcaneal joints, as outlined shortly.

Films taken in plantar flexion at any age will distinguish quickly between the true (rigid) congenital vertical talus and a similar flexible deformity, because the latter condition nearly always exhibits normal tarsal ossification centers. Thus, a paralytic vertical talus or a moderately severe pes valgoplanus or plantarflexed talus, on roentgenographic examination, exhibits normal tarsal bone relationships whether the foot is in repose or in forced plantar flexion (Fig. 3-2).

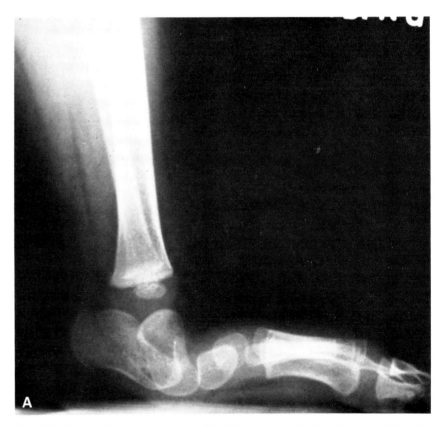

FIG. 3-9. **A,** Lateral roentgenogram of the Type I congenital vertical talus. Note the reasonably well preserved calcaneocuboid relationships.

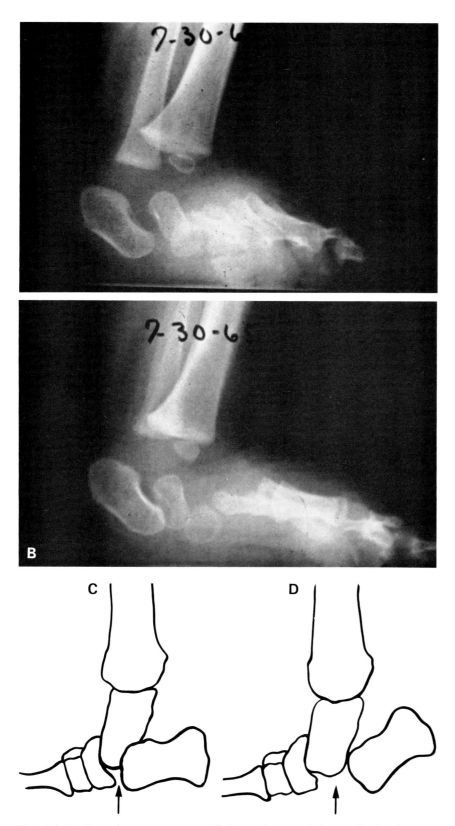

FIG. 3-9. **B,** Lateral roentgenograms of a Type II congenital vertical talus. Observe the major alteration in the calcaneocuboid relationships. These differences are illustrated diagrammatically in **C** and **D**.

TABLE 3-1. *Anomalies Associated with Congenital Vertical Talus*

| | |
|---|---|
| Arthrogryposis Multiplex Congenita | Congenital Hip Dislocation |
| Myelodysplasia | Neurofibromatosis |
| Sacral Agenesis | Trisomy 13-15 and Trisomy 18 |
| Mental Retardation | Contralateral Congenital Equinovarus |
| Turner's Syndrome | Contralateral Calcaneovalgus |
| Pollex Varus | Syndactyly |

On the other hand, in true congenital vertical talus, films taken in either repose or forced plantar flexion divulge a persistently abnormal relationship of the hindfoot structures, demonstrated by Eyre-Brook.[9] These two deformities must be distinguished, of course, because the treatment of each is radically different. Thus, properly performed roentgenograms are important diagnostic aids to the surgeon, not only in establishing the presence or absence of a congenital vertical talus, but also in clearly distinguishing it from other conditions that may simulate it.

*Associated Abnormalities*

Although the cause and pathogenesis of congenital vertical talus remain somewhat obscure, I have observed, as noted earlier, that this foot deformity is accompanied by other skeletal, visceral, and neurologic abnormalities in a high percentage of cases. In fact, my experience dictates that finding a true congenital vertical talus mandates a thorough search for other congenital and developmental disorders. Of the more than 40 cases I have treated during the past 20 years, only 2 did *not* have other substantial musculoskeletal or visceral abnormalities. In one child, no abnormality existed at all, and in the other, only a moderately severe flexible flatfoot was present on the opposite side. The deformity is often associated with contralateral clubfoot, a variety of musculoskeletal syndromes, arthrogryposis, and other overt skeletal deformities (Table 3-1 and Fig. 3-10). This observation, however, *excludes* congenital vertical talus associated with myelomeningocele, in which paralytic and other factors may play a causal role.

*Treatment*

Even though one may encounter a rare case of true congenital vertical talus that can be treated nonoperatively, as noted previously, it has been rather well established that once this condition is diagnosed, surgical treatment of some sort is essential to correct it satisfactorily. The type and success of the operation depend largely on the age of the patient, since the older the child, the greater the degree of established adaptive change in the articulations and shapes of the bones.

Furthermore, a prewalking infant is easier to treat than a weight-bearing child. Contrary to congenital clubfoot, weight bearing tends to reproduce or encourage recurrence of congenital vertical talus, and it is difficult to keep a young ambulatory infant from walking in a cast, even a hip spica. Therefore, I find it convenient to divide the treatment program into four broad age categories: (a) prewalking age, (b) onset of walking age through age $2\frac{1}{2}$ years, (c) age $2\frac{1}{2}$ through 6 years, and (d) over age 6 years. These divisions are somewhat arbitrary, but are made for specific reasons, as discussed in the following sections.

If one is fortunate enough to diagnose a true congenital vertical talus when the patient is still a neonate or prewalking infant, the treatment is simpler and the results usually more predictable and far more rewarding than those of treatment administered at any later age. Even though surgical treatment is almost always required for satisfactory correction, the operation necessary for this age group is often less complicated than that required later.

PREWALKING AGE

PRELIMINARY NONOPERATIVE CORRECTION. Initially and upon first diagnosis, one should try to correct the deformity passively in the hope (usually futile) of reducing it nonoperatively. Since the foot is so rigid and has such a paradoxic deformity, however, it is virtually never corrected satisfactorily by this means. Nonetheless, such efforts are essential and can be helpful because the foot can be gradually forced into plantar flexion, thus stretching out the soft-tissue structures over the dorsum of the foot. These structures include the skin, subcutaneous tissues, ligaments, and capsules of the tarsal and ankle joints. As described in the following section, this nonoperative, corrective maneuver also aids in the subsequent surgical correction.

An above-knee cast should be applied with the foot held gently in maximum equinus (Fig. 3-11). The cast should be changed weekly or

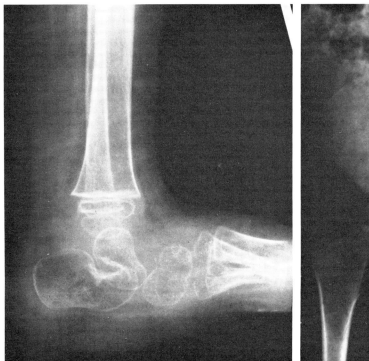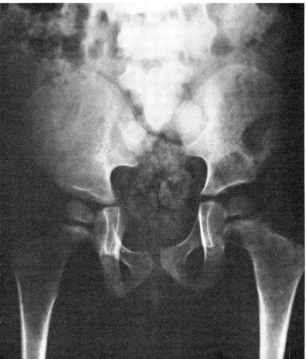

FIG. 3-10. An example of the many associated abnormalities that can be seen in patients with congenital vertical talus: in this case, a congenital absence of the sacrum.

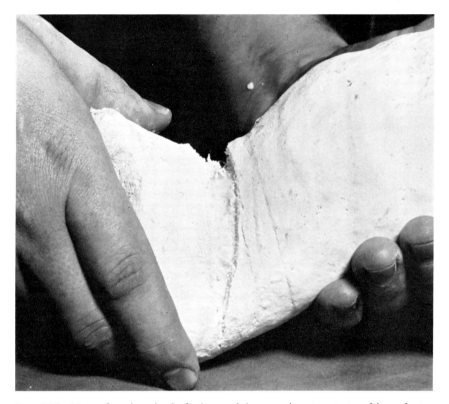

FIG. 3-11. My preferred method of using wedging casts in attempts to achieve plantar flexion in congenital vertical talus. Alternatively, the foot can be manipulated gently into plantar flexion, and then the cast can be applied. Either a below-knee cast, applied with skin adhesive, or an above-knee cast may be employed.

biweekly; at each change, the foot and ankle are gently placed into further plantar flexion. The foot's response to these preliminary corrective efforts should be monitored periodically (every week or so) by means of lateral roentgenograms taken with the foot held in maximum plantar flexion. The foot should also be examined physically to determine whether or not the navicular (forefoot) is being reduced to its normal position over the head of the talus. If the foot is being corrected, the plantar flexion cast program should be continued. In rare instances, it may be possible to correct the deformity without resorting to a subsequent operation, but I have never been successful in this effort in the case of a *true* congenital vertical talus.

Usually, one can determine whether or not the foot is being corrected within 4 to 6 weeks. In nearly all instances, the bony deformities will not be corrected, and surgical correction therefore will be clearly indicated. No well established guidelines govern the age at which the operation should be done. In theory, however, once it is clear that nonoperative cast correction has failed, it is reasonable to proceed with the appropriate surgical procedure. In general, I prefer to wait until the infant is at least 3 months old. The reason for any delay (if the nonoperative treatment was begun early) is simply to wait for the infant's foot to increase in size and to ensure that the infant can safely undergo general anesthesia. It is important to correct the abnormality surgically as early as possible, once the indications and safety of the procedure are established. As noted previously, the basic indication for the operation is simply the failure of nonoperative measures.

OPERATIVE CORRECTION. The ultimate objectives of the operation are to achieve and maintain correction of the disturbed bone and joint relationships and to restore to as normal as possible any existing muscle imbalance as outlined previously in the section on pathology. This means that the contracted extensor tendons may require elongation, the talonavicular dislocation must be reduced and stabilized, and the talocalcaneal subluxation and the equinus attitude of the talus must be corrected. In the case of Type II lesions, the calcaneocuboid joint must also be reduced and stabilized. It is also advisable to re-establish and strengthen the integrity of the plantar calcaneonavicular (spring) ligament.

Whether complete correction requires one or two operative stages depends upon the surgeon's experience and judgment of the extent of surgical intervention the infant's foot can safely undergo in one operation. From my own experience, it seems safer and more effective to employ two stages, with the first stage designed to correct the foot and the second to correct the ankle equinus and to repair and reinforce the plantar-medial joint structures.

*First Stage.* A dorsolateral oblique incision is placed over the dorsum of the foot, centering over the sinus tarsus and extending from the peroneal tendons posterolaterally to the anterior tibial tendon medially (Fig. 3-12). This incision permits complete access to all long extensor and dorsiflexor tendons of the ankle and toes, as well as to the capsules of the talonavicular and subtalar joints. Furthermore, the neurovascular bundle (dorsalis pedis artery) can be easily identified and protected.

The incision is deepened and the extensor digitorum brevis dissected from its origin and retracted distally. The sinus tarsus is evacuated of all fatty tissues, and the talocalcaneal interosseous ligament is sectioned. The anterior tibial, extensor hallucis longus, and extensor digitorum longus tendons are sectioned and lengthened in a "Z" fashion. (The degree of lengthening that they require largely reflects both the effectiveness of the preoperative plantar flexion manipulations described earlier and the age of the patient.)

In exposing the tendons, the retinacula, which are often thick and inelastic, must be sectioned. The anterior tibial and long extensor tendons are tagged and retracted proximally and distally, and the underlying dense intertarsal ligaments and capsule of the talonavicular joint can be identified. The navicular will be encountered on the dorsal aspect of the neck of the talus. Identification of the separation between the navicular and the neck of the talus requires careful, sharp dissection. This can be facilitated by placing a small, sharp rake retractor into the navicular bone and exerting gentle, distal traction. The ligaments and capsular connections are usually thick and contracted, and

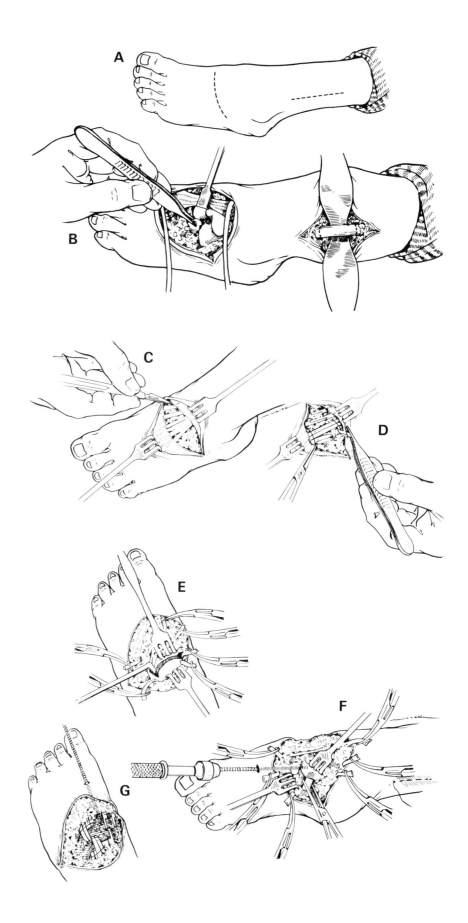

one often encounters great difficulty in defining the plane of dissection. Considerable care is therefore required to avoid damaging the articular surfaces of these bones when sectioning the talonavicular capsule.

Once released, the navicular usually can be gently pulled distally over the head of the talus. In this maneuver, the talus usually must be elevated upwards from its displaced position on the calcaneus. This requires evacuation of the dense fibrous tissue in the sinus tarsus, as well as sectioning of the talocalcaneal interosseous ligament. Once the talonavicular and talocalcaneal joints have been acceptably reduced, the talonavicular joint is stabilized by a smooth Kirschner wire of appropriate size. As the forefoot is placed into its new position, the posterior tibial tendon often assumes a more normal position in the plantar-medial aspect of the head and neck of the talus, in contrast to its previous dorsomedial position caused by the upward dislocation of the navicular on the talar neck.

In the uncommon Type II deformity, it is advisable to expose the calcaneocuboid joint to ensure that this joint has been satisfactorily reduced. This is done through the same incision, using subcutaneous dissection distal to the calcaneocuboid joint. Once established, reduction is maintained by a smooth Kirschner wire placed across this joint, using the same technique as that employed with a talonavicular joint.

In the infant prewalker, it is *not* necessary to stabilize the subtalar joint by means of a subtalar bone block, because the talonavicular (and calcaneocuboid, where necessary) transfixion will adequately stabilize the triple joint. Furthermore, with the rapid growth and remodeling of the bones of the foot characteristic in prewalkers, intrinsic bony stability usually occurs rapidly (Fig. 3-13).

The tendons are then repaired and the skin is closed. Usually skin closure is not a problem if the skin and soft tissues have been adequately stretched in the preoperative plantar flexion manipulations. In rare circumstances, I have done a percutaneous heelcord lengthening

Fig. 3-12. The first stage in correction of a rigid, congenital vertical talus. **A**, the dorsolateral incision centers over the sinus tarsus; the other incision, over the distal end of the fibula, is used in the case of older children (over 18 months) who require a subtalar bone block for stabilization. **B**, The sinus tarsus is emptied of its fat and capsular tissues; the talocalcaneal ligament also must be cut to permit correction of the talocalcaneal relationship. A fibular graft is removed at this time if necessary. **C** and **D**, The extensor tendons are identified, freed up, and lengthened in step-cut fashion. **E**, By gentle distal traction on the navicular bone, and after complete talonavicular capsulotomy, the navicular is pulled forward and in the plantar direction about the head of the talus. This usually permits easy reduction of both the talonavicular and talocalcaneal joints. With these three bones in their appropriate position, a smooth or threaded Steinmann pin of appropriate size is placed across the talonavicular joint. In young children (prewalkers), this is usually all the stabilization that is necessary. **F**, In older children, however, especially those over 18 months, a subtalar bone block is accomplished to stabilize the talocalcaneal joint. **G**, The extensor tendons are then repaired in their lengthened position. The wounds are then closed, and an above-knee cast is applied with the foot and ankle in equinus. My preferred method for performing the subtalar bone block is seen in Figure 5-7. (Redrawn from Coleman, S. S., Stelling, F. H., and Jarrett, J.: Pathomechanics and treatment of congenital vertical talus. Clin. Orthop., *70*:65, 1970.)

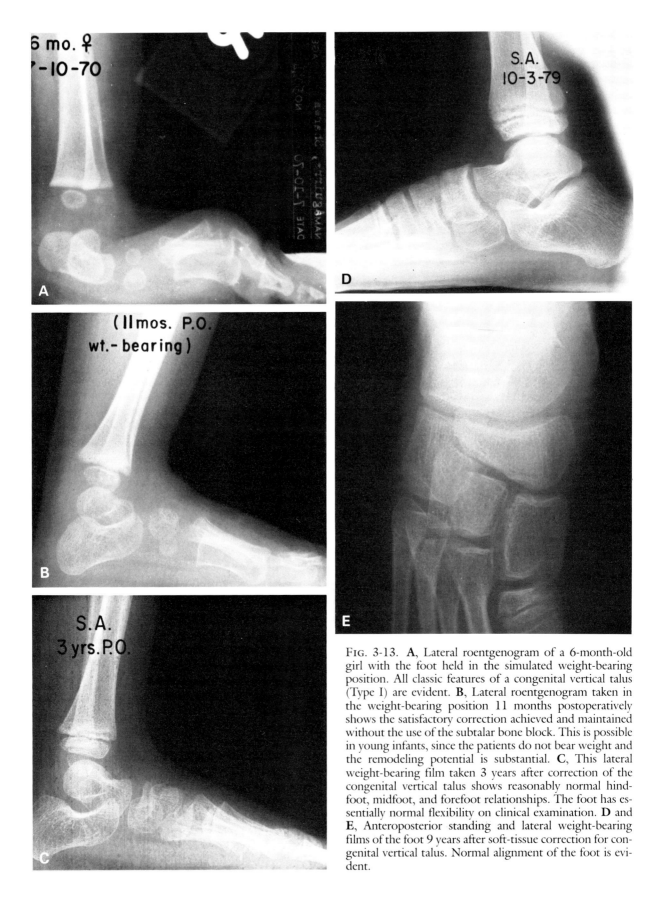

FIG. 3-13. **A,** Lateral roentgenogram of a 6-month-old girl with the foot held in the simulated weight-bearing position. All classic features of a congenital vertical talus (Type I) are evident. **B,** Lateral roentgenogram taken in the weight-bearing position 11 months postoperatively shows the satisfactory correction achieved and maintained without the use of the subtalar bone block. This is possible in young infants, since the patients do not bear weight and the remodeling potential is substantial. **C,** This lateral weight-bearing film taken 3 years after correction of the congenital vertical talus shows reasonably normal hindfoot, midfoot, and forefoot relationships. The foot has essentially normal flexibility on clinical examination. **D** and **E,** Anteroposterior standing and lateral weight-bearing films of the foot 9 years after soft-tissue correction for congenital vertical talus. Normal alignment of the foot is evident.

to permit some slight degree of ankle dorsiflexion. This can often relieve any worrisome or threatening tension on the skin over the dorsum of the foot. Complete correction of ankle equinus requires a full posterior ankle capsulotomy, a procedure I prefer to delay until a second stage. Some surgeons believe it is safe to accomplish the entire procedure at one operation; as mentioned earlier, however, I feel that the staged sequence is safer and, for me, more effective because it is possible at the time of the second stage to reef or plicate the medial capsular structures and to translocate the posterior tibial tendon under the head of the talus, as described by Kidner (see Chapter 6).[15]

After skin closure, a well padded, above-knee cast is applied with the foot in as much equinus as necessary to maintain good alignment but at the same time to avoid any undue tension on the skin. At the conclusion of the first stage, the following have been accomplished: (1) The talonavicular dislocation has been reduced and stabilized, (2) the talocalcaneal subluxation has been reduced, (3) some degree of muscle balance has been restored, and (4) the foot alignment has been restored as completely as possible. The entire foot remains in some degree of equinus; however, it remains so only until the second stage is accomplished.

*Second Stage.* Six weeks after the first stage, the cast is removed and the transfixion pin extracted from the talonavicular joint. The foot and ankle are kept in a removable splint until the operative wounds and pin tract sites are completely healed. Then the second stage is accomplished, consisting of a complete posterior release of the ankle joint and plantar translocation of the posterior tibial tendon under the head of the talus, as described in the following section.

A posterior release is accomplished first by a conventional medial curvilinear vertical incision placed over the distal portion of the Achilles tendon. The tendon is lengthened in a stepcut "Z" fashion, and the ankle capsule is incised in the same manner as in the posterior release for congenital equinovarus (Fig. 3-14) (see also Chapter 2). This usually permits satisfactory dorsiflexion of the entire foot at the ankle joint. The surgeon should decide whether the tibiofibular syndesmosis should also be sectioned. The Achilles tendon is repaired in the lengthened position, and the wound is closed.

A second incision is made over the medial aspect of the foot at the level of the talonavicular joint. The posterior tibial tendon is identified and freed up as far proximally as the medial malleolus. Its insertion on the navicular and its more distal insertion on the medial cuneiform and first metatarsal are left intact, but the tendon itself is translocated and sutured into the periosteum and the ligamentous structures under the head and neck of the talus, using the technique described by Kidner. The medial talonavicular capsular ligaments can also be plicated or reefed.

At this time, a smooth Kirschner wire or small Steinmann pin again may be placed across the talonavicular joint to maintain stabilization of the joint and thus protect the tendon transfer and the ligamentous repair. The wound is closed, and a well padded, above-knee

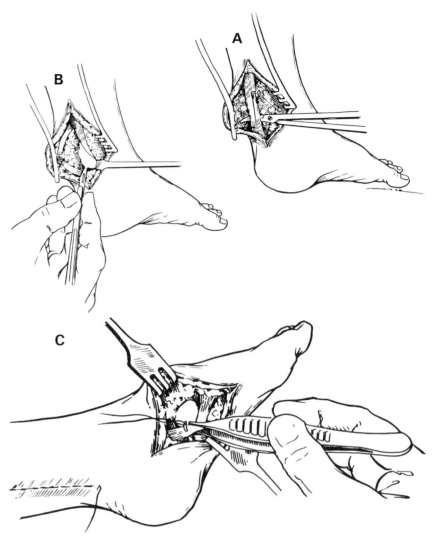

FIG. 3-14. The second stage in correction of congenital vertical talus requires (**A**) lengthening of the Achilles tendon, in addition to (**B**) posterior ankle capsulotomy. **C**, Also, as a means of reinforcing the ligamentous structures under the head of the talus (spring ligament), a modified Kidner procedure is accomplished by translocating the posterior tibial tendon beneath the talar head.

cast is applied, with the foot in at least 10° of dorsiflexion. This cast is removed in 6 weeks; the pin is extracted and a polypropylene or plastic UCB-type splint is prescribed (Fig. 3-15). This is worn both day and night until the patient becomes ambulatory and stability of the previously dislocated and subluxated joints can be demonstrated.

Complete anatomic restoration is sometimes not possible because of the previous long-term disturbance (ante- as well as postnatal) of these bony relationships. In some cases, the forefoot will remain abducted, and the arch will not be restored as fully as desired, although the functional and anatomic results are usually far better than if the foot had been left untreated. As in the case of congenital clubfoot (see Chapter 2), however, the parents should be advised that such a foot can never be expected to be indistinguishable from normal.

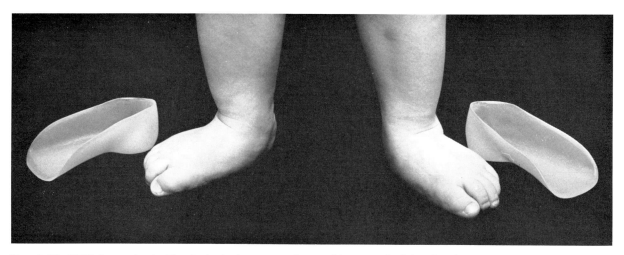

FIG. 3-15. UCB foot orthosis. The device is the same as that used in severe flexible valgoplanus feet in young children. It is versatile because it can be placed in any kind of shoe.

As the child grows and develops, efforts at normal use will usually strengthen all the muscles and increase foot mobility; the foot may require protection by some form of orthosis, however, for many months or even a year or two.

The only difference in the therapeutic approach for this age group, as compared to the infant prewalker, is the question of the need for a subtalar extra-articular arthrodesis.[10] The age at which this arthrodesis becomes necessary is not well established, and the decision to employ it must be based largely on clinical judgment and intuition, since no well established guidelines can predictably or reliably answer this question. Hopefully, in the future, the question itself will arise less often as our improved diagnostic acumen makes it possible to treat these youngsters during the first few months of postnatal life, which is the ideal time. It must be emphasized that the subtalar bone block (extra-articular arthrodesis) is *not* totally innocuous; considerable deliberation therefore should be exercised before the need for such a procedure is established.

When the bone block is deemed necessary, it is done during the first stage at the time that the sinus tarsus is evacuated and the talocalcaneal interosseous ligament is severed, as described previously and illustrated in Figure 3-12. At this time, the subtalar bone block can be inserted and can effectively stabilize the subtalar joint. I prefer to use a small segment of the distal fibula, taken through an incision centered over the lateral aspect of the fibula that is just above the lateral malleolus. Other donor sites are equally appropriate, however, as long as the bone is an isograft and not an allo- or heterograft. In my experience, these latter two types of grafts often fail because of nonunion or graft reabsorption. I have had no instances in which the fibular donor site failed to regenerate as long as the length of graft did not exceed a length of 2.0 cm, which is more than adequate for the block and of ideal size and shape. It is important not to *over*correct the

ONSET OF WALKING
THROUGH AGE
$2\frac{1}{2}$ YEARS

talocalcaneal reduction, because this will create a deformity that is difficult to correct subsequently.

Except for this variation, the other aspects of surgical correction are identical with the two stages described earlier in this chapter. The postoperative care is also the same, except that ambulation must await thorough incorporation of the subtalar bone block, if used. Also, because the patient is older, the bracing program may require more time.

AGE 2½ TO 6 YEARS    This age group is separated from the previous two because a subtalar bone block is necessary in all instances to stabilize the subtalar joint (Fig. 3-16). It has been my experience that when the subtalar bone block is not employed in this age group, the deformity inevitably recurs to some degree (Fig. 3-17). The facet joints and other supporting structures have undergone such extensive adaptive change that ligamentous repairs and tendon transfers cannot provide the stability necessary to maintain correction. The only exception to this might be the transfer of the anterior tibial tendon to the neck of the talus as prescribed by Sharrard and Cowell.[7,23] I have had no experience with this procedure, and a published follow-up report on a substantial series of patients is not available from which to draw meaningful conclusions regarding its effectiveness.

The principal objections to the use of the subtalar bone block are those inherent in the procedure itself: (1) the hindfoot is made rigid and, in essence, an iatrogenic talocalcaneal coalition is produced, (2) with growth, the heel may gradually develop either a varus or valgus configuration, possibly requiring later correction, (3) with skeletal growth, a "ball-and-socket" ankle joint may be produced, especially if the hindfoot is in any substantial degree of varus, and (4) later hypertrophic changes often develop at the talonavicular joint (Fig.

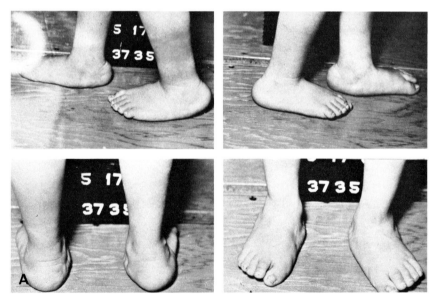

FIG. 3-16. An example of a patient requiring subtalar bone block procedures to stabilize the hindfoot. **A,** Standing photographs.

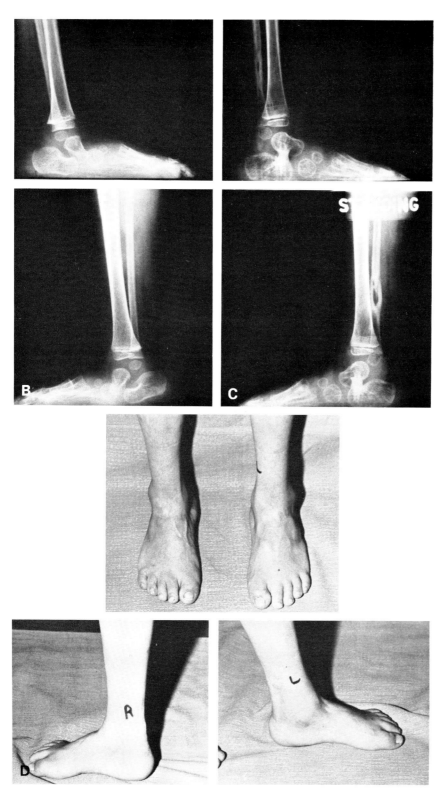

FIG. 3-16. (**B**) Preoperative standing roentgenograms of a 3-year-old boy with typical bilateral congenital vertical talus deformities. **C** and **D**, The postoperative standing radiographic and physical features 2 years later. The feet are plantigrade and have excellent function, even though there is some weakness of push-off. Note regeneration of the region of the fibular donor graft.

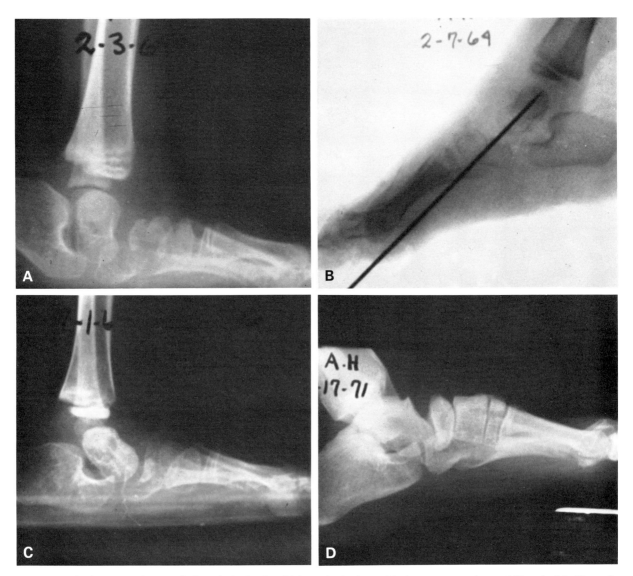

FIG. 3-17. An instance of congenital vertical talus in which a subtalar bone block was not used to stabilize the hindfoot. **A**, Standing preoperative lateral weight-bearing roentgenogram in a 5-year-old female who also had a congenital scoliosis. **B**, A Polaroid film taken intraoperatively shows acceptable reduction of the talonavicular and talocalcaneal joints. Note absence of subtalar bone block. **C**, Five months later, the correction has been partially maintained. **D**, Seven years later, substantial recurrence of the deformity is evident. This case emphasizes the need for hindfoot stabilization in the older child (over 2 years of age). (Courtesy of Dr. Robert Carson, Salt Lake City, Utah.)

3-18). Thus, it must be recognized that one abnormality (the talocalcaneal coalition) is being accepted in place of another; namely, an untreated foot that becomes a rigid, possibly painful flatfoot and that usually becomes a progressively more serious and difficult shoe-fitting problem in adult life.

In our review of over 40 cases, with follow-up as long as 20 years and in which a subtalar bone block was used for this condition in this age group, I found no discernible changes directly attributable to aseptic osseous necrosis of the talus, although some remodeling of the talus occurred with growth.[4] Clearly, however, one must be careful in dissecting about the dorsal talotibial capsule and ligaments because of this possibility.

Other than the routine need for a subtalar bone block, the entire treatment program for this group is identical to that for the first two age groups. As one approaches the fifth and sixth years, however, much more extensive and radical procedures will be required, as outlined in the following section.

When the child has been walking on a foot with congenital vertical talus for 6 years or more, the treatment becomes complicated. The configuration of the facet joints, and even the bones themselves, have undergone such extensive and irreversible changes that they cannot be corrected without major bone and joint surgery. The questions that arise are how extensive and what kind of a surgical procedure is required for correction.

From a review of the literature, it is evident that many operations recommended in the past were done on older children, because the list of procedures is extensive and somewhat awesome. As noted earlier, these have been thoroughly reviewed and tabulated by Outland.[20] Most of these operations were done because, owing to the age of the patient, the medial column of the foot was relatively overgrown in length. Thus, because of the longstanding talonavicular dislocation, any effort to reduce these joints was virtually futile unless or until the navicular and/or the talus were resected to some degree. Anyone who

OVER AGE 6 YEARS

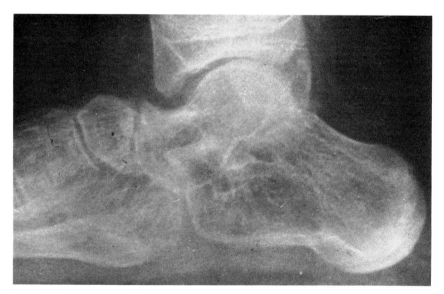

FIG. 3-18. Lateral standing roentgenogram of a foot treated for congenital vertical talus 9 years before when the patient was 2 years old. A subtalar bone block was accomplished, as described in the text. Note hypertrophic changes present in the talonavicular joint (see also Figure 9-9). (Coleman, S. S., Stelling, F. H., and Jarrett, J.: Pathomechanics and treatment of congenital vertical talus. Clin. Orthop., *70*:65, 1970.)

has attempted to reduce the bones of this foot deformity in this older age group has quickly encountered this difficulty. It is obvious that the deformity must be corrected before any type of stabilization is accomplished, but the best way to reduce the deformity represents a major dilemma for the surgeon.

In the younger children, Clark and associates feel that complete excision of the navicular bone is the only effective way to reduce the disturbed bony relationships and to stabilize the foot.[5] In this procedure, the medial column is clearly shortened, but an important set of tarsal articulations is eliminated in the process. The long-range effects of the procedure are not well established, and the ability to accomplish a subsequent triple arthrodesis, if necessary, is obviously compromised. This salvage procedure may be the most effective method of correction at this age, and although I have no strong objections to it in this age group, I have had only one experience with the procedure (Fig. 3-19).

In treating this age group, unless there is a substantial reason to operate on the foot earlier, I prefer simply to provide appropriate shoe wear until the patient is old enough to undergo a corrective triple arthrodesis. This is the most certain way to achieve and maintain correction, even though it can be done only with substantial sacrifice in the length of the foot. In bilateral cases, triple arthrodesis is probably not clinically significant, but in instances of unilateral involvement, a major discrepancy in foot size may result. It should be emphasized that triple arthrodesis is difficult to accomplish and, for satisfactory correction, best done through two incisions, medial and lateral (see p. 217).

Although I have not had occasion to attempt a modified approach to correction of this severe deformity in the older age group, it appears that one might consider a solution comparable to that employed to correct the overgrown lateral column seen in older children with congenital equinovarus. In this situation, either the talonavicular joint may be partially resected (reverse Lichtblau procedure) or the talonavicular joint may be fused (reverse Evans procedure). Intuitively, I would prefer this approach in contrast to complete naviculectomy, but I emphasize again that I have done neither of these procedures.

## VERTICAL TALUS IN MYELODYSPLASIA

Vertical talus in the myelodysplastic patient poses a special set of problems. On the one hand, the deformity may be a straightforward congenital vertical talus, simply one manifestation of several congenital anomalies. In this instance, the approach to correction follows the same concepts and principles as outlined in earlier sections of this chapter. On the other hand, it can represent a paralytic vertical talus, in which a substantial number of muscles are paralyzed, and the deformity involves not only a true intrauterine abnormality, but also a major degree of muscle paralysis and imbalance.

In such situations, Sharrard recommends correction of the foot, followed by or in conjunction with tendon transfers when active motor units are available. He proposes transferring the anterior tibial

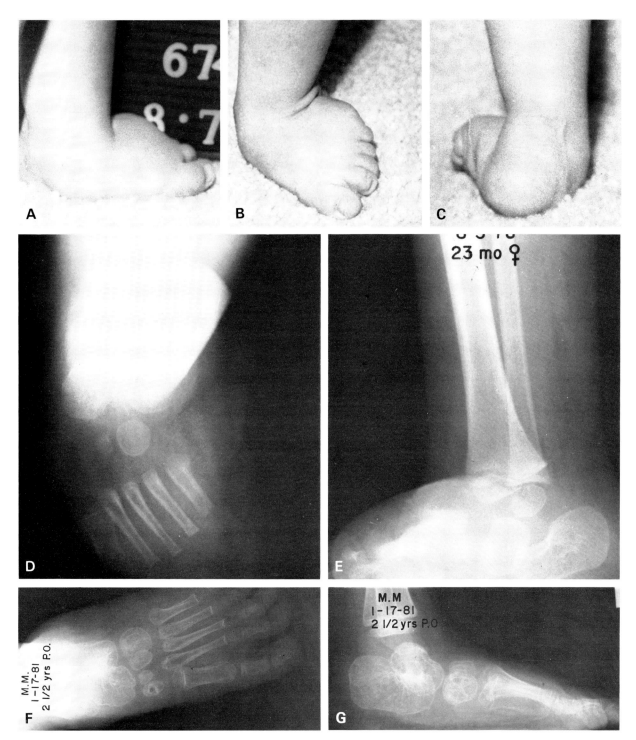

FIG. 3-19. **A**, **B**, and **C**, Standing photographs show a severe deformity of the left foot due to congenital vertical talus. This 23-month-old female initially was operated on elsewhere at age 7 months; however, exactly which operative procedure she underwent could not be determined. The postoperative casts were left on for only 5 weeks, after which "corrective" shoes were prescribed. The scars are evidence of the prior operation. **D** and **E**, Roentgenograms, also taken at age 23 months, show the persistent marked plantar prominence of the talar head, the severe abduction of the forefoot, and the excessive valgus of the heel. **F** and **G**, Weight-bearing radiographs, taken 2½ years after the accomplishment of a subtalar bone block and complete excision of the tarsal navicular necessitated by the relatively "overgrown" medial column. Despite the relatively acceptable result of this procedure, I feel that excision of the navicular should be considered a "salvage" procedure in the treatment of congenital vertical talus.

muscle to the neck of the talus and transferring the peroneus brevis or longus posterolaterally into the posterior tibial tendon. A subtalar bone block seems optional. I have not had occasion to perform this combination of procedures in myelodysplastic vertical talus, because the program outlined in earlier sections has proven eminently satisfactory.

In the final analysis, in view of my own experience and from a review of the literature, the following issues seem axiomatic: (1) Conservative therapeutic measures usually fail, (2) the talonavicular joint must be restored to as much anatomic normality as possible, (3) the subtalar joint must be reduced as far as possible, (4) a posterior ankle release nearly always must be performed, and (5) these bones must be held in position by some means until they become stable, or the deformity will recur. In brief, by paying particular attention to detail, one can usually deal with this deformity satisfactorily and can produce a painless and plantigrade foot.

## References

1. Armkriech, P., cited by Tachdjian, M. O.: *Pediatric Orthopedics.* Philadelphia, W. B. Saunders, 1972, p. 1359.
2. Aschner, B., and Engelmann, G., cited by Tachdjian, M. O.: *Pediatric Orthopedics.* Philadelphia, W. B. Saunders, 1972, p. 1359.
3. Batchelor, J., cited by Eyre-Brook, A. L.: Congenital vertical talus. J. Bone Joint Surg., *49B*:618, 1967.
4. Bigos, S. J., and Coleman, S. S.: Unpublished data, 1980.
5. Clark, M. W., D'Ambrosia, R. D., and Ferguson, A. B., Jr.: Congenital vertical talus, treatment by open reduction and navicular excision. J. Bone Joint Surg., *59A*:816, 1977.
6. Coleman, S. S., Stelling, F. H., and Jarrett, J.: Pathomechanics and treatment of congenital vertical talus. Clin. Orthop., *70*:62, 1970.
7. Cowell, H. H.: Personal communication, Houston, Texas, April, 1981.
8. Ellis, J., and Scheer, G. E.: Congenital convex pes valgus. Clin Orthop., *99*:168, 1974.
9. Eyre-Brook, A. L.: Congenital vertical talus. J. Bone Joint Surg., *49B*:618, 1967.
10. Grice, D. S.: Extra-articular arthrodesis of the subastragalar joints for correction of paralytic flatfeet in children. J. Bone Joint Surg., *34A*:927, 1952.
11. Hark, F. W.: Rocker-foot due to congenital subluxation of the talus. J. Bone Joint Surg., *32A*:344, 1950.
12. Harrold, A. J.: Congenital vertical talus in infancy. J. Bone Joint Surg., *49B*:634, 1967.
13. Henken, R.: Contribution a l'etude des formes osseuses du pied plat valgus congenital. Theses de Lyon, 1914.
14. Herndon, C. H., and Heyman, C. H.: Problems in the recognition and treatment of congenital convex pes valgus. J. Bone Joint Surg., *45A*:413, 1963.
15. Kidner, F. C.: The pre-hallux (accessory scaphoid) in its relation to flatfoot. J. Bone Joint Surg., *11*:831, 1929.
16. Lamy, L., and Weissman, L.: Congenital convex pes valgus. J. Bone Joint Surg., *21*:79, 1939.
17. Lange, F.: Plattfussbeschwerden und Plattfussbehandlung. MMW, *59*:300, 1912.
18. Ogata, K., Schoenecker, P. S., and Sheridan, J.: Congenital vertical talus and its familial occurrence. Clin. Orthop., *139*:128, 1979.
19. Osmond-Clarke, H.: Congenital vertical talus. J. Bone Joint Surg., *38B*:334, 1956.

20. Outland, T., and Sherk, H. H.: Congenital vertical talus. Clin. Orthop., *16:*214, 1960.
21. Patterson, W. R., Fitz, D. A., and Smith, W. S.: The pathologic anatomy of congenital convex pes valgus. J. Bone Joint Surg., *50A:*458, 1968.
22. Rocher, H. L., and Pouyanne, L.: Pied plat congenital par subluxation sousa-tragalienne congenitale et orientation verticale de l'astragale. Bourdeaux Chir., *5:*249, 1934.
23. Sharrard, W. J. W., and Grosfield, J.: Management of deformities in paralysis of the foot in myelomeningocele. J. Bone Joint Surg., *50B:*456, 1968.
24. Storen, H.: Congenital convex pes valgus with vertical talus. Acta Orthop. Scand., Suppl. 94, 1967.

# 4

# The Cavovarus Foot

The cavovarus foot is one of the most perplexing and challenging of all foot deformities. In this condition, as contrasted to such abnormalities as congenital clubfoot and congenital vertical talus, multiple etiologic factors are involved, and in some instances, the exact cause is never accurately established. This latter group is the most puzzling because, in most cases, the deformity is not present at birth, but instead gradually becomes apparent as the child's foot grows and matures.

Prior to 1960, most procedures designed to treat this condition employed resection or osteotomy of various bones of the hindfoot or midfoot. For example, Cole believed that the principal deformity was in the midfoot, and he performed a dorsally based tarsal-wedge resection, excising the naviculocuneiform joint and carrying the osteotomy in the plantar direction into the cuboid bone.[3] Japas suggested a modified tarsal osteotomy.[11] Dwyer felt that the varus of the heel was the principal problem and therefore proposed either an opening medial or a closing lateral osteotomy of the calcaneus.[5] Fowler, Brooks, and Parrish accomplished an osteotomy of the medial cuneiform bone in the belief that the deformity was located predominantly in the first ray.[7] Hammond, McElvenney, and Caldwell elevated the first metatarsal by different techniques, believing that a plantarflexed first metatarsal is the principal deformity.[9,13] These operations all resulted in clinical improvement, but by themselves did not achieve anatomic correction.

Since 1960, soft-tissue releases have assumed greater importance in treatment. Abrams, Bost, Schottstaedt, Larsen, Evans, Turco, and Westin all believed that the residual cavus component of clubfoot was managed most appropriately by a plantar release of some kind.[1,2,6,18,19] Westin, Guyer, and Fagan all believed that the plantar release was the most important element in correcting the cavovarus deformity, irrespective of cause.[8,19]

Unfortunately, in most instances, neither the bony procedures nor the commonly used soft-tissue operations have uniformly and completely considered the multiplicity of factors that can exist in the cavovarus foot. These include the tight, contracted plantar structures, the muscle imbalance, and the issue of whether the hindfoot varus is fixed or flexible. Failure to fully consider these factors has frequently led to unsuccessful or incomplete correction. The results have also been inconsistent. Since the degree of severity and the location of the deformity in cavovarus vary greatly from one case to another, it is evident that all feet with this deformity should not undergo the same operation. The surgical procedure should be appropriate for the existing pathologic features. Therefore, it is axiomatic that the problem must be defined accurately and thoroughly prior to planning any surgical treatment program.

## Etiology

A substantial number of feet with cavovarus deformity represent residual stigmata of congenital clubfoot, but the largest group are due to some form of muscle imbalance stemming from a variety of neuromuscular disorders, in which almost any level of the neuromuscular unit may be involved. Some are progressive; often they are familial. Specific examples include Charcot-Marie-Tooth's peroneal muscle atrophy and Friedreich's ataxia. These conditions present special problems because of their usually progressive though somewhat predictable nature.

In view of these diversified etiologic patterns, the complexity of the problem becomes clearly evident. At the present state of our knowledge and technical skill, a consistently satisfactory solution to all ramifications of this fascinating foot deformity is not readily apparent. When considering the conditions that may simulate it, one must exclude such abnormalities as "pes cavus" (cavus deformity without heel varus) and calcaneocavus (see Chapter 5). Calcaneocavus is seen most commonly following poliomyelitis or in myelodysplasia. As will be seen, these particular conditions represent substantially different problems, both diagnostically and therapeutically.

## Pathology and Pathogenesis

Even though the exact mechanism by which this deformity develops is not easily established, one can postulate a series of events that may adequately explain its evolution. Some degree of tightness of the heelcord and posterior ankle structures is usually found; also, although difficult to prove, it is reasonable to suspect a varying degree of anterior tibial muscle weakness. The long toe extensors attempt to compensate and assist in dorsiflexion of the foot against a somewhat tight heelcord by elevating (dorsiflexing) the digits. Instead of dorsiflexing the foot, however, the metatarsals, especially the first, are forced into plantar flexion by a "windlass" mechanism (Fig. 4-1). The forefoot plantar flexion then elevates the arch, the plantar structures become foreshortened, and a vicious cycle develops. This scheme for the pathogenesis of this deformity is open to challenge, but it serves as a good starting point for synthesis of a treatment plan.

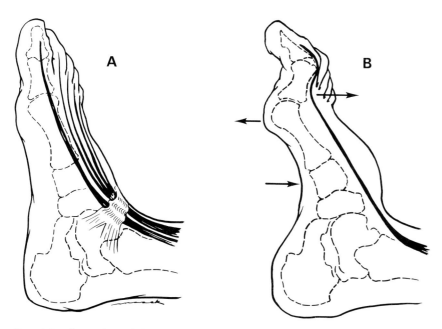

Fig. 4-1. Illustration of the "windlass" mechanism involved in producing the cavovarus foot deformity. **A**, The normal musculotendinous and osseous relationships. **B**, In the presence of a tight heelcord and a weak anterior tibial tendon, the long toe extensors compensate by dorsiflexing the proximal phalanx. This then depresses the first metatarsal, which in turn elevates the longitudinal arch.

As can be seen from the preceding discussion, the cavovarus foot presents major problems for both the patient and the treating surgeon. For the patient, it causes varying degrees of disability resulting from painful callosities under the first metatarsal head and also over the dorsal aspect of the clawtoe deformities usually present. Shoes break down, become deformed, and wear out rapidly. If the deformity is uncorrected, the late adolescent or adult ultimately is left with a misaligned, painful, rigid foot.

*Clinical Features*

Irrespective of cause, the basic clinical abnormalities characteristic of the cavovarus foot are consistently evident. As outlined subsequently, abnormalities are present in both the forefoot and the hindfoot. Furthermore, in no foot abnormality are the hindfoot and the forefoot so clearly interdependent and their relationships so essential to establish as in the cavovarus foot. Basically, the forefoot is pronated; that is, all metatarsal bones, and especially the first, are excessively plantarflexed; also, the hindfoot is in varus (supinated), and the longitudinal arch is elevated (Fig. 4-2).

As a result of this abnormal configuration, the base of the fifth metatarsal and the head of the first metatarsal beneath the sole of the foot are unusually prominent and readily identified because of the callosities that are usually present over these bony prominences. In more advanced and longstanding deformities, a clawtoe configuration develops, accompanied by contraction and foreshortening of the plantar fascia and the intrinsic musculature of the foot. The abductor hal-

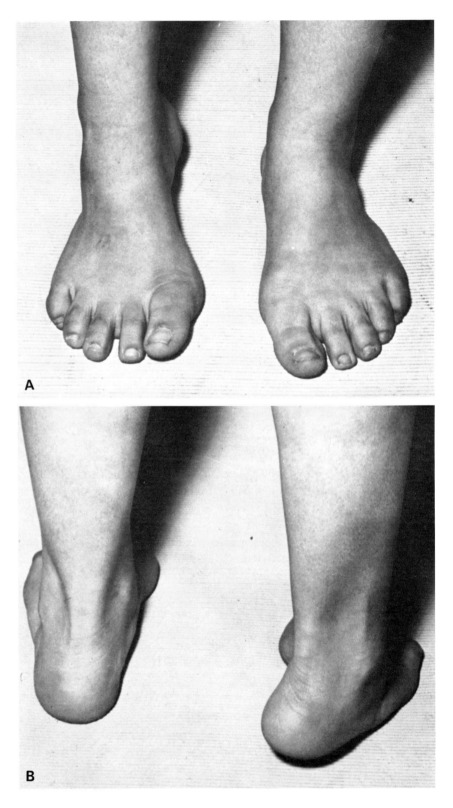

FIG. 4-2. Standing photographs show a typical cavovarus foot due to mild spastic encephalopathy. Note the varus of the heel, the prominent head of the first metatarsal, the elevated longitudinal arch, and the prominent head of the base of the fifth metatarsal.

lucis and flexor digitorum brevis are especially important in this latter consideration (Fig. 4-3).

As noted earlier, Hammond, and later McElvenny and Caldwell, proposed that an excessively plantarflexed first ray is a substantial element in the basic pathology of the cavovarus foot.[9,13] This concept is now well accepted, even though some controversy exists as to whether or not it is the primary component of the deformity. Nevertheless, either rigid or dynamic plantar flexion of the first metatarsal produces a pronated forefoot, and a flexible hindfoot, upon weight bearing, will

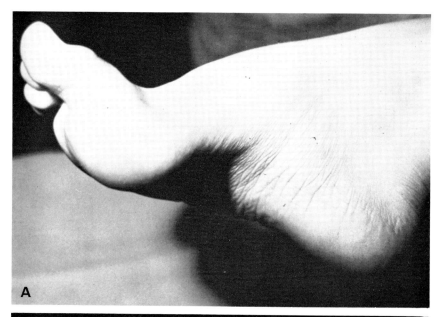

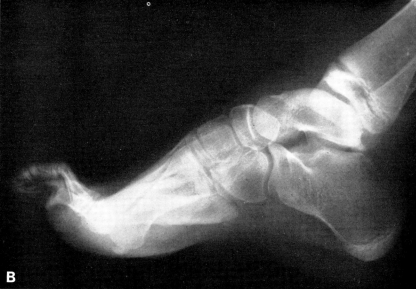

FIG. 4-3. **A**, Photograph (nonweight-bearing) of the typical high longitudinal arch, prominent first metatarsal head, and cock-up of the toes typical of the cavovarus foot. **B**, Lateral radiograph of the same foot. Note the marked degree of plantar flexion of the first metatarsal and the thickened cortices of the fifth metatarsal. This fifth metatarsal sustained a stress fracture, an occurrence that is not rare in severe cavovarus feet.

be forced into varus (or supination) owing to the "tripod effect" (Fig. 4-4). It is important to clarify this concept of *pronation* of the forefoot and *supination* of the hindfoot in order to avoid any confusion in subsequent discussions.

## *Evaluation of Flexibility*

Gradually, if untreated, and often in the case of residual stigmata of congenital equinovarus, adaptive changes occurring in the foot result in fixed bony abnormalities of both the hindfoot and the forefoot. This then results in two major problems, a structural deformity of the forefoot (pronation) and a rigid hindfoot varus (supination). Thus, in the clinical evaluation of the cavovarus foot, the most important determination is an accurate assessment of whether (a) the forefoot is rigidly held in pronation with a flexible hindfoot, (b) the hindfoot is in fixed varus, with a flexible forefoot (a rare condition), or (c) the forefoot and hindfoot are both rigid. These determinations assume critical value when attempting to establish the surgical treatment program.

We have developed a rather simple test for hindfoot and forefoot flexibility that can be readily documented both photographically and radiographically, consisting of a standing lateral block test.[4,15] A wooden block of variable height (usually 1 to 1½ inches) is placed under the lateral aspect of the foot and the heel. This permits the first metatarsal to hang freely and thus negates any effect it may have upon the hindfoot by eliminating or neutralizing the tripod mechanism. In the standing posture, a flexible hindfoot will assume its normal valgus position, and the correction of the previous heel varus can be readily documented (Fig. 4-5). In addition to routine photographs and standing roentgenograms, the degree of correction can also be quantified using special hindfoot roentgenograms (see the following).

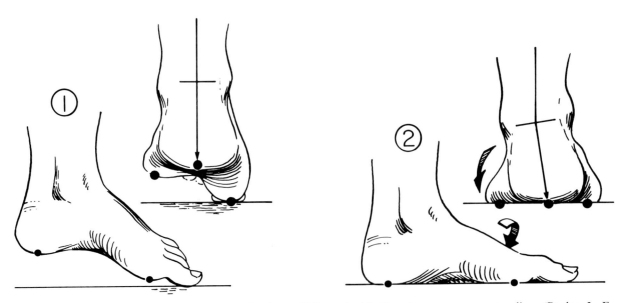

FIG. 4-4. The tripod effect. A rigid, pronated forefoot will force the hindfoot into varus upon standing. (Paulos, L. E., Coleman, S. S., and Samuelson, K. M.: Pes cavovarus: Review of a surgical approach using soft-tissue procedures. J. Bone Joint Surg., *62A*:942, 1980.)

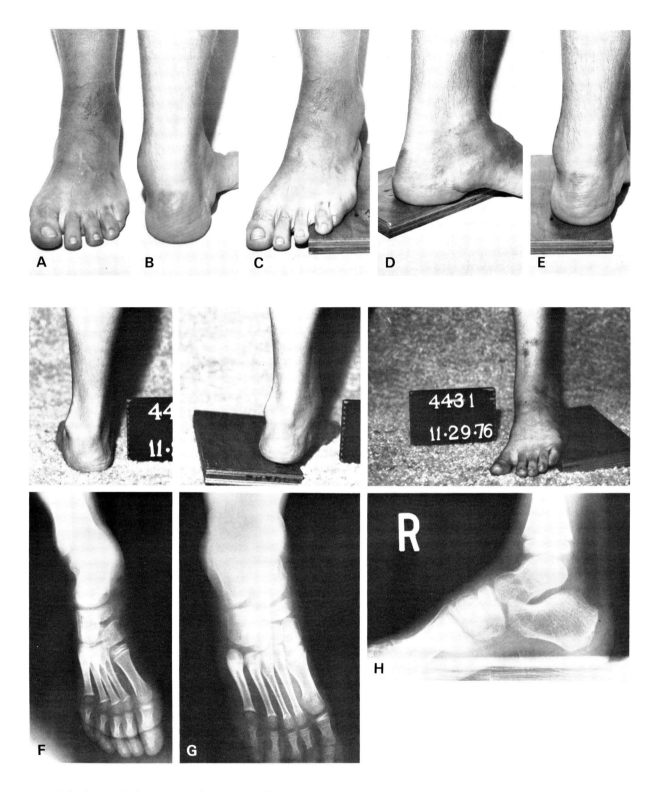

FIG. 4-5. **A** and **B**, Anteroposterior and lateral photographs show the typical cavovarus foot. **C, D,** and **E,** Hindfoot flexibility is illustrated by means of the block test. The heel and outer border of the foot are placed upon a 1-inch block of wood (or higher if necessary) so that the first metatarsal head and remainder of the forefoot can fall freely to the floor. A supple hindfoot will then go into valgus. The alteration in the roentgenogram of the foot when using the block test is well illustrated. **F,** The uncorrected hindfoot. **G** and **H,** The talus and calcaneus assume a more normal relationship when the effect of the forefoot on the hindfoot is eliminated.

On the other hand, if the hindfoot is not corrected, it can be assumed to be rigid; the surgeon must therefore plan a treatment program that will correct both a rigid, pronated forefoot and a rigid varus (supinated) hindfoot.

The degree of cavus present in the routine standing films can be estimated by the method of Meary as shown in Figure 4-6.[14] Attempts to quantify varus using Kite's angle, however, are almost impossible owing to the difficulty of accurately reproducing the data from one observer to the next. Thus, even though estimates of the amount of existing varus can be made radiographically, the lack of consistency in this observation prompted the development of a technique that permits reproducible data. This has been called a "hindfoot view," and I am indebted to Samuelson for its concept and development.[16] (It has already been described in detail in Chapter 1.) By this means, the clinical evaluation can be quantitated and verified radiographically. This radiographic examination and evaluation is an attractive scientific exercise, but from a practical point of view it is not critically necessary for effective treatment in all cases.

The second major consideration in the clinical evaluation of the

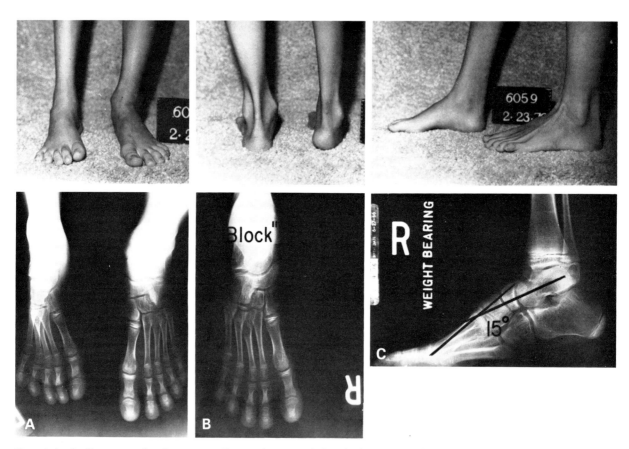

FIG. 4-6. **A,** One example of cavovarus foot and a normal foot is demonstrated in these standing clinical photos and roentgenograms. **B,** The varus of the heel is demonstrated in the posterior view; the normal bony relationships of the hindfoot are seen in the standing anteroposterior roentgenogram taken with the foot undergoing the block test. **C,** The angle of Meary in this patient is 15°.

cavovarus foot is the muscle balance. It must be assumed that, unless the deformity clearly represents residual stigmata of clubfoot, or until proven otherwise, some form of muscle imbalance must exist in the foot in order for the deformity to develop. Careful muscle testing may simply support the obvious observation that a neuromuscular defect is present, but it is important to record such findings accurately because of their implications for treatment, as they relate to subsequent muscle and tendon transfers when needed. The surgeon should not be dismayed, however, if no obvious muscle imbalance can be demonstrated, because, as noted earlier, in a small number of these feet, the deformities never have a clearcut causal explanation.

Once the deformity has been recognized, the flexibility (or rigidity) of the forefoot and the hindfoot established, and muscle balance and neurologic function thoroughly evaluated, a decision then can be made as to the need for further, more sophisticated diagnostic studies. If the deformity is not clearly the result of either an established, proven neuromuscular disease, the residual stigmata of congenital equinovarus, or an infantile (congenital) deformity, then it is wise to proceed with a more extensive and detailed diagnostic program. This requires consultation with a qualified pediatric neurologist, and in most instances, it should include an electromyogram as well as nerve conduction studies of the lower limb. These studies are especially necessary in cases of unilateral cavovarus deformities (Fig. 4-7).

Once these data have been gathered, the need for even more sophisticated studies, such as a lumbar myelogram or a lower-spine CAT (computerized axial tomography) scan can then be assessed. It is important to recognize that unusual foot deformities, especially cavovarus, may be the only early finding in lesions of the lower spine; thus, as with all complex foot deformities in children, it is axiomatic that plain films of the pelvis and the lumbosacral spine should be accomplished at the time of the initial radiographic examination (see p. 17).

## Principles of Treatment

Synthesis of an appropriate treatment program depends upon the cause of the cavovarus foot deformity. If a lower spinal or central-nervous-system deficit exists, the basic neurologic abnormality must first be accurately identified to ascertain (a) whether the primary neurologic problem can be corrected and (b) whether the deformity is likely to be progressive.

In the event that a lower spinal problem can be corrected, it is reasonable to expect that appropriate neurosurgical treatment will interrupt progression of the neurologic deficit. Any uncorrected muscle imbalance that remains, however, clearly will influence the configuration of the foot that develops as a result of additional growth. The combination of the presence of a muscle imbalance and continued growth mandates operative treatment in the cavovarus foot. Nonoperative methods (e.g., braces, shoes) are not effective in correcting this foot deformity or preventing it from worsening under these circumstances.

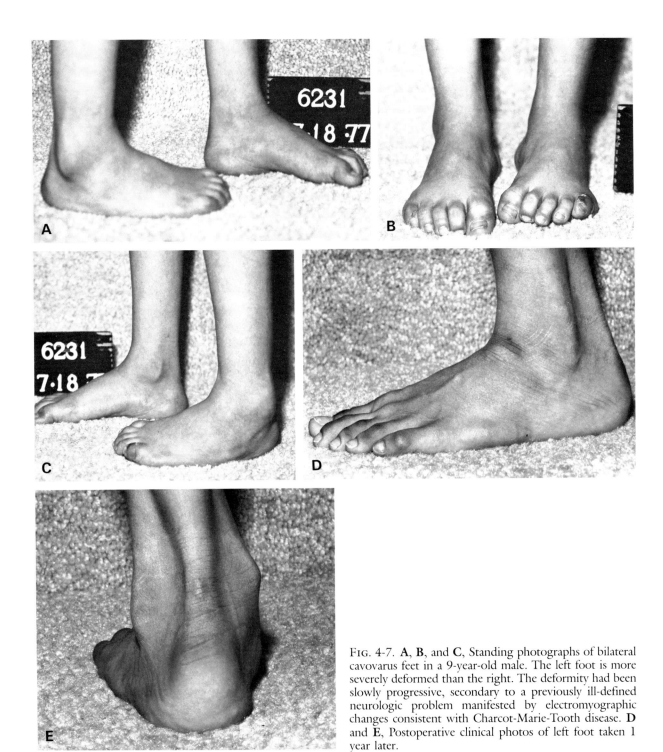

FIG. 4-7. **A**, **B**, and **C**, Standing photographs of bilateral cavovarus feet in a 9-year-old male. The left foot is more severely deformed than the right. The deformity had been slowly progressive, secondary to a previously ill-defined neurologic problem manifested by electromyographic changes consistent with Charcot-Marie-Tooth disease. **D** and **E**, Postoperative clinical photos of left foot taken 1 year later.

The natural history of any underlying, basic neurologic problem should guide one in deciding whether or not, and at what age, to administer surgical treatment. The principles involved in *correcting* the foot are the same as for all cavovarus deformities. The type of muscle transfers that should be used, however, will depend largely on the nature of the *disease process*, especially as it relates to whether or not progressive paralysis of certain muscles or muscle groups will take place. For example, in such conditions as Charcot-Marie-Tooth's neuromuscular atrophy, the posterior tibial tendon ultimately may be the only tendon that can be effectively transferred, because all dorsiflexors and evertor muscles usually become either grossly weakened or totally paralyzed.

In instances of cavovarus deformity associated with congenital equinovarus, functional muscle imbalance may or may not be demonstrable, and in many cases, the clubfoot deformity will not necessarily worsen, although it surely will not respond to any nonoperative corrective measures. In these instances, one therefore must evaluate the severity of the existing deformity and determine whether or not it justifies operative correction.

The so-called "idiopathic" cavovarus foot represents a special challenge because, by definition, the problem has no clearcut, definable cause. The deformity is nearly always bilateral. Muscle imbalance is not evident. Neurologic studies are almost always normal, but the deformity is usually progressive. Fortunately, this is an uncommon situation, but the therapy is conceptually the same as for the deformities mentioned earlier; namely, that if treatment is indicated, the deformity must be corrected first, and then some type of subsequent muscle-balancing procedure will be essential to maintain the correction.

Anyone who has treated this foot deformity has found that special shoes or orthoses are uniformly ineffective. The deformity usually worsens and progresses inexorably unless surgically corrected. The type of surgical correction required depends upon three major factors: the cause of the deformity, the age of the patient, and the degree of bony deformity. The cause provides practical information relative to the behavioral characteristics of the deformity; the age of the patient provides some concept of the degree of adaptive change that may have occurred in the bones and joints; and quantitation of the existing bony deformity assists in evaluating the need for bone surgery. Fundamentally, the earlier the progressive cavovarus deformity can be diagnosed, the less complicated will be the required treatment.

In most children under 7 to 8 years of age, the deformity can be corrected satisfactorily solely through soft-tissue procedures. Also, if muscle-balancing operations are needed, the patient can readily cooperate during the process of muscle testing so that relatively accurate and predictable muscle and tendon transfers can be planned and accomplished. In older children, on the other hand, because of the adaptive structural changes in the foot, osteotomies of some sort often will be required for correction. Table 4-1 presents a flowsheet outlining the diagnostic studies necessary and the indicated treatment.

Once the cause of the deformity has been established, the flexibility or rigidity of the various parts of the foot must be determined. Documentation requires clinical as well as radiographic evaluation. As noted earlier, one must determine whether (a) the forefoot is rigidly

*Definition of the Problem*

TABLE 4-1. *Flowsheet summarizing the analysis to which each individual problem is exposed and the resulting recommended surgical procedure. (Paulos, L. E., Coleman, S. S., and Samuelson, K. M.: Pes cavovarus: Review of a surgical approach using soft-tissue procedures. J. Bone Joint Surg., 62A:942, 1980.)*

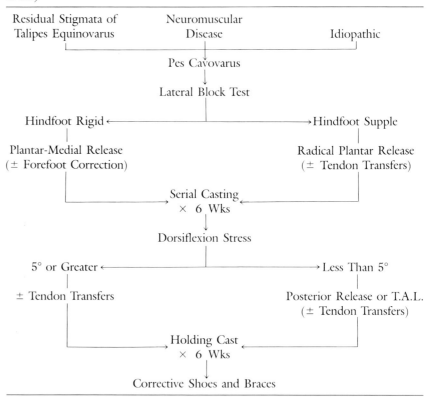

held in pronation with a flexible hindfoot, (b) the hindfoot is in fixed varus, with a flexible forefoot (a rare condition), or (c) the forefoot and hindfoot are both rigid. These determinations can be made through appropriate clinical and radiographic examinations and readily documented from a practical standpoint by the simple block test described earlier. It is also essential to accurately appraise muscle function.

It is convenient to consider treatment under *three* categories, because each has its own special conditions, namely, (a) fixed pronated forefoot with a flexible hindfoot, (b) fixed pronated forefoot with rigid varus (supinated hindfoot) and (c) conditions requiring salvage procedures (triple arthrodeses).

## FIXED PRONATED FOREFOOT AND FLEXIBLE HINDFOOT

The major problem in correcting this type of foot lies in the plantar flexion of the first metatarsal, which is almost always accompanied by contracture of the plantar fascia, along with corresponding foreshortening of the first layer of intrinsic pedal musculature. These latter structures all originate from the os calcis and insert into the digits. In younger children with flexible tarsal and tarsometatarsal joints and minimal secondary adaptive changes, a simple radical plantar release is usually sufficient to correct the foot satisfactorily. This release must be done thoroughly and must be followed by postoperative cast changes that exploit the soft-tissue-releasing procedures.

It is often impossible to correct the foot completely at the time of operation. Indeed, in older children, it is often not advisable to attempt full correction at the time of operation because wound healing and soft-tissue viability may be compromised. Westin has emphasized the need for postoperative cast corrections, and in keeping with the philosophy of Lloyd-Roberts, one should view the surgical release as simply an integral part of the continuum of nonoperative correction.[12] Thus, casts should be changed weekly or biweekly to maximize the correction achieved by the surgical release. The surgical procedure and the method of cast correction are described in the following section.

SURGICAL TECHNIQUE. The plantar release that I prefer is a variation of that recommended by Williams and Tachdjian.[17,20] A generous, curved incision is made over the medial aspect of the foot, extending anteriorly from the os calcis as far as the base of the first metatarsal bone (Fig. 4-8). The entire origin of the abductor hallucis is then identified and separated from its bony and soft-tissue attachments both proximally and distally, but initially it is left attached at its origin and insertion. The neurovascular bundle is identified as it divides into its medial and lateral branches and enters the intrinsic musculature of the foot.

At the point where the neurovascular bundle bifurcates, a substantial tendinous origin of the abductor can be identified as it attaches to the calcaneus *between* the medial and lateral plantar branches of the nerve and artery. This attachment must be cut in order to free up the origin of the abductor hallucis. The long toe flexors are then identified as they course along the plantar aspect of the foot, and the retinaculum of these tendons (Henry's knot[10]) is sectioned.

The origins of the plantar aponeurosis, the abductor hallucis, and the short flexors are then severed from their attachments to the os calcis, and this entire musculotendinous mass is gently dissected distally, *extraperiosteally,* as far as the calcaneocuboid joint. At this juncture, a complete plantar release has been achieved. The wound is closed and a well padded, below-knee cast is applied, with the hindfoot (heel) held in valgus and the forefoot held in some degree of supination. Great care must be exercised so that the foot is not corrected completely, since this might compromise healing of the surgical wound.

POSTOPERATIVE CARE. We believe that this is an important aspect of the procedure because it is that part of the operation that capitalizes upon the soft-tissue release just described. One week postoperatively, the entire cast is changed, the wound inspected, and a new cast applied. If the wound is sufficiently healed and the skin edges are healthy, a greater degree of correction can be attempted if indicated. Again, the

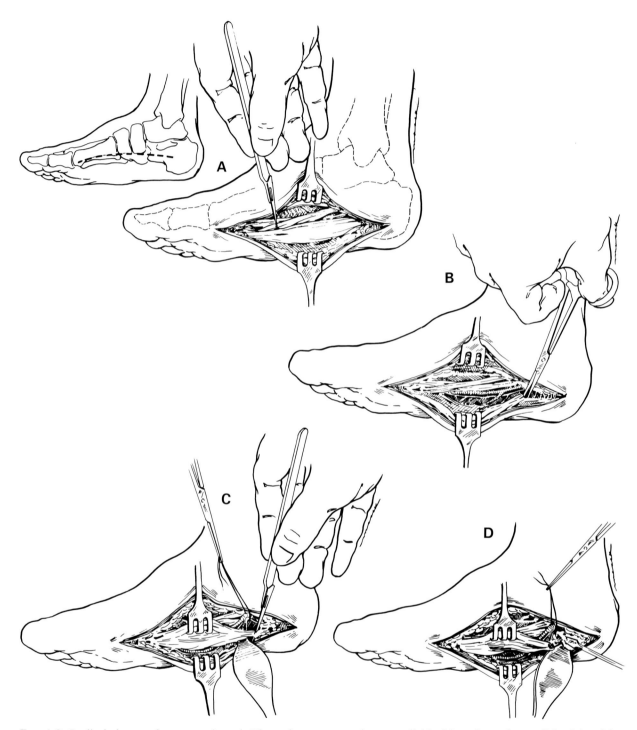

FIG. 4-8. Radical plantar release procedure. **A**, Through a generous plantar medial incision, the entire medial origin of the abductor hallucis is exposed and released from its underlying fascial and osseous origins. In the process, the two long flexors of the toes are exposed. The medial and lateral plantar branches of the neurovascular bundle are identified, and (**B**) the dense, heavy origin of the abductor that separates these two neurovascular branches is carefully sectioned. **C**, The short abductor, the plantar aponeurosis, and the other plantar muscles arising from the os calcis are completely separated from the overlying skin and subcutaneous tissue from the medial to the lateral side of the foot, and the origins of these structures are completely severed from the os calcis. **D**, With the neurovascular branches carefully protected, the plantar musculotendinous structures are then dissected distally extraperiosteally from their origins on the os calcis as far as the calcaneocuboid joint. When metatarsal or cuneiform osteotomy is deemed necessary for more complete correction, it can be done easily by a simple distal extension of this incision.

heel is placed into a greater degree of valgus and the forefoot is further supinated (see Fig. 2-22). This tends to flatten the longitudinal arch, thus correcting the previously existing cavovarus deformity. Weekly or biweekly cast changes similarly applied can add further correction. Six weeks postoperatively, a holding (walking) cast can be applied, in preparation for anticipated tendon transfers.

In older children in whom substantial bone and joint adaptive changes have occurred, it may be necessary to perform an extension (dorsiflexion) osteotomy either of the first cuneiform bone, as described by Fowler, or of the base of the first metatarsal, in order to correct the fixed plantarflexed deformity of the first ray (Fig. 4-9). Again, before deciding to perform either of these osseous procedures, one must demonstrate hindfoot flexibility, such that if one dorsiflexes and supinates the forefoot, the hindfoot will be flexible enough that the foot, upon stance, will be plantigrade postoperatively.

The technique used in either of these osteotomies must be tailored to the underlying problem. If the medial column of the foot is foreshortened, an opening-wedge osteotomy of the cuneiform or metatarsal could possibly provide needed foot length. In the opposite (rare) instances in which the first ray is not shortened, a dorsiflexion closing-wedge osteotomy would be acceptable. In either case, the osteotomy must be transfixed by a Steinmann pin (preferably threaded), and the transfixion must be retained until bony union is evident. This is especially true in the case of the opening-wedge osteotomy, in which a bone graft is required.

The same postoperative cast procedure is used as in those instances in which an osteotomy is not done. In some situations, the foot may be adequately corrected at the time of the initial combined plantar release and first-ray osteotomy, so that tendons may be transferred in the same procedure. This is only possible, however, if posterior ankle release has been deemed unnecessary. One must therefore demonstrate that the ankle can be passively dorsiflexed. If not, tendon transfers should *not* be done at the time of foot correction.

Factors that enter into the decision to perform any postcorrection tendon transfers are difficult to establish. The judgment involved in making this decision must be based on a sound knowledge of the results of a thorough preoperative muscle test, a reasonable awareness of the behavioral characteristics of the underlying neurologic condition producing the deformity, and a considerable degree of clinical intuition. Most often, I transfer the extensor hallucis longus to the neck of the first metatarsal and the extensor digitorum longus to the second or third cuneiform bones.

Whether or not the posterior tibial tendon should be lengthened is a matter of judgment. In some situations (see p. 237), the posterior tibial tendon should be transferred anteriorly. At this time, the surgeon must also decide whether posterior ankle release is necessary. In most cases it is, but I find it difficult to establish specific guidelines governing this decision. Following tendon transfer, a below-knee walking cast must be used for at least 6 weeks.

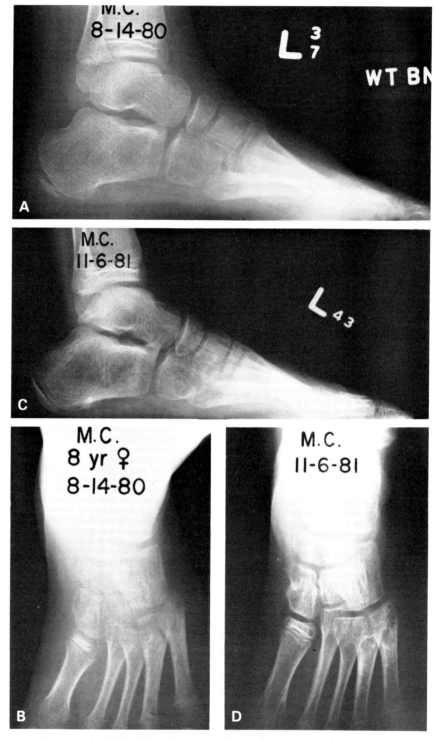

FIG. 4-9. **A** and **B**, Standing anteroposterior and lateral roentgenograms give an example of the need for plantar fasciotomy and biplane opening-wedge osteotomy for cavovarus in this 8-year-old girl. Note the adduction of the forefoot in the anteroposterior view, and the hindfoot varus, elevated longitudinal arch, and plantarflexed first metatarsal in the lateral view. **C** and **D**, Fifteen months later, following a radical plantar-medial release and biplane opening-wedge osteotomy of the medial cuneiform, the improved hindfoot, midfoot (longitudinal arch), and forefoot relationships can be seen.

Postcast Care. Postcasting care is the same whether or not osteotomy is done. After removal of the second cast following tendon transfers, a below-knee, spring-loaded, dorsiflexion-assist brace is prescribed. This is worn for a minimum of 6 to 12 weeks or until the tendon transfers demonstrate good, active function. A program of muscle-strengthening exercises is then prescribed to strengthen the transferred muscles and improve muscle balance. Follow-up examinations are conducted at regular intervals until it can be determined that lasting surgical correction has been achieved, which usually requires follow-up through the age of skeletal maturity. In some situations, the deformity may gradually recur, in which case the surgeon must reappraise the entire situation in the light of the foregoing concepts and principles of treatment. Just as often, the deformity may be *over*corrected, but this is usually a more acceptable situation, and the residual stigmata can be treated more effectively by nonoperative measures such as shoe inserts and arch supports.

This situation usually occurs either in older children with longstanding deformities or in patients with residual congenital equinovarus (Fig. 4-10). Pronounced rigidity of the foot is the important issue, especially as it applies to the hindfoot. If the rigid hindfoot is not corrected on clinical examination, and if the block test shows it to be inflexible, it, as well as the forefoot, must be corrected surgically. In young children, the procedure necessary to correct this problem is called the plantar-medial release (see Chapter 2). In children under age 6 or 7 years with cavus residual stigmata of equinovarus (equinocavovarus), the operation usually can be accomplished by soft-tissue procedures alone as outlined in Chapter 2. In older children with more established bony deformities, however, most often osseous procedures will be required, either in the forefoot, the hindfoot, or both.

The forefoot bony corrective procedures available to the surgeon have been described earlier and apply in either case. The approach to the hindfoot problem requires further discussion because, in this situation, it is important to determine whether or not any deformity of the calcaneus is present. This can be established by taking the axial or so-called "ski-jump" view of the calcaneus (see Fig. 9-7). In unusual circumstances, a true varus deformity of the calcaneus may exist, and, in my opinion, this is the one (and only) indication for a medial opening- or lateral closing-wedge osteotomy of the calcaneus as described by Dwyer. Such an osteotomy places the hindfoot in valgus, while at the same time correcting an established and proven bony deformity. Any deformity of the forefoot must be dealt with either at the same time or as a separate procedure, depending upon the individual problem.

If, on the other hand, the deformity is in the subtalar joint, and the patient has a substantial degree of fixed, bony deformity so that soft-tissue releases are contraindicated or deemed ineffective, the rigid, supinated hindfoot is best corrected through a triple arthrodesis (Fig. 2-39). If necessary, the forefoot can be corrected at the same time by

FIXED PRONATED FOREFOOT
WITH RIGID VARUS
(SUPINATED HINDFOOT)

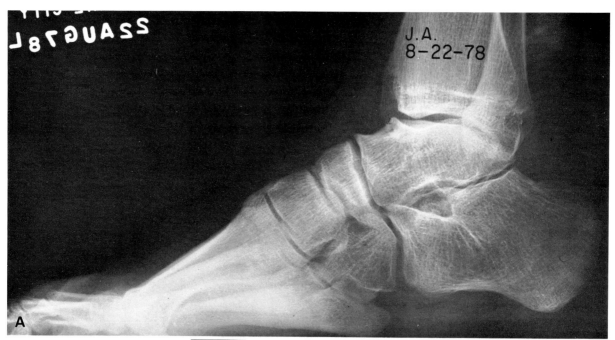

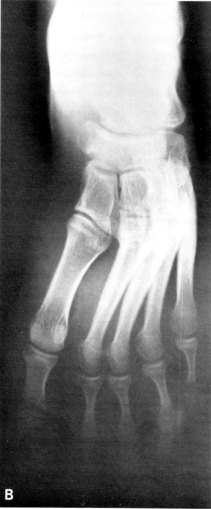

Fig. 4-10. **A** and **B**, Roentgenograms give an example of the established bony deformities that can occur following longstanding congenital equinovarus showing the typical features of the equinocavovarus deformity. Both anteroposterior and lateral views clearly show the plantarflexed, adducted first metatarsal, the parallelism of the talus and calcaneus, and the high arch.

osteotomy of the medial (first) cuneiform bone or the first metatarsal (Fig. 2-39).

The technique of triple arthrodesis is well established, and as long as one has fully identified the deformity, the achievement of a plantigrade foot simply reflects the technical expertise of the surgeon. In all such patients, and especially in those in whom skeletal growth is still occurring, it is critical that the corrective triple arthrodesis be followed by appropriate tendon transfers; otherwise, with growth, the deformity will probably recur to some degree even in the presence of a well performed, solid, triple arthrodesis (see Chapter 7).

**TRIPLE ARTHRODESIS**

*References*

1. Abrams, C. R.: Relapsed clubfoot, the early results of an evaluation of Dillwyn Evans' operation. J. Bone Joint Surg., *51A*:270, 1969.
2. Bost, F. C., Schottstaedt, E. R., and Larsen, L. J.: Plantar dissection. An operation to release the soft tissue in recurrent or recalcitrant talipes equinovarus. J. Bone Joint Surg., *42A*:151, 1960.
3. Cole, W. H.: The treatment of clawfoot. J. Bone Joint Surg., *22A*:895, 1940.
4. Coleman, S. S., and Chesnut, W. J.: A simple test for hindfoot flexibility in the cavovarus foot. Clin. Orthop. Rel. Res., *123*:60, 1977.
5. Dwyer, F. C.: The treatment of relapsed clubfoot by the insertion of a wedge into the calcaneum. J. Bone Joint Surg., *45B*:67, 1963.
6. Evans, D.: Relapsed clubfoot. J. Bone Joint Surg., *43B*:722, 1961.
7. Fowler, S. B., Brooks, A. L., and Parrish, T. F.: The cavovarus foot. Proc. AAOS, J. Bone Joint Surg., *41A*:757, 1959.
8. Guyer, W. D., and Fagan, C. A.: Cavus deformity of the foot. Proc. West Orthop. Assoc., J. Bone Joint Surg., *41A*:564, 1959.
9. Hammond, G.: Elevation of the first metatarsal bone with hallux equinus. Surgery, *13*:240, 1943.
10. Henry, A. K.: *Extensile Exposure*. 2nd Edition. New York, Churchill Livingstone, 1970, pp. 300–309.
11. Japas, L. M.: Surgical treatment of pes cavus by tarsal V-osteotomy; preliminary report. J. Bone Joint Surg., *50A*:927, 1968.
12. Lloyd-Roberts, G. C.: Seventh Annual International Pediatric Orthopedics Seminar, Chicago, 1978.
13. McElvenney, R. T., and Caldwell, G. D.: A new operation for correction of cavus foot, fusion of first metatarsocuneiformnavicular joints. Clin. Orthop., *11*:85, 1958.
14. Meary, R.: On the measurement of the angle between the talus and the first metatarsal. Symposium: Le Pied Creux Essentiel. Rev. Chir. Orthop., *53*:389, 1967.
15. Paulos, L. E., Coleman, S. S., and Samuelson, K. M.: Pes cavovarus: Review of a surgical approach using soft-tissue procedures. J. Bone Joint Surg., *62A*:942, 1980.
16. Samuelson, K. M.: Unpublished data.
17. Tachdjian, M. O.: Pes cavus. In *Pediatric Orthopedics*. Philadelphia, W. B. Saunders, 1972, pp. 1300–1322, 1378–1397.
18. Turco, J. V.: Surgical correction of the resistant clubfoot. One-stage posteromedial release with internal fixation. A preliminary report. J. Bone Joint Surg., *53A*:477, 1971.
19. Westin, W.: Personal communication, 1980.
20. Williams, P.: Personal communication, Melbourne, Australia, 1975.

# 5

# Calcaneocavus Foot Deformity

Since the incidence of poliomyelitis has been reduced in the United States, the problems posed by the calcaneocavus foot deformity have substantially decreased. On the other hand, because this particular foot abnormality is most often the result of a multiplicity of neurologic abnormalities, a *thorough* discussion of its causation and treatment will probably always be necessary. This is one of the most interesting and challenging of all complex foot deformities in children. Basically, it usually results from some central or peripheral neurologic defect. The deformity is always debilitating, nearly always progressive, and, according to Whitman, "far more important as a disability than a deformity."[23] In fact, Hoke felt that a patient with this deformity often walked with more difficulty "than a patient with an artificial limb."[11] Irwin wrote that patients with calcaneocavus foot deformity "walk as though they are wearing a prosthesis on the involved side."[12]

This deformity was one of the first for which a tendon transfer was employed. Thus, in 1881, Nicoladoni transferred both peroneal tendons to the Achilles tendon in an effort to correct the calcaneus deformity.[17] Other surgical procedures have been employed in attempts to solve this ostensibly difficult problem. Trendelenburg suggested complex osteotomies of the tibia and foot to correct the deformity.[20] Gleich had previously described a calcaneal osteotomy designed to correct paralytic deformities of the hindfoot, but did not specifically refer to the calcaneocavus deformity.[8]

During the earlier years of the century, this challenging foot deformity was treated in a number of ways. Whitman advocated astragalectomy and posterior displacement of the remaining portion of the foot on the tibia. Jones described a two-stage tarsal resection and ankle fusion.[13] Davis proposed a plantar fasciotomy, a midtarsal osteotomy, and tendon transfers.[4] Dunn supported and further developed this therapeutic approach.[6] In 1921, Hoke recognized the need for and the value of a corrective triple arthrodesis in correcting the deformity in the older child in whom advanced bony adaptive change necessitated radical resection of the head and neck of the talus (Fig. 5-1). Cholmeley gave credit to Elmslie as having subsequently recognized not only that corrective stabilization was essential, but that tendon transfers were also vital in order to achieve anatomic and functional correction.[2] Peabody also recognized the need for tendon transfer and, along with Herndon, Strong, Heyman, Turner, and Cooper, suggested transfer of the anterior tibial tendon posteriorly through the tibiofibular interosseous membrane to the os calcis in order to provide some degree of heel pushoff.[10,18,21]

If the child is too young for major joint or stabilization surgery and already has an established deformity of the calcaneus, I have used a posterior displacement "crescentic osteotomy" of the os calcis since 1965 (Fig. 5-2).[3] The concept is designed to elongate the os calcis and

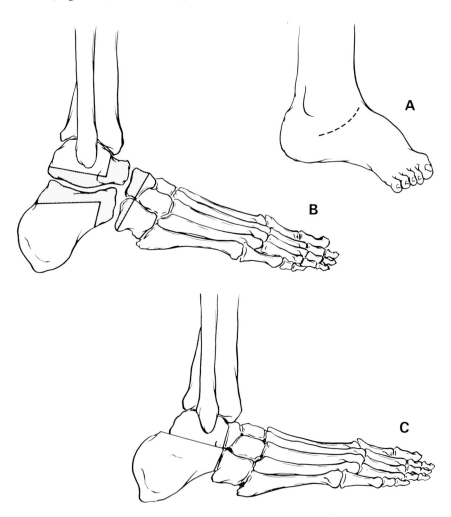

FIG. 5-1. Corrective triple arthrodesis for severe calcaneocavus foot deformity. **A,** An oblique incision is placed over the sinus tarsus. **B,** Stippling shows the appropriate size and shape of bone and joint resection; **C,** the corrected foot. In order to maintain this correction, either internal fixation (staples or screws) or transfixion (threaded pins) are necessary.

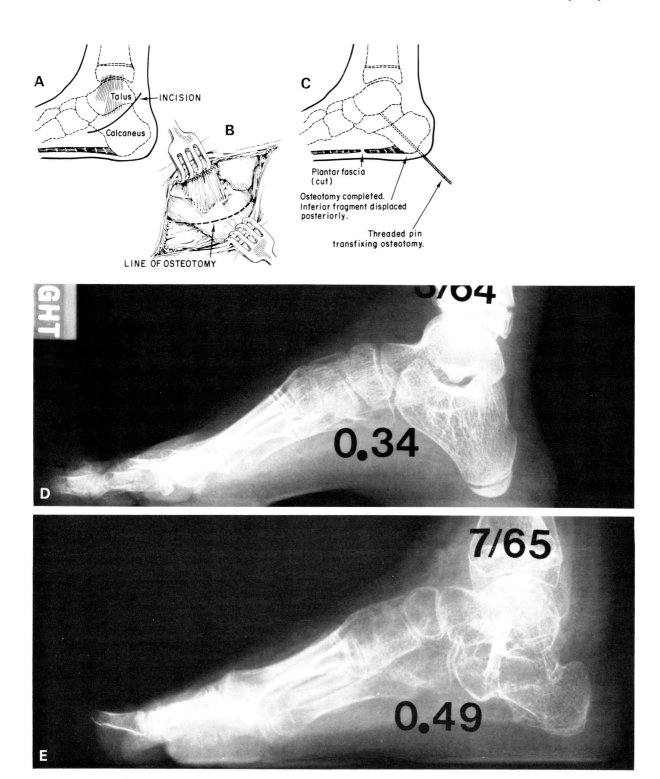

FIG. 5-2. My preferred method of performing a crescentic, posterior displacement osteotomy of the calcaneus for older children with calcaneocavus foot deformity. **A,** The incision is made over the medial aspect of the calcaneus. **B,** The neurovascular bundle is retracted upward, exposing a generous distance of the calcaneus, and the line of the cut in the calcaneus is identified. **C,** The plantar fascia and short plantar muscles are sectioned to permit posterior and upward displacement of the proximal fragment of the calcaneus. The corrected posterosuperior position is held by means of a transfixion threaded wire. **D** and **E,** Pre- and postoperative standing roentgenograms of a sample patient. Note flattening of the longitudinal arch and elongation of the calcaneus. (Bradley, G. W., and Coleman, S. S.: Treatment of the calcaneocavus foot. J. Bone Joint Surg., *63A*:1161, 1981.)

thereby to improve the lever arm for plantar flexion. Tendon transfers are accomplished at a second stage. Samilson and Mitchell have used a similar osteotomy of the calcaneus.[16,19]

From this historical sketch, three basic issues become evident. First, the deformity is usually secondary to some form of neurologic disturbance. Second, the deformity must be corrected by either soft-tissue or major bone and joint procedures. Third, some effort must be made to balance the muscle function to avoid persistence or recurrence of the deformity.

## Etiology and Pathogenesis

As already mentioned, the most common cause of the calcaneocavus foot is a flaccid paralysis of the calf musculature, either congenital or acquired. The vast majority of these feet result from a paralytic muscle imbalance in which the triceps surae is partially or completely paralyzed, with the remaining dorsiflexors and forefoot plantar flexors varying in strength. The paralysis can have many causes, but poliomyelitis still remains the most common throughout the world.

In the United States and other countries that are at present relatively free from the ravages of poliomyelitis, the deformity is more often encountered in other neurologic conditions such as cerebral palsy, myelomeningocele, Charcot-Marie-Tooth's disease, Friedreich's ataxia, Roussy-Lévy syndrome, diastematomyelia, post-traumatic fibrosis of the posterior compartments of the calf, overzealous lengthening of calf musculature in equinus deformities, Refsum's syndrome, and a multiplicity of other rare neurologic disorders. In some, the deformity is familial, according to Lloyd-Roberts,[15] and, rarely, the cause is unknown, in which case the deformity is seen in early infancy and, with growth and development, will usually be slowly corrected (Fig. 5-3).

The important issues that govern treatment are (a) the underlying neurologic cause, (b) the exact nature of the muscle imbalance, and (c) the age of the patient. If the deformity is the result of a progressive neurologic deficit, clearly one would delay or defer treatment depending upon the ultimate functional result of the neurologic disorder. On the other hand, in a static, stabilized situation, one may plan and execute a well designed surgical therapeutic treatment program.

The nature of the muscle imbalance is an important factor in the choice of correction procedures. For example, if the foot has only one functioning normal muscle (i.e., anterior tibial) it is treated differently than if all other muscles except for the triceps surae are intact, even though the deformities are almost indistinguishable from each other. The age of the patient is important because, in older children and young adults, corrective bone and joint procedures are often necessary, whereas in younger children, substantial remodeling can be expected from corrective muscle transfers.

All of these factors must be considered thoroughly because of their obvious effect upon the synthesis of a surgical therapeutic program. Finally, it is apparent from this brief discussion that as long as the

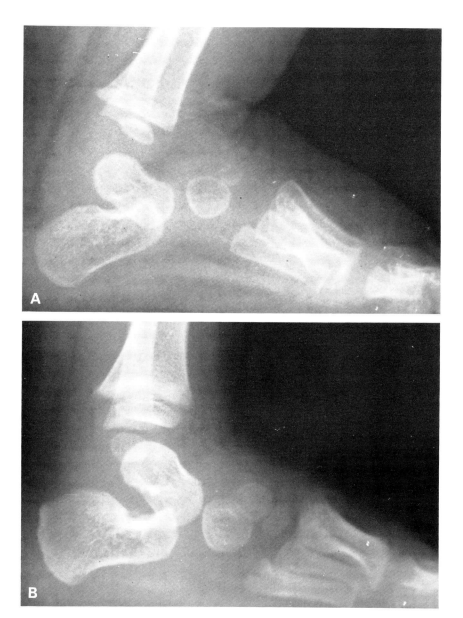

FIG. 5-3. **A**, Simulated standing lateral roentgenogram of the foot of a 6-month-old girl, showing the characteristic features of a calcaneocavus foot. This deformity was noted at birth; there was no evident neurologic cause, and no treatment was administered. **B**, Observe the decided improvement in the foot seen in the standing lateral weight-bearing film taken 17 months later.

basic, underlying problem is a muscle imbalance, any form of nonoperative treatment most likely will be ineffective and futile.

If one agrees that the basic cause of the calcaneocavus deformity is a muscle imbalance and that the major site of muscle weakness is the triceps surae, it is easy to explain the mechanism by which the deformity develops and why it does not respond to nonoperative treatment.

    Whitman aptly described the calf musculature as the "principal lifting and propelling force of the body."[23] The loss of strength of this

*Pathomechanics*

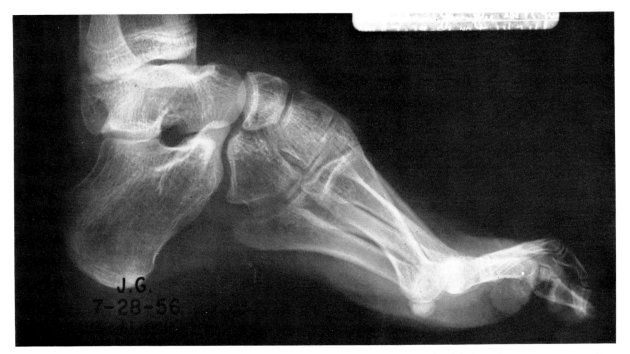

FIG. 5-4. The typical pistol-grip deformity of the calcaneus and hindfoot is seen in this lateral roentgenogram of an 11-year-old girl with a calcaneocavus foot due to poliomyelitis.

calf musculature allows the gradual development of a "vertical calcaneus," which, in the adult, results in a pistol-grip deformity (Fig. 5-4). This deformity shortens the lever arm upon which the triceps surae acts, thus creating the basis for a vicious cycle. That is, the weaker the calf musculature, the less the force that is exerted upon the calcaneal apophysis. This reduced force, when acting upon a growing calcaneus, leads to a shorter lever arm and a weaker pushoff (Fig. 5-5). The verticality of the calcaneus elevates the longitudinal arch of the foot, and the forefoot, because of either the effects of gravity or the action of the forefoot plantar flexors, assumes an absolute as well as a relative plantarflexed posture. The combination results in the calcaneocavus foot deformity (Fig. 5-6).

As a secondary phenomenon, extension of the metatarsophalangeal joints is often increased, accompanied by plantar flexion of the interphalangeal joints, leading to clawtoes (Fig. 5-6). The most extreme manifestation results from triceps surae paresis, plus the unopposed action against that muscle, namely, the forefoot plantar flexors and midfoot dorsiflexors.

## Pathologic and Clinical Features

From the foregoing discussion of pathogenesis, the pathology of this deformity becomes clear and easy to comprehend. The hindfoot is in calcaneus, the forefoot is in excessive plantar flexion, and the arch is excessively high, such that the foot is reduced in length, and the toes may be clawed. If the plantar flexors of the forefoot are strong enough, the deformity will be more severe than if the foot is totally flail. This analysis of the problem is essential when formulating a surgical solution. Briefly, but importantly, the deformity must be corrected *first;* thereafter, any existing muscle imbalance must be corrected as completely as is technically feasible.

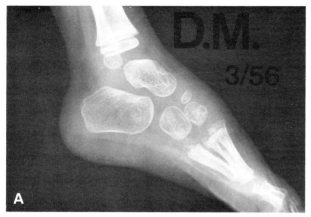
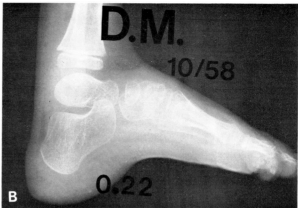

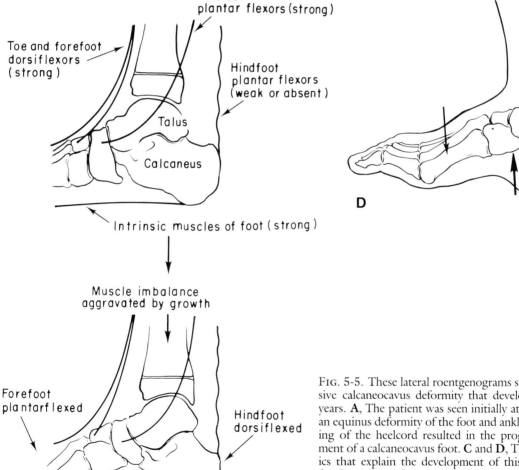

FIG. 5-5. These lateral roentgenograms show the progressive calcaneocavus deformity that developed in just 2½ years. **A**, The patient was seen initially at age 4 years with an equinus deformity of the foot and ankle. **B**, A lengthening of the heelcord resulted in the progressive development of a calcaneocavus foot. **C** and **D**, The pathomechanics that explain the development of this deformity. The forefoot plantar flexors (posterior tibial and peroneals) are strong, thus permitting the calcaneus (hindfoot) to go into dorsiflexion. The anterior tibial muscle is usually strong, thus elevating the midfoot, and the common toe extensors further plantarflex the metatarsals by the "windlass" action they exert as they dorsiflex the toes. In addition, the intrinsic muscles undergo contracture, as growth accentuates the effect of this muscle imbalance on the skeleton. (Bradley, G. H., and Coleman, S. S.: Treatment of the calcaneocavus foot deformity. J. Bone Joint Surg., *63A*:1165, 1981.)

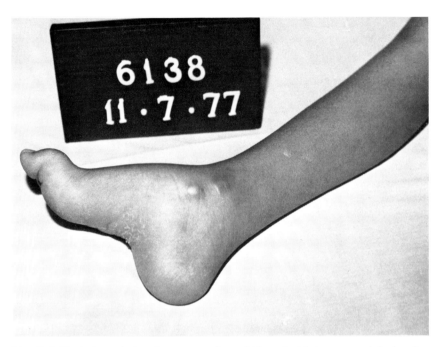

FIG. 5-6. Typical paralytic calcaneocavus foot. Although this is not a weight-bearing photograph, the characteristic and diagnostic features—prominent heel, high arch, plantarflexed forefoot, and cock-up toes—are plainly evident.

## Treatment

Dunn enunciated the thrust of the therapeutic problem in 1919 when he wrote, "Once the deformity is established, treatment by splintage is difficult and usually ineffective."[5] This observation has been borne out by all who have treated this complex deformity. Bracing the primary osseous deformity, namely, the severe progressive dorsiflexion of the calcaneus, is fruitless, and the remainder of the deformity cannot be effectively braced because it is secondary to muscle imbalance. Therefore, successful treatment of this deformity must be surgical. The brief historical review given earlier outlines some of the considerations that have been employed in attempting to solve this difficult problem. This section attempts to put into perspective the various therapeutic approaches and to present a treatment regimen that can be applied to different age groups.

For this particular discussion, it is essential to define these age groups, even though the definition is somewhat arbitrary. Generally, children under age 3 to 5 years with a calcaneus or calcaneocavus foot deformity are not candidates for surgical treatment, for the following reasons: First, substantial bony deformity has not yet become manifest; second, muscle strength and thus imbalance are difficult to assess accurately at this age; and third, the deformity usually is not so disabling in this age group that it justifies surgical correction.

In patients above 5 years of age, the bony deformity becomes progressively more evident, the muscle strengths can be more easily established, and the deformity usually becomes progressively more disabling. These are the patients who require major therapeutic efforts, and they comprise two groups. The first group includes patients between age 5 and 12 years (the "pre-triple arthrodesis group"), and the second, those over 12 years of age. This arbitrary division is based upon the commonly held view that a triple arthrodesis should rarely be done in patients under skeletal age 12 (girls) or 13 (boys). For both groups, it is assumed that the underlying neurologic problem has been clearly defined and that surgical correction of the foot is therefore justified.

The child in this age group has a demonstrable neurologic deficit, as noted earlier. The plantar aspect of the heel is prominent, but posterior projection of the os calcis is scant because the heel is in calcaneus. As Irwin wrote, "These patients have a large callused or mushroomed heel."[12] The longitudinal arch is exaggerated, thus producing a cavus configuration of the foot. Irwin also observed that the dorsum of the foot is elongated as compared to the plantar surface, which is concave. The gait characteristically exhibits little or no pushoff, and sometimes the forefoot does not touch the floor even at the time of "toe-off." This gives the gait a "pegleg" appearance. On muscle testing, the triceps surae is weakened, and, depending upon the underlying neurologic problem, other muscles are preserved to varying degrees.

AGES 5 THROUGH 12 YEARS

    Radiographically, the os calcis exhibits an increase in the calcaneal "pitch." This nearly always exceeds 30°, with the normal upper limits about 15° to 20°. The apophysis of the os calcis does not become ossified until about age 9 or 10 years, but ossification may be delayed in this deformity. The longitudinal arch is elevated, and the entire foot is substantially shorter than normal.

TREATMENT CONSIDERATIONS. Because of the muscle imbalance and the resultant instability of the foot, it is essential first of all to stabilize the hindfoot. This is necessary not only to eliminate subtalar instability, but also because transfers of the lateral stabilizers of the foot (posterior tibial and peroneals) are often required, and thus, lateral (subtalar) stability is essential. The first step in surgical correction, therefore, is the subtalar or extra-articular arthrodesis by means of a talocalcaneal bone block.[9] My preferred technique is illustrated and described in Figure 5-7. Following the bone graft, an above-knee, nonweight-bearing cast is applied for 6 weeks, at the end of which period the graft is usually well incorporated. A below-knee walking cast may then be needed for an additional 6 weeks to restore bone stock and to enable the graft to hypertrophy (Fig. 5-8D).

    The second stage consists of the tendon transfers, with or without the posterior displacement (crescentic) osteotomy of the os calcis. The decision as to whether the osteotomy is necessary is based largely on the estimate of the degree of deformity or upward pitch of the calcaneus. The age of the patient also is a major factor, because a 5-year-old has a much greater remodeling capacity than a 10-year-old. Therefore, if tendons can be transferred to the calcaneus in the younger patient, it

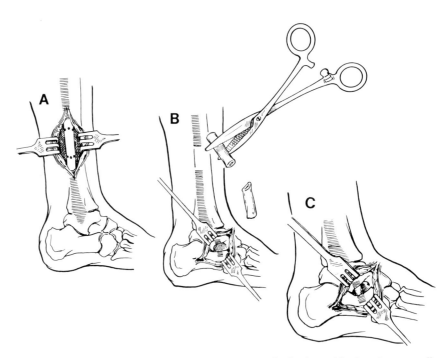

FIG. 5-7. My preferred method of performing a subtalar bone block, using a small, full-thickness segment of the fibula. The bone segment must be removed subperiosteally so that regeneration of the fibula will occur. The removed portion is approximately 1 inch long, and one end is bevelled to facilitate its placement into the slots (shaded areas) created in the talus and calcaneus. Note the oblique angle of the graft placement. In growing children between the ages of 3 and 12 years, I have had no failures of talocalcaneal fusion or of regeneration of the area of fibular resection.

is reasonable to expect a substantial degree of remodeling of a mild or moderate calcaneal deformity with growth, or at least enough to eliminate the need for calcaneal osteotomy (Fig. 5-9).

On the other hand, an older child (age 10 years or older) has minimal remodeling capacity, and a calcaneal osteotomy therefore will probably be necessary to restore the lever arm to an acceptable degree. Obviously, an area of uncertainty exists in which the need for crescentic calcaneal osteotomy will be difficult to determine. One can use only judgment and clinical experience to make that decision.

When one has a solid extra-articular subtalar arthrodesis, it is possible to transfer appropriate tendons to the calcaneal apophysis. Clearly, the strength of the remaining calf musculature will govern which tendons are transferred. In cases in which strong anterior tibial and common toe extensors are available for transfer, but minimal if any lateral stabilizer function is evident, then the most appropriate procedure is transfer of the anterior tibial tendon to the calcaneal apophysis as described by Peabody (Fig. 5-10). This provides at best an active plantar flexor and at worst an effective tenodesis effect.

At the time of tendon transfer, one must address the cavus component of the deformity. In nearly all instances, the plantar fascia and intrinsic musculature of the foot will be contracted and must be lengthened in order to correct the cavus element of the deformity.

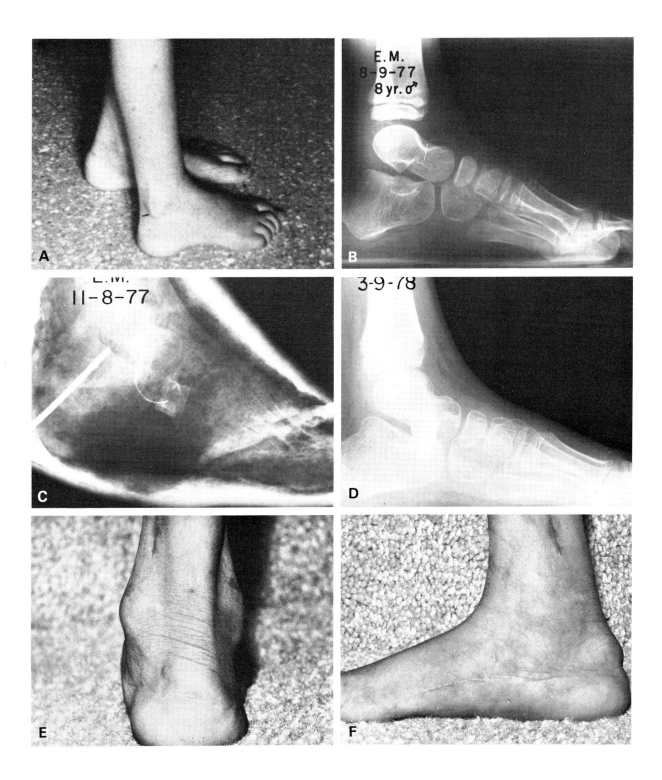

FIG. 5-8. **A**, Preoperative standing photograph and **B**, lateral roentgenogram of a 10-year-old patient with calcaneocavus foot due to poliomyelitis. Muscle strength was Grade IV to V in all groups except the triceps surae, which had a Grade 0. The patient underwent a two-stage operation as described in the text. Initially, a subtalar bone block was done, followed 8 weeks later by transfer of the posterior tibial and peroneal tendons into the os calcis apophysis. **C**, The postoperative roentgenogram after the second stage; **D**, the standing roentgenogram 1 year later. **E** and **F**, In the postoperative photos, the greatly improved plantigrade appearance of the foot is evident. Though the patient continued to have weak push-off, his gait was much improved. Note hypertrophy of the subtalar bone block.

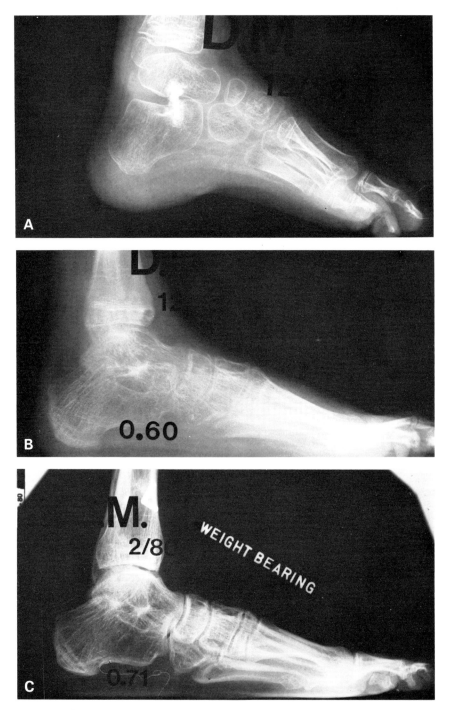

Fig. 5-9. **A**, Preoperative lateral standing roentgenogram of a 6-year-old boy with calcaneocavus deformity. A subtalar bone block had been accomplished 8 weeks earlier. A two-stage procedure was accomplished, transferring the posterior tibial and peroneus longus and brevis tendons to the calcaneus. Because of his young age, a calcaneal osteotomy was not done. **B**, Progressive improvement in the configuration of the foot is seen 7 years later and (**C**) 22 years later. The presence of the screw seen in **B** is the result of a tibial lengthening procedure that was done at an earlier age. This case illustrates that the calcaneus lever arm can still be corrected substantially if the tendon transfers are done early, while considerable growth remains in the foot and if the tendons are placed into the apophysis of the calcaneus. The posterior displacement osteotomy is unnecessary under these circumstances.

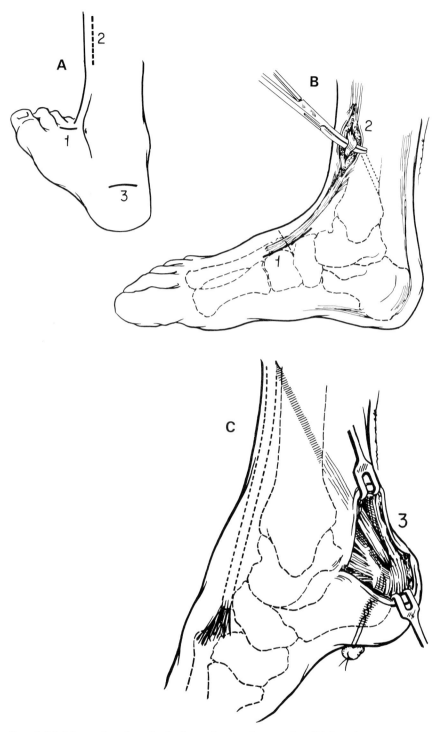

F IG. 5-10. My preferred method of transferring the anterior tibial tendon posteriorly through the tibiofibular interosseous membrane into the calcaneus. **A,** The three necessary incisions. The anterior tibial tendon is sectioned at its insertion through the first incision (1), and (**B**) it is extracted through the second (counter) incision (2). The tendon is retracted along with the anterior tibial vessels and nerves, and a generous "window" is made in the tibiofibular interosseous membrane. Through the third incision, placed transversely over the calcaneus (3), the anterior tibial tendon is rerouted to the calcaneal apophysis, and (**C**) is implanted into bone in the same fashion as described in Figure 5-12.

Also, in order to maximally correct the cavus, the calcaneus must be stabilized in some degree of equinus by means of a transfixion pin (Fig. 5-11). If the calcaneus is not fixed, efforts at flattening the longitudinal arch by dorsiflexing the forefoot will be fruitless. This is essential whether or not the crescentic osteotomy is performed. It is important to emphasize that posterior displacement of the proximal fragment of the os calcis is impossible without a release of the plantar structures.

Subsequent transfer of the common toe extensors to the midfoot may be indicated in order to give the foot improved dorsiflexion power. It must be emphasized, however, that this transfer (of the extensors) must be done at a *later* stage when the foot can be brought out of plantar flexion. Clearly, when the anterior tibial tendon is transferred posteriorly into the os calcis, the foot must be placed into a cast postoperatively in maximum equinus. Slowly thereafter, the foot can be brought out of equinus, and then the extensor tendons can be transferred.

In the event that lateral stabilizers are present and strong (Grade IV or better), these phasic transfers are preferred. These transfer procedures use forefoot plantar flexors and convert them to hindfoot or ankle plantar flexors. No change of phase is necessary, and the patient automatically uses the transferred tendons as intended. In my experience, this is the most effective tendon transfer in the muscle-balancing program. It must be recognized, however, as emphasized by Irwin, that the function of the triceps surae can never possibly be replaced by any combination of transfers to the os calcis.

Irrespective of which tendon or tendons are transferred, the tech-

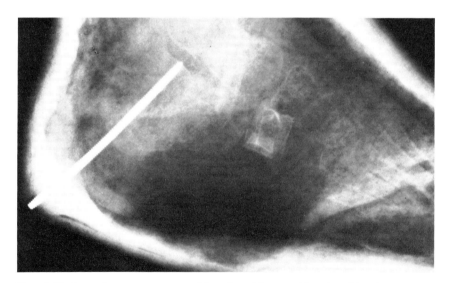

FIG. 5-11. Lateral roentgenogram of foot in a 10-year-old male with calcaneocavus deformity. Following a subtalar bone block, tendon transfers to the calcaneus were accomplished, in conjunction with a plantar fasciotomy. In order to stabilize the heel, a transfixion threaded Steinmann pin was placed into the calcaneus and incorporated into the cast. The forefoot was then dorsiflexed on the hindfoot, and the forepart of the cast was added and attached to the leg and heel portions of the cast.

nique deserves special consideration. It is essential to emphasize that any tendon transferred to the calcaneus that is designed to replace the function (in part) of the triceps surae must be implanted directly into bone in the calcaneal apophysis (Fig. 5-12). Irwin emphasized this point and also recommended that if the tendons are not placed into the calcaneal apophysis, not only will the transfers fail to provide effective pushoff, but they will also fail to stimulate subsequent posterior growth and elongation of the calcaneus. Above all, Irwin continued, these tendons should *not* be attached directly to the Achilles tendon, because they will elongate or pull away from their attachment. Also, according to Irwin, they should be put into the os calcis more on the lateral side in order to promote the development of the more stable valgus hindfoot.[12]

If, in the surgeon's judgment, the calcaneal deformity requires correction, then the crescentic or posterior displacement osteotomy should be done to lengthen the calcaneus and thus to improve the calcaneal lever arm. In the process, the effectiveness of the tendon transfers is increased or enhanced. The technique for this osteotomy is demonstrated and described in Figure 5-2.

Whether tendon transfers are accomplished alone or in combination with the calcaneal osteotomy, the foot and leg are placed in an above-knee cast postoperatively, with the foot and the ankle in equinus. In 6 weeks, the cast and the calcaneal pin are removed. A below-knee brace is applied, attached to a shoe with a tapered, elevated heel. The brace has a dorsiflexion stop to prevent excessive stretching of the transferred tendons and also has a spring-loaded *plantar* flexion assist (Fig. 5-13). This brace is worn for at least 12 weeks or until the transferred tendons demonstrate satisfactory plantar flexion function. Whether or not a rigid polypropylene brace should be employed thereafter is a matter of judgment. If the transferred tendons are phasic, usually they will convert automatically to plantar flexors. Therefore, little, if any, formal physiotherapy will be necessary. On the other hand, if the anterior tibial tendon is transferred to the os calcis, physical therapeutic assistance is often essential in order to achieve conversion.

OVER AGE 12 YEARS

In this age group, the foot looks essentially the same as that of the younger child with a calcaneocavus deformity. Virtually no heel prominence is found posteriorly, and the heel pad is hypertrophied (Fig. 5-14). The gait abnormality, muscle testing, and other clinical features are the same as in the younger child. Because the deformity is of longer duration, the foot is even more foreshortened.

Roentgenographically, the typical calcaneocavus foot at this age shows a calcaneus with a pronounced "pistol grip" deformity (Fig. 5-4). Even more advanced adaptive bony changes have occurred in all of the bones of the foot, and the foot will have attained a more mature appearance. As with the calcaneocavus foot in younger children, the longitudinal arch is exaggerated, the forefoot is plantarflexed, and the toes exhibit a clawtoe deformity.

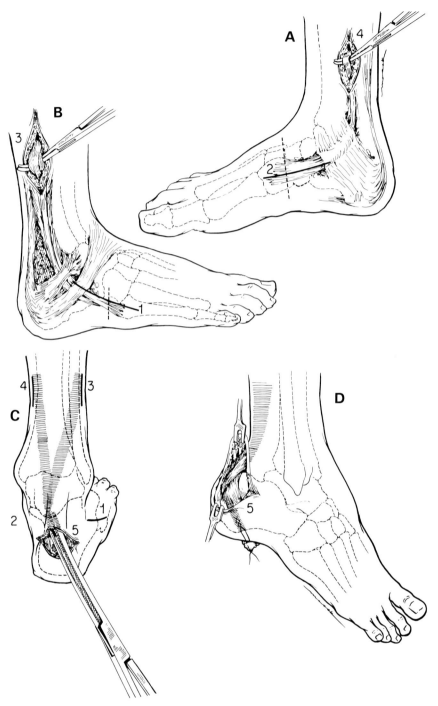

Fig. 5-12. My preferred method of transferring the peroneal and posterior tibial tendons to the calcaneus. **A** and **B**, Incisions 1 and 2 are used for exposing the tendon insertions; the counter incisions are necessary for extracting the peroneal and posterior tibial tendons. **C**, Utilizing a long uterine-packing forceps, these tendons are rerouted subcutaneously through a generous transverse incision (5) that is placed over the calcaneus in the vicinity of the insertion of the Achilles tendon. A drill hole of appropriate size is then made into the calcaneus, beginning in the calcaneal apophysis and extending in a plantar direction into the sole of the foot. The tendons are sewn together and then implanted into the calcaneus through the drill hole. **D**, The foot and ankle are held in maximum plantar flexion, and the sutures used to route the tendon into the calcaneus are then tied over a dental cotton.

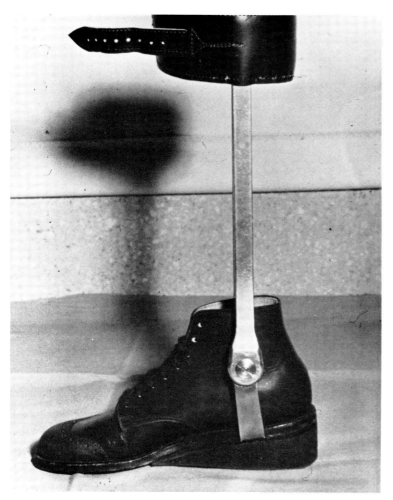

FIG. 5-13. Brace that is used for at least 3 months following the second stage (muscle transfer) correction of a calcaneocavus foot. Note the equinus of the foot created by the wedge-shaped heel lift. The stirrup ankle has a dorsiflexion stop, but free plantar flexion.

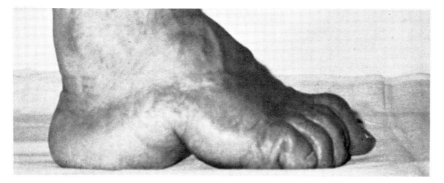

FIG. 5-14. In the adolescent and adult patient, the features of the calcaneocavus deformity are even more pronounced. This is a lateral standing photograph of the foot of a male physician who contracted poliomyelitis in early childhood. Total triceps surae paralysis produced the typical calcaneocavus foot, showing the "mushroom" heel, the absence of any calcaneal lever arm, an elevated longitudinal arch, and flexed toes.

TREATMENT CONSIDERATIONS. Because these children are eligible for triple arthrodesis, this is the first surgical procedure to be performed. It is essential that one correct all components of the foot deformity in the process of performing the triple arthrodesis. In my opinion, this is a most difficult triple arthrodesis to perform if it is to be accomplished correctly. It must be accompanied by percutaneous plantar fasciotomy in order to correct the abnormally elevated longitudinal arch. This triple arthrodesis must: (1) correct the vertical pitch of the calcaneus, (2) restore the lever arm of the calcaneus, and (3) flatten the longitudinal arch.

This procedure is illustrated and described in Figure 5-1, and Figure 5-15 gives an example of a patient who has undergone the operation. I have not been able to perform this operation without using some form of internal fixation (staples) or transfixion (threaded wires) in order to maintain the surgical correction. Postoperatively, an above-knee cast is preferred; however, if the internal fixation is sufficiently sound, one may possibly use a below-knee cast.

The operative cast is removed in 6 weeks. The surgical wounds should be well healed. If the transfixion pins have been used, they should be removed at this time and the pin tracts allowed to heal. A roentgenogram usually shows good union of the triple arthrodesis. Once the skin can be rendered surgically clean, the appropriate tendon transfers can be accomplished.

The same principles regarding tendon transfers used in treating the younger child apply here. Clearly, one must deal with whatever muscles and tendons are available and strong enough for transfer (Grade IV or better). The most attractive transfers use the posterior tibial and peroneus longus and brevis tendons. If the anterior tibial is the only good muscle, however, it can be transferred to the calcaneus through the interosseous membrane as described earlier. Often this results in a dropfoot, but this deformity responds readily to a dorsiflexion-assist brace or simply a polypropylene dropfoot brace (Fig. 5-16). Upon completion of the transfers, a below-knee cast is applied, with the foot and ankle in equinus. It is removed in 6 weeks, and the same postcasting program used for the younger child with calcaneocavus foot is implemented. Depending on the strength of the transferred tendons, a reasonably satisfactory gait can be expected.

It should be emphasized that determining which musculotendinous units should be transferred requires an accurate test of muscle strengths *before* any program of surgical correction is begun. A muscle should rate at least Grade IV to qualify for transfer, since a muscle with this strength can carry a joint through a full range of motion against gravity and some degree of resistance. Also, no matter how skillfully the tendon is transferred, it nearly always loses some degree of strength, even as much as one grade.

Although the results of these correcting and stabilizing tendon transfer procedures have uniformly improved appearance and function in the foot, we have devised a radiographic method to calculate the improvement on a more accurate and biomechanically sound basis.[1] A

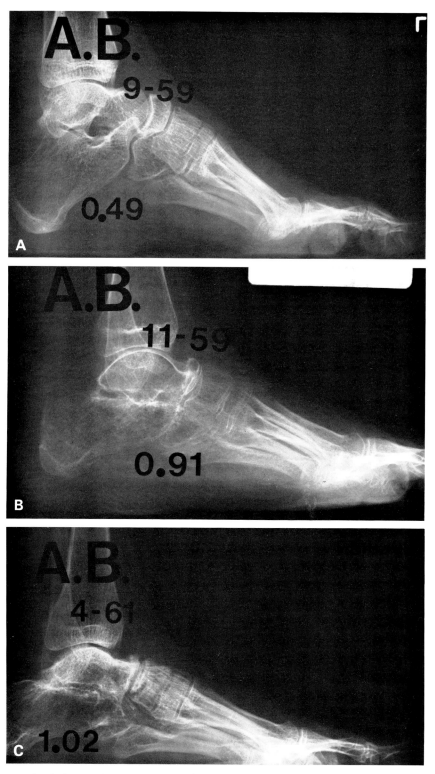

FIG. 5-15. **A**, Standing, preoperative lateral roentgenogram of a 12-year-old girl with calcaneocavus due to poliomyelitis. She had good to normal strength in all muscle groups except for the triceps surae, which was rated Grade 0. A corrective triple arthrodesis was done, as depicted in Figure 5-1. This was followed by transfer of the peroneal and posterior tibial tendons into the calcaneus. **B**, The immediate postoperative result; **C**, the result 1½ years later.

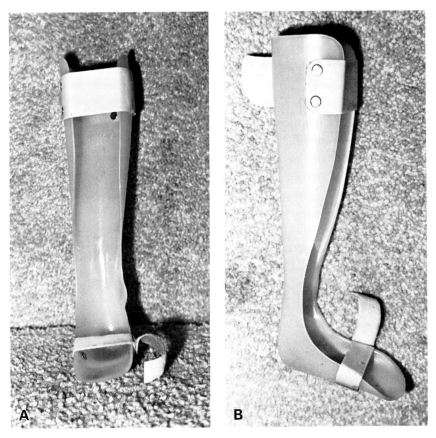

FIG. 5-16. **A,** Front and (**B**) lateral photographs of a typical polypropylene ankle-foot orthosis (AFO). The device is custom made, utilizing Velcro straps for suspension. The device can be worn in any shoe and at night as a splint without the shoe.

ratio [R] is computed between the distance from the ankle joint to the most prominent, weight-bearing portion of the calcaneus and the triceps surae lever arm.

(1) Using a lateral roentgenogram of the foot and ankle in one standing position, a perpendicular line is drawn from the vertical axis of the tibia to the distal, most plantar aspect of the calcaneus. (2) A second line is drawn, perpendicular to the first line, from the center of the tibial plafond to the posterior end of the os calcis; this line represents the triceps surae lever arm. The ratio is computed by dividing the length of the first line into the length of the second. The lines are illustrated in Figure 5-17, and the equation is as follows:

$$[R] = \frac{(2)\ \text{center of tibia to posterior end of calcaneus}}{(1)\ \text{ankle joint to bottom of calcaneus}}$$

The results of this computation are interpreted as follows: An [R] greater than 0.65 indicates an increased distance from the ankle to the posterior aspect of the calcaneus, plus a decreased distance from the ankle to the plantar aspect of the calcaneus, and thus a favorable biomechanical relationship. The converse relationship, with [R] less than

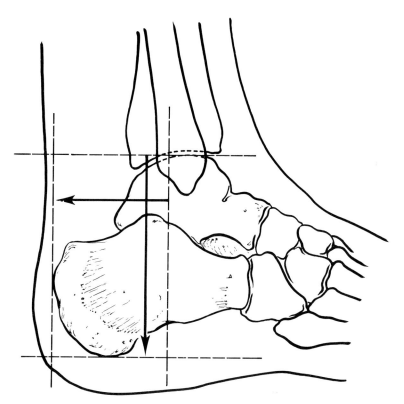

FIG. 5-17. My preferred method of evaluating surgical correction. A weight-bearing film is necessary so that the tibia is perpendicular to the ground. A horizontal line is then drawn at the level of the dome of the talus, and a perpendicular line is drawn at the most posterior aspect of the calcaneus. A third line is drawn parallel to the weight-bearing surface of the calcaneus, and a perpendicular line is drawn centering over the axis of rotation of the talus in the ankle joint. Using these reference points, it is simple to calculate the relationship [R] between the vertical distance, or height, of the hindfoot and the horizontal distance, representing the lever arm. (Bradley, G. W. and Coleman, S. S.: Treatment of the calcaneocavus foot deformity. J. Bone Joint Surg., *63A*:1162, 1981.)

0.50, suggests a less favorable biomechanical situation. This ratio represents a determination that can be documented quite accurately and that is directly and consistently related to the appearance of the foot and patient's ability to wear standard shoes. In addition, a *substantially* consistent relationship is found between the mathematical and functional result, which includes evaluation of such determinants as gait and pushoff. Since function of a partially paralyzed foot and ankle is so difficult to document, however, and because many other factors often are involved in appraising the functional capacity of a paralyzed lower limb, it is not possible to precisely correlate these objective and subjective data.

In some circumstances, the therapeutic regimen just described will be neither appropriate nor adequate. Specific situations may deny the surgeon the opportunity to perform the operations as described. These include the totally flail foot and ankle and the foot that has substan-

SPECIAL
CONSIDERATIONS

tially impaired sensation. In the former, no muscles are available for transfer, and thus no surgical procedure should probably be considered until age 12 or 14, when a pantalar arthrodesis would be the most appropriate corrective procedure. This operation should not be done, however, if the foot is insensitive, as is often the case in myelomeningocele or other neurologic problems accompanied by lack of sensation. A pantalar arthrodesis is not performed in such situations because of the overwhelming likelihood of fracture, through either the distal tibial physis or some portion of the previously fused joints.

When performing a pantalar arthrodesis in calcaneocavus feet that have normal sensation, one must make every effort to correct all aspects of the deformity as mentioned earlier in order to provide the most plantigrade foot possible and to render shoe fitting more appropriate. The closer to skeletal maturity that the procedure is performed, the more permanent and predictable will be the result (Fig. 5-18).

In some calcaneocavus feet in which the predominant deformity is in the calcaneus, a tenodesis of the Achilles tendon to the tibia may be advantageous. The operation, originally described by Gallie for the calcaneus and calcaneocavus foot due to poliomyelitis, consisted of a tenodesis of the proximal cut end of the Achilles tendon into the tibia.[7] Even though the procedure did not produce effective toe rise or pushoff, Gallie claimed that it could either halt or substantially reduce progression of the deformity. Knight, however, found that the effect of the tenodesis lasted no more than 1 or 2 years in a growing child and would then stretch out.[14] This procedure seems to be most appropriate in instances of myelomeningocele with similar paralytic causes of the deformity. Westin learned by serendipity that tenodesis of the Achilles tendon was better done to the fibula (Fig. 5-19) than to the tibia, because this stimulated growth of the fibula and thus reduced the valgus of the ankle joint that usually develops in myelomeningocele.[22] This is a most unusual procedure, and I have not yet had occasion to perform it, nor have I had any experience with the Gallie procedure.

## References

1. Bradley, G. W., and Coleman, S. S.: Treatment of the calcaneocavus foot deformity. J. Bone Joint Surg., *63A*:1159, 1981.
2. Cholmeley, J. A.: Elmslie's operation for the calcaneus foot. J. Bone Joint Surg., *35A*:46, 1953.
3. Coleman, S. S., and Lee, G.: Unpublished data, 1965.
4. Davis, G. G.: The treatment of hollow foot (pes cavus). Am. J. Orthop. Surg., *11*:234, 1913.
5. Dunn, N.: Calcaneocavus and its treatment. J. Orthop. Surg., *1*:711, 1919.
6. Dunn, N.: Stabilizing operations in the treatment of paralytic deformities of the foot. Proc. R. Soc. Med., *15*:17, 1921.
7. Gallie, W. E.: Tendon fixation in infantile paralysis—A review of one hundred and fifty operations. Am. J. Orthop. Surg., *14*:18, 1916.
8. Gleich, A.: Beitrag zur Operativen Plattfuss Behandlung. Arch. Klinesche Chir., *46*:358, 1893.
9. Grice, D. S.: An extra-articular arthrodesis of the subastragalar joint for correction of paralytic flat feet in children. J. Bone Joint Surg., *34A*:927, 1952.

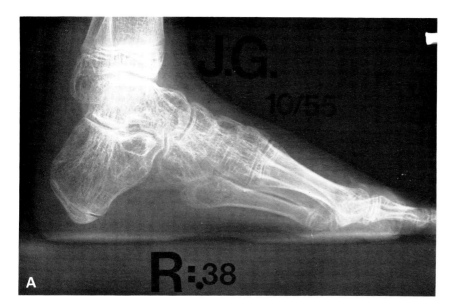

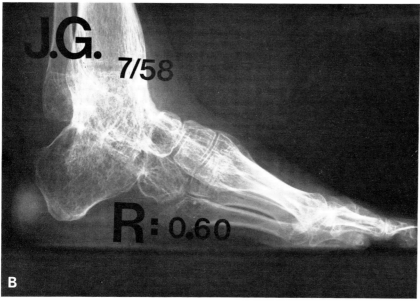

Fig. 5-18. **A,** Preoperative lateral roentgenogram in an 11-year-old girl with a calcaneocavus deformity due to poliomyelitis. Except for minimal intrinsic toe flexion
power, her foot and ankle were flail. Thus, a pantalar arthrodesis was done. **B,** Her
standing roentgenogram, with a functional [R] of 0.60. Twenty-two years later, it had
remained relatively unchanged. A calcaneocavus foot can develop even in the absence
of muscle power and is best treated by corrective pantalar arthrodesis, which improves
shoe wear, eliminates a brace, and improves gait.

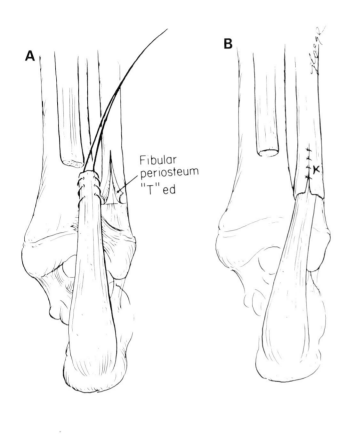
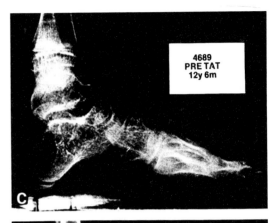
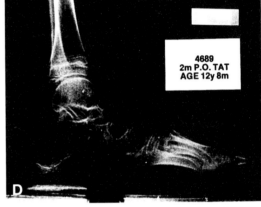
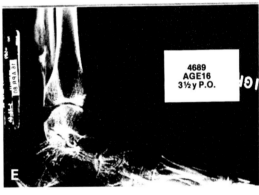

Fig. 5-19. Method of performing tenodesis of the Achilles tendon to the fibula in calcaneocavus deformity in myelodysplasia. **A** and **B**, Tenodesis to the fibula following sectioning of the contracted plantar musculotendinous structures. **C**, Preoperative, (**D**) 2 months postoperative, and (**E**) 3½ years postoperative lateral standing roentgenograms. **F**, Preoperative and (**G**) postoperative anteroposterior roentgenograms of the ankle in the same patient. Note the improved relationship of the bones comprising the ankle mortise, especially the elongation of the distal end of the fibula. (Courtesy of G. Wilbur Westin, M.D., Los Angeles, California.)

10. Herndon, C. H., Strong, J., and Heyman, C. H.: Transposition of the tibialis anterior in the treatment of paralytic talipes calcaneus. J. Bone Joint Surg., *38A:*751, 1956.

11. Hoke, M.: An operation for stabilizing paralytic feet. J. Orthop. Surg., *19:*494, 1921.

12. Irwin, C. E.: The calcaneus foot. South. Med. J., *44:*191, 1951.

13. Jones, R.: Certain operative procedures in the paralysis of children with special reference to poliomyelitis. Br. Med. J., *11:*1520, 1911.

14. Knight, R., in *Campbell's Operative Orthopaedics.* 2nd Edition. Edited by J. S. Speed and H. Smith. St. Louis, C. V. Mosby, 1949, p. 1348.

15. Lloyd-Roberts, G. C.: *Orthopaedics in Infancy and Childhood.* London, Butterworths, 1971, p. 301.

16. Mitchell, G. P.: Posterior displacement osteotomy of the calcaneus. J. Bone Joint Surg., *59B:*233, 1977.

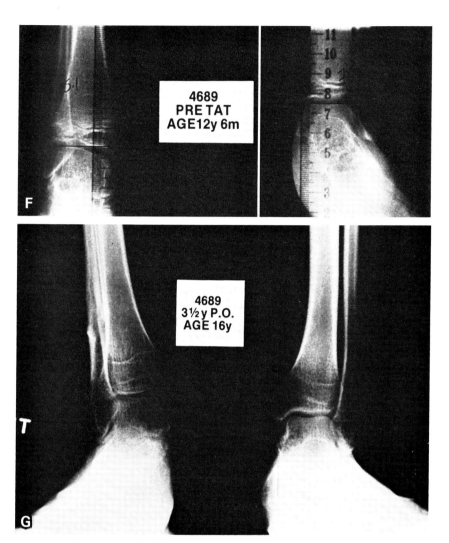

Fig. 5-19. *continued*

17. Nicoladoni, C.: Nachtrag zum pes calcaneus und zur transplantation der peronealsehnen. Arch. Chir., *27:*660, 1881.

18. Peabody, C. W.: Tendon transposition. An end-result study. J. Bone Joint Surg., *20:*193, 205, 1938.

19. Samilson, R. L.: Crescentic osteotomy of the os calcis for calcaneocavus feet. In *Foot Science.* Edited by J. E. Bateman. Philadelphia, W. B. Saunders, 1976, pp. 18–25.

20. Trendelenburg, F.: Ueber Plattfussoperationen. Arch. Klin. Chir., *39:*751, 1889.

21. Turner, J. W., and Cooper, R.: Posterior transposition of tibialis anterior through the interosseous membrane. Clin. Orthop., *79:*71, 1971.

22. Westin, G. W.: Personal communication, 1980.

23. Whitman, R.: The operative treatment of paralytic talipes of the calcaneus type. Am. J. Med. Sci., *122:*593, 1901.

# 6

# Severe, Flexible Planovalgus Foot (Flatfoot)

This chapter primarily discusses those uncommon and occasional flatfoot problems that produce sufficient symptoms or handicaps so as to justify surgical correction. This condition is also referred to as a pronated foot, a relaxed flatfoot, and congenital planovalgus. Much has been written concerning theories of etiology and the treatment of this frequently encountered condition. A consensus has not been reached with respect to either of these issues; if one does exist, however, it is that the large majority of these feet are asymptomatic and will remain so. Many feel that conservative care is usually sufficient in the vast majority of cases; most who advocate surgical intervention emphasize the need to limit such treatment to feet with substantial symptoms or severe deformity. The literature does not contain long-term studies on the asymptomatic flatfoot that has received either no treatment or various forms of nonoperative treatment.

Since most flexible flatfeet in children and adolescents are usually asymptomatic, surgical correction is rarely needed, and the indications for operative correction therefore must be highly individualized. Furthermore, no firmly established or well accepted objective parameters are available at present that can be used as indications for surgical correction; thus, the surgeon is usually faced with a complex series of subjective and objective data that must be coupled with experienced judgment when deciding for or against surgical intervention.

Varying degrees of flexible flatfoot are common in young children, and no clear distinction is found between normal and abnormal in the young child as long as the foot has normal musculature and flexibility (see Chapter 1). Blount stated that the feet of the normal child are pronated until the age of 6 years or later.[7] Ozonoff has stated that almost all children under 18 months of age appear to have a flatfoot with no medial longitudinal arch, but that by age 10, only 4% of children have this configuration.[51] As noted previously, only a few of these feet will develop symptoms of pain, disability, or abnormal shoe wear sufficient to warrant surgical correction. This is supported by Crego's long-term study, in which he found that only about 1 child in 40 with flexible flatfeet ever required a surgical procedure.[13]

As will be evident in the ensuing discussion, it therefore must be accepted that the simple presence of an *asymptomatic* flexible flatfoot in a child or adolescent does *not* indicate any particular form of therapy, either operative or nonoperative. The ultimate goal of this chapter is to develop a rationale for the management of this condition and to put the role of surgical correction into perspective. In a situation in which the problems are so individualized, my conservative biases probably will be clearly discerned. Because of the controversial nature of this foot deformity, I will allude to nonoperative methods of treatment; also, because of the intriguing and provocative concepts of its etiology and pathogenesis, a more detailed review of these issues appears in the following section.

## Etiology and Pathogenesis

As with most complex foot deformities, two broad etiologic categories of flexible flatfoot can be defined: (1) neurologic and (2) developmental or "idiopathic." In the neurologic type, the basic cause is paralytic, in which muscle function is compromised. In the developmental category, the flexible flatfoot deformity has no well defined cause, but the muscular function of the foot and ankle is normal. The obvious difference between these two *anatomically* similar deformities is that in paralytic flatfoot, any treatment program must employ joint stabilization and muscle transfers (when possible), whereas with the idiopathic flatfoot, the therapy program is less well defined and most likely calls for a substantially different approach. Paralytic flatfoot is discussed in Chapter 7.

The literature is replete with theories concerning the cause of flexible idiopathic or developmental flatfoot. No agreement has been reached on the essential lesion that might cause this condition. Defects of the muscles, the bones, the ligaments, and various combinations of these have been considered.

### THE MUSCLES

Over 100 years ago, Duchenne showed that by Faradic stimulation of the peroneus longus, he could always produce a progressive increase in height of the plantar arch.[15] Keith agreed that the supporting muscles of the foot are the most important factors in maintaining the longitudinal arch and felt that the ligaments of the foot came into play only after the muscles had failed.[34] Jones, Haraldsson, and Niederecker also supported the concept that the muscles were the most important factors in maintaining the longitudinal arch.[25,33,48] Hoke based his operative procedure on the concept that muscle weakness was the primary cause of the flatfoot. He stated that "The human foot can be held up in an arched position only by the power of muscles acting coordinately the instant weight is borne. No mechanical substitute can be found for the arch-lifting power of the tibialis posterior, tibialis anterior, and flexor hallucis longus."[29]

Morton stated that appreciable muscle exertion is needed only when the center of gravity moves beyond the margins of structural stability.[46] Only acute, heavy, transient forces, such as in the take-off phase of walking, required dynamic muscle action. Jones estimated that the posterior tibial and peroneal muscles bear only 15 to 20% of the tension stress on the foot.[32] He concluded that both passive elasticity of ligaments and active contractility of muscles controlled the normal longitudinal arch, with the plantar aponeurosis and plantar tarsal ligaments holding together the anterior and posterior pillars of the arch.

Hicks demonstrated the windlass mechanism of the foot, in which passive extension of the great toe resulted in (1) elevation of the longitudinal arch, (2) inversion of the hindfoot, (3) lateral rotation of the leg, and (4) tightening of the plantar aponeurosis (see Fig. 4-1).[28] The arch was thus elevated without true muscle force, but rather by simple mechanical depression of the first metatarsal head. Chapter 4 further reviews this complex series of biomechanical principles.

Basmajian strongly challenged the theories supporting the concept that active contraction of muscles maintains the longitudinal arch of the foot.[2,3] His electromyographic studies showed little or no muscular activity in the intrinsic or extrinsic muscles of the normal foot when standing at rest. The muscles tested were the tibialis anterior, the tibialis posterior, the peroneus longus, the flexor hallucis longus, the abductor hallucis, and the flexor digitorum brevis. These muscles showed no electrical activity in reaction to loads that actually surpassed those normally applied to the static plantigrade foot. These observations support the concept that in a strong foot, muscles are primarily used to maintain balance, to adjust the foot to uneven ground, and to propel the body. In a structurally weak foot, it is probable that muscles are called upon to maintain the normal shape of the foot at rest.

Many authors have felt that planovalgus feet do not have normal bony architecture and ligamentous supports. Jack felt that the medial longitudinal arch of the foot depended upon the intrinsic structure of the bones, the joints, and the integrity of the plantar ligaments.[31] He agreed with Basmajian that muscles were concerned solely with balance and with protecting the ligaments from abnormal stress. He also believed that the musculature of the foot can lift a sagging arch temporarily, but cannot constantly maintain an arch that has a ligamentous or bony defect. Butte agreed that the shape of the bones and the strong ligaments that bind them together and limit motion determine the integrity of the normal transverse and longitudinal arches of the foot.[8]

THE BONES AND LIGAMENTS

THE BONES    Others have felt that the bones themselves are mainly responsible for the planovalgus deformity. Harris and Beath believed that the function of the foot and its shape under the stress of weight bearing depended chiefly upon the design and configuration of the tarsal bones and their position relative to each other.[26] They stated that the strong foot is one in which the tarsal bones are so well articulated with each other that they bear the weight of the body without appreciable movement between them. Gleich, Lord, and Chambers concluded that the altered relationships between the calcaneus and the talus were important in the cause of the flatfoot and that excessive forefoot abduction resulted in flattening of the longitudinal arch, thereby stretching the ligaments as a secondary rather than primary cause.[10,21,40]

*Pathomechanics*    From the foregoing discussion, it is reasonable to conclude that the structural and functional characteristics of the flexible flatfoot are determined by the integral relationship of the osseous architecture of the foot, the relative strength of supporting ligamentous and capsular structures, the muscle balance about the foot, and the functional stress brought to bear about the foot. Inman states that with eversion of the heel, all articulations in the midfoot become unlocked, and maximum motion occurs in the talonavicular and calcaneocuboid joint.[30] Conversely, if the heel is inverted, the foot is then converted to a more rigid structure. Therefore, the everted foot is mechanically less stable than the inverted foot.

In the planovalgus deformity, the patient presumably tends to shift the body weight medially, as mentioned earlier; this shift, it is postulated, places excessive stress on the ligaments that support the longitudinal arch. This alters the normal pattern, in which the lateral border of the foot and the first and the fifth metatarsal heads bear weight more or less equally. Tachdjian feels that this medial shift in weight bearing, rather than the flatness of the longitudinal arch, produces foot strain and symptoms.[62]

In the flexible flatfoot, the talar head loses its support because the calcaneus assumes a more valgus position; therefore, the talus becomes more vertically disposed, and the longitudinal arch consequently flattens. With this combination of the flattened longitudinal arch and valgus deformity of the heel, the Achilles tendon is shortened and acquires an evertor action that accentuates or contributes to the overall deformity. It is also believed that some associated factors, such as genu valgum and obesity, can increase the gravity of the deformity.

Although it is difficult to summarize these concepts and to discuss them all adequately, certain consistent features continue to surface. At the present state of our knowledge, the following conclusions appear justified: (1) In flexible flatfoot, the plantar ligamentous structures that bind the tarsal and metatarsal bones together must be excessively lax, (2) an asymptomatic flatfoot that has normal muscle strength does not require any treatment in the form of muscle transfers; (3) abnormal bone configuration most likely is a late, adaptive change and not a primary causal deformity; and (4) any surgical treatment program therefore must be directed towards some form of joint stabilization and ligament reconstruction rather than a muscle-balancing or transfer operation. Thus, whether heelcord lengthening, muscle and tendon advancements, or transfers are necessary seem to be optional and highly individualized issues.

The term planovalgus describes a foot in which the medial longitudinal arch has lost height and the hindfoot assumes a valgus or pronated orientation upon weight bearing (Fig. 6-1). Also, the forefoot is abducted. This, coupled with the valgus of the heel, results in the loss of

*Clinical Features*

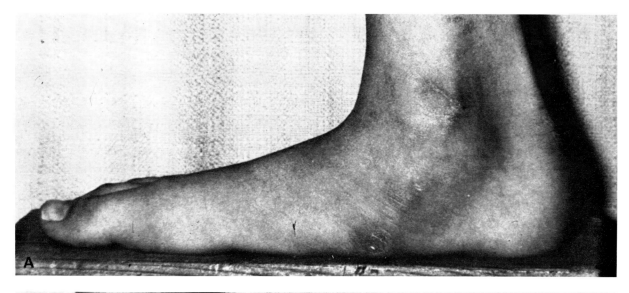

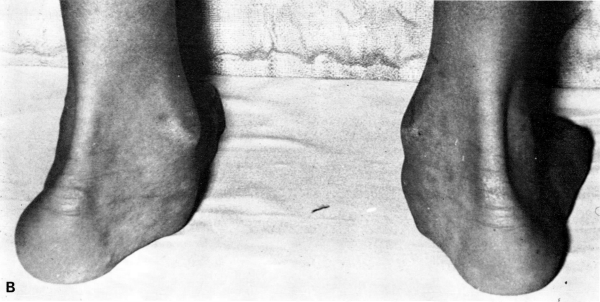

FIG. 6-1. Standing photographs show an example of severe flexible planovalgus feet. **A,** Note absence of the longitudinal arch and callosities over the medial aspect of the foot. **B,** The posterior view shows the marked valgus of the hindfoot and the fullness of the medial plantar aspects of both feet.

the longitudinal arch, and upon weight bearing, the center of gravity ultimately comes to lie directly over or medial to the first metatarsal. When not bearing weight and in repose, these feet have a normal contour and a normal longitudinal arch. Subtalar motion is normal or may even be increased. The condition is often associated with generalized ligamentous laxity, and many authors feel it is often a familial trait.

The term "pronated" foot is probably neither accurate nor appropriate for this condition. This is because, with the heel in *valgus* upon weight bearing, the lateral side of the forefoot cannot be in contact with the ground unless the forefoot *supinates* to some degree in relationship to the hindfoot. Thus, even though the hindfoot is pronated, in the flexible weight-bearing flatfoot, the forefoot is truly supinated in relation to the hindfoot.

Abduction and eversion are concomitant motions. As the calcaneus is everted, its anterior portion is displaced laterally and posteriorly with respect to the talus, resulting in loss of the normal support beneath the head of the talus. The talus thus drops into equinus and shifts anteriorly with respect to the calcaneus.

Tachdjian postulates that a child with planovalgus feet may toe-in actively in an effort to shift the body weight laterally upon weight bearing. He feels that such toeing-in may be a natural protective mechanism for the child's foot. Frequently, as the heel goes into valgus, the Achilles tendon is shortened and consequently acts to evert the hindfoot. Thus, heelcord tightness must be carefully assessed when evaluating the planovalgus foot.

## Radiographic Features

It must be emphasized that in order to be valid, roentgenograms must be made with the foot in the weight-bearing position. With planovalgus deformity, the following roentgenographic changes are noted. On the anteroposterior film, the hindfoot is in valgus, as evidenced by an increased talocalcaneal angle of Kite (Fig. 6-2).[36] If the long axis of the talus diverges more than 35° from the calcaneus, excessive heel valgus is considered to be indicated. The midtalar line passes substantially medial to the first metatarsal base. The navicular is also displaced laterally from its usual position opposite the head of the talus.

On the lateral projection, hindfoot valgus is again noted, with the talus being much more vertical than normal (Fig. 6-2). The calcaneus and the metatarsals are also more horizontal than normal because of the flattening of the longitudinal arch, which is accompanied by a sag in the normal straight line of the talus, navicular, medial cuneiform, and first metatarsal, as described by Meary.[43] This sag may occur at any one of the joints between these bones or at more than one of the joints (Fig. 6-2).

## Treatment: General Considerations

A large portion of flatfeet in young children are normal or represent a variation of normal; therefore, no treatment is warranted other than reassurance to the parents and the patient. Multiple forms of nonoperative and operative therapy have been recommended, however, for

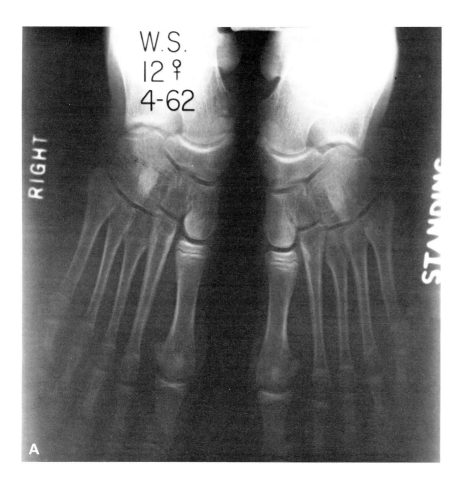

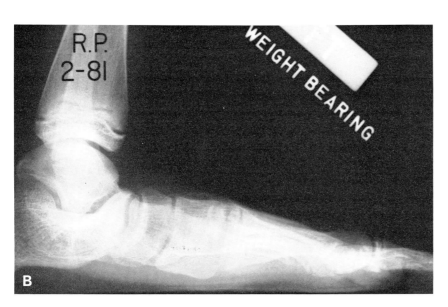

FIG. 6-2. The principal roentgenographic changes include a substantial increase in the divergent talocalcaneal angle of Kite. **A**, This patient with severe flexible flatfeet had a greatly increased divergent angle. **B**, In the lateral weight-bearing view, the talocalcaneal angle in another patient, as measured in the lateral projection, shows substantial depression of the talar head, along with clearly evident flattening of the longitudinal arch.

flexible flatfeet persisting into late childhood and adolescence and for symptomatic feet with a planovalgus deformity, especially those experiencing pain or fatigue with activity or producing rapid and uneven shoe wear.

NONOPERATIVE
TREATMENT

Those who believe that muscle weakness is an etiologic factor in this deformity have recommended various exercise programs designed to strengthen the musculature of the foot and ankle. Bettman stated that, phylogenetically, the human foot was intended to be a gripping organ and that properly functioning muscles would prevent the lowering and sagging of the arch.[4] He believed that "in the treatment of flatfoot, exercise is of equal importance with, if not more important than, mechanical supports" and developed several ingenious devices to be used in his recommended exercise program. Chandler recommended exercises for toe flexor strengthening and heelcord stretching.[11] Hoke and Zadek each recommended exercises as valuable adjuncts to other conservative treatment programs.[29,66]

As noted earlier, many investigators do not believe that weak muscles play a role in flexible flatfeet and therefore do not include exercises as part of their treatment program. More specifically, Tachdjian, Lowman, and Milch believed that exercises are therapeutically futile;[42,44,62] I tend to agree with them. Not only are exercises ineffective, but children rarely do them consistently or effectively.

More commonly prescribed conservative, nonoperative treatment includes a wide variety of corrective shoes, arch supports, and heel inserts designed to hold the foot in a corrected position. Shoe modifications in vogue at present include built-up arch supports, scaphoid pads, medial heel and sole wedges, extended medial heel counters, and below-knee braces with medial T-straps. The purpose of medial heel and sole wedges supposedly is to tilt the calcaneus out of valgus, a mechanism that conceptually would indirectly improve the longitudinal arch. Rose and Helfet did not believe that arch supports or scaphoid pads help correct the deformity, and Helfet even believed that the institution of shoe modifications in children increased the likelihood of symptoms occurring later in life when the modifications were discontinued.[27,52]

Shoe modifications that hold the foot in a corrected position rely on a strong shoe in which the uprights of the heel must grasp the calcaneus snugly; otherwise, the heel will simply twist into eversion. To overcome this problem, several shoe inserts have been devised to hold the foot in the desired position. Among these are the Whitman plate, the Schwartz meniscus, the Helfet cup, and the UCB insert (Fig. 6-3). These inserts have several advantages over prescribed shoe modifications because they are rigid and custom made and in most instances can be transferred from one shoe to another.

Bleck studied 2000 feet in 1000 children who ranged in age from 6 months to 16 years.[5] The studies included standing anteroposterior and lateral roentgenograms of the feet, standing molds of the feet constructed from polyfoam plastic, and similar plastic molds of the

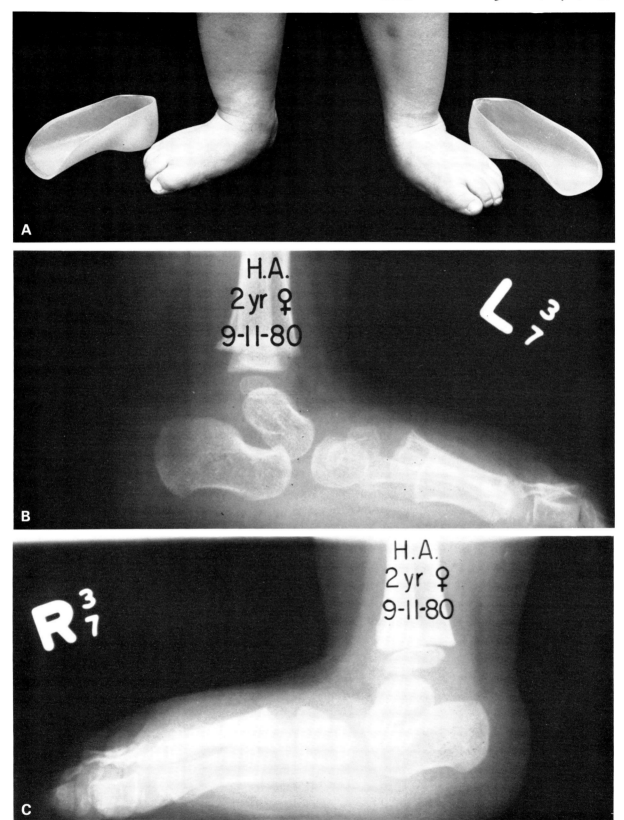

FIG. 6-3. An example of severe, flexible planovalgus feet with a plantarflexed talus is seen in this 2-year-old girl. These feet were completely correctable passively, and lateral roentgenograms confirmed correction. Normal ranges of motion and muscle strength were present. **A,** The clinical appearance of the feet, with the UCB custom-made insert. **B** and **C,** Lateral standing roentgenograms. The UCB splint is used to support the foot and to prevent shoe breakdown.

children's shoe outlines. After a thorough analysis of the results, he concluded that "prescribing special shoes has, for the most part, been based upon unobjective data." On the other hand, Bleck and Berzins believed that the Helfet heel cup and the UCB shoe insert both improved the clinical and radiographic appearance of the foot when the plantarflexed angle of the talus in the weight-bearing position exceeded 35 to 45°.[6]

Staheli and Giffin polled orthopedic surgeons, pediatricians, and pediatric orthopedists and found that a large number of "corrective" shoes were still being prescribed, but that such prescriptions had little scientific basis.[60] They further concluded that shoe modifications are "rarely appropriate." In an earlier publication, Staheli felt that greater effort should be exercised in educating parents than in prescribing expensive corrective shoes for children with otherwise normal flexible flatfeet.[59]

Unquestionably, the prescription of shoe modifications or inserts for the nonoperative treatment of the asymptomatic flexible flatfoot in children has been based largely upon the arbitrary concept that a sagging longitudinal arch in a growing foot deserves some form of mechanical support. No reliable control studies have been done to show that such modifications or inserts influence the ultimate adult configuration in such feet. As previously mentioned, Bleck and Staheli have already studied this issue in depth, and at the present state of the art and science, no scientific proof has been offered to support the value of these devices in the *asymptomatic* flexible flatfoot that has (a) a normal configuration (arch) in repose, (b) normal function or muscle power, and (c) normal ankle dorsiflexion. This is *not* to say that such prescriptions are necessarily wrong, only that their therapeutic value remains unproven.

OPERATIVE TREATMENT A small minority of patients with symptomatic planovalgus foot deformity fail to respond to the conservative measures just described and, because of continued pain or dissatisfaction with shoe prescriptions, eventually request surgical correction. Although it is obviously difficult to establish firm guidelines, most would agree with the following indications for surgical treatment: (1) pain and/or fatigue sufficient to prevent the patient from taking part in normal activities and failure to respond to nonoperative measures, and (2) deformity so great that it causes rapid, abnormal shoe wear.

A multitude of surgical procedures have been proposed for the treatment of the flexible flatfoot. They can be divided into three categories: (a) soft-tissue procedures, (b) bone and joint procedures, and (c) operations on the bones, joints, and soft tissues. Many of those described in the following sections have been discarded and are mentioned mostly for historical interest.

SOFT-TISSUE PROCEDURES. Phelps divided, shortened, and plicated all of the soft structures on the medial side of the foot, a procedure similar in reverse to the medial release operation performed for clubfoot.[53]

Muller proposed drawing the tendon of the anterior tibial through a canal created in the scaphoid in order to elevate the arch.[47] Legg subsequently suggested a modification of this procedure.[38] Ryerson transferred both peroneals dorsally into the first cuneiform.[56] Fisher proposed a free graft of the peroneal tendons from the navicular to the tibia.[19] The operation was designed to provide a check-rein to support the longitudinal arch (tenodesis).

Roberts recommended transplanting the extensor hallucis longus to the tibialis anterior, a procedure intended to strengthen its supposed action of elevating the arch.[54] Gocht advocated medialization of the Achilles tendon in order to improve its inverting or varus-producing effect upon the os calcis.[13] Numerous authors have lengthened the Achilles tendon, either alone or in combination with other procedures. The results of all of these soft-tissue procedures performed in the absence of concomitant bony operations have been highly variable, largely reflecting the fact that the exact etiology and pathology of flexible flatfoot is not yet established.

BONE AND JOINT PROCEDURES. Even more numerous procedures on the bones and joints have been developed for the treatment of symptomatic flexible flatfoot. Some have operated primarily on the hindfoot valgus and some on the bones comprising the medial longitudinal arch. Gleich performed an oblique osteotomy of the os calcis and displaced the posterior fragment forward, medially, and downward in an attempt to restore the normal angle between the os calcis and the floor. Dwyer performed a laterally based opening-wedge osteotomy of the calcaneus and inserted a tibial graft in the outer side of the calcaneus.[17] Koutsogiannis reported improvement in 17 of 19 patients using a simple calcaneal osteotomy designed to improve the shape of the foot and to prevent abnormal shoe wear.[37] It consisted of an osteotomy of the os calcis and medial displacement of the posterior fragment to restore normal weight bearing.

Armstrong suggested elongating the lateral column of the foot, just the reverse of the procedure used by Evans and Lichtblau to treat residual equinovarus deformity.[1,18,39] Armstrong's procedure consisted of a wedge osteotomy of the calcaneus just proximal to the calcaneocuboid joint. Perthes advocated a closing-wedge osteotomy of the scaphoid, the wedge of bone being inserted into an opening-wedge osteotomy in the os calcis.[52] This combination of procedures was designed to elongate the lateral border of the foot and to shorten the medial border. Trendelenburg believed erroneously that the major problem was in the ankle and recommended a supramalleolar osteotomy designed to tilt the ankle into varus.[63]

More extensive bone operations *of historical interest* include the following. Golding-Bird completely excised the navicular.[23] Davy carried this a step further and removed the head of the talus in addition to the navicular.[14] Stokes recommended a closing-wedge osteotomy of the head and neck of the talus.[61] Weinlechner even performed a talectomy to correct flatfoot.[64] Ogston performed a talonavicular fusion after resecting the head of the talus.[50] Ogilvy and Soule also recommended arthrodesis of the talonavicular joint.[49,58]

Clark advocated a closing-wedge osteotomy of the neck of the talus to correct the abduction of the foot, combined with a closing-wedge osteotomy of the bone and cartilage from the inferior talus to correct hindfoot pronation.[12] He avoided a subtalar fusion by leaving the cartilage of the facets of the calcaneus undisturbed. Wilms took a wedge of bone from the head of the talus and used it in an opening-wedge fusion of the calcaneocuboid joint, at the same time fusing the talonavicular joint.[65] Almost exclusively, these operations have become obsolete in recent years.

Hoke believed that the naviculocuneiform and the internal-middle cuneiform joints had the greatest abnormal joint laxity and that this interfered with the arch-lifting power of the posterior tibial, anterior tibial, and flexor hallucis longus tendons.[29] He therefore recommended arthrodesis of the navicular to the first and second cuneiforms in order to increase the lever arm of these muscles, combining this fusion with lengthening of the Achilles tendon. Hoke initially reported good results, but Butte's later follow-up revealed deterioration in the ultimate functional results, with 50% rated as either fair or poor.[8]

Operations on the subtalar joint have included both an intra-articular arthrodesis in older children and adolescents and an extra-articular arthrodesis of the subtalar joint for young, immature patients with *paralytic* flatfeet. In the past, many surgeons attempted this procedure as a direct surgical method of treating *idiopathic* planovalgus in young children. Fortunately, this practice was rapidly abandoned. It is important to emphasize this issue because, if one accepts the fact that the great majority of nonparalytic, flexible flatfeet in children never require surgical correction, such a *major* procedure that eradicates the major hindfoot articulation (the subtalar joint) should be viewed with great caution.

Grice felt that in older children with flexible flatfeet, the most successful procedure for correction of the severe flatfoot deformity was a triple arthrodesis in which appropriate wedges are resected to correct the deformity.[24] Most surgeons now reserve the triple arthrodesis only for symptomatic, rigid flatfeet (see later section on triple arthrodesis for rigid flatfoot), preferring to use some form of reconstructive procedure for the flexible flatfoot. (These arthrodesing procedures are described in Chapter 7.)

OPERATIONS ON BONES, JOINTS, AND SOFT TISSUES.   Several procedures have been devised that combine both soft-tissue and bone operations to correct the flatfoot deformity. Schede tightened the medial ligaments, in addition to performing a talonavicular arthrodesis.[57] Giannestras advocated a naviculocuneiform fusion, with advancement of a fascial sling coupled with transposition of the tendons of the tibialis anterior and tibialis posterior into the plantar surface of the navicular.[20]

The best known and most effective variations of these procedures that have surfaced recently are the Miller, the "Scottish Rite," and the Durham procedures.[16,41,45] These three, in addition to the Kidner procedure,[35] are those I consider most appropriate for the surgical treatment of a symptomatic flexible flatfoot; they are described and illustrated in the following sections.

*The Miller Flatfoot Operation.* Miller proposed fusion of the naviculo-cuneiform and the cuneiform-first metatarsal joints, combined with shortening and capsulorrhaphy of the medial joint capsules.[45] He used a proximally based flap of the posterior tibial tendon, its accompanying fascia and capsule, and osteoperiosteal slivers of the navicular and medial cuneiform bone, which are advanced distally (Fig. 6-4). The details of the procedure are described as follows.

An incision is made over the medial aspect of the foot, extending from the head of the talus to the base of the first metatarsal. The insertion of the posterior tibial tendon is exposed, and an osteoperiosteal flap of this tendon, along with its ligamentous attachments, is elevated. Beginning at the base of the first metatarsal where the tendon is sectioned transversely, an osteotome is used to elevate the flap that contains thin slices of the inner surfaces of the medial cuneiform and navicular bones, along with their associated ligaments and periosteum. The distal portion of the anterior tibial tendon must be protected in the dissection.

The osteoperiosteal flap is reflected proximally beneath the anterior tibial tendon. The articular cartilage and subchondral bone of the naviculocuneiform and cuneiform-first metatarsal joints are excised, and the underlying bone is roughened with a gouge to create an appropriate bed for fusion of these joints. The heelcord is lengthened if indicated, and the osteoperiosteal flap is then advanced beneath the anterior tibial tendon so that the thin slices of the navicular and medial cuneiform bones span the underlying joints that were prepared for fusion.

I depart from this procedure in that I prefer to leave the cuneiform-first metatarsal joint undisturbed, and I use a staple or a transfixion-threaded wire (Fig. 6-5); more recently I have used a small-fragment compression cancellous screw to stabilize the naviculocuneiform joint. Otherwise, on the rare occasions that I have performed this operation, the technique is essentially the same as that described by Miller.

The plantar and medial ligamentous structures are tightened with heavy sutures, and the wound is closed. A below-knee cast is applied with the foot and ankle held in the same position as in the Durham or Scottish-Rite operation. An example of this operation is seen in Figure 6-5.

*The Scottish-Rite Procedure.* This operation, championed by Lovell and associates, embodies certain features of the Miller procedure, deviating from it principally in two ways, namely, that only the naviculo-cuneiform joint is fused, and a dorsally based opening-wedge osteotomy of the medial cuneiform is accomplished in an effort to improve

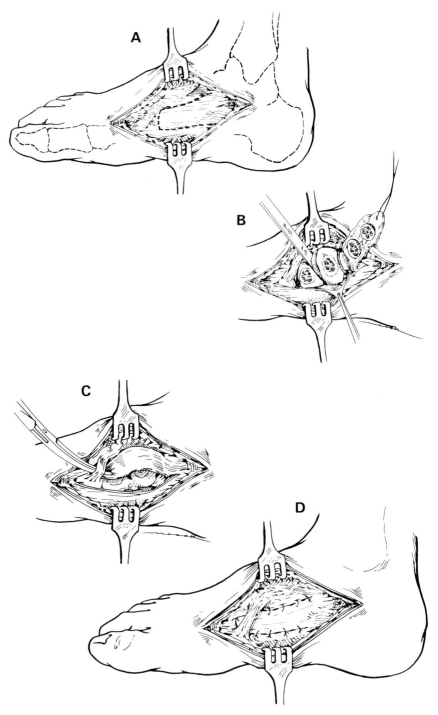

Fig. 6-4. Salient features of the Miller flatfoot plasty as originally described. The incision is the same as for the Durham or "Scottish Rite" procedure. **A,** An osteoperiosteal, proximally based flap of the posterior tibial tendon and its insertion is raised from the medial cuneiform and navicular bones, thus exposing the naviculocuneiform and cuneiform-first metatarsal joints. **B,** The cartilage from these two joints is excised, and the bony surfaces are roughened. **C,** The osteoperiosteal flap is then advanced distally beneath the anterior tibial tendon, so that the osseous portions of the flap bridge the two joints to be fused. **D,** The flap is then sutured to the surrounding deep fascia and periosteum. I prefer a modification of the operation, in which only the naviculocuneiform joint is fused, using internal (staple or screw) fixation.

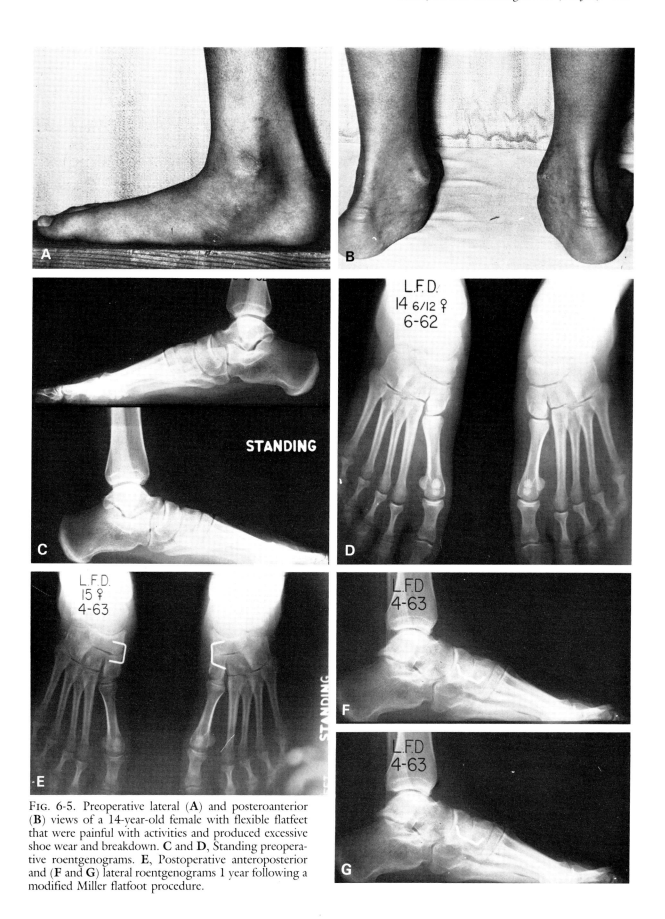

FIG. 6-5. Preoperative lateral (**A**) and posteroanterior (**B**) views of a 14-year-old female with flexible flatfeet that were painful with activities and produced excessive shoe wear and breakdown. **C** and **D**, Standing preoperative roentgenograms. **E**, Postoperative anteroposterior and (**F** and **G**) lateral roentgenograms 1 year following a modified Miller flatfoot procedure.

the height of the longitudinal arch.[41] The details of the procedure are described as follows and illustrated in Figure 6-6.

The incision is the same as that employed in the Miller and Durham procedures (see Figs. 6-4 and 6-8). The insertion of the posterior tibial tendon is exposed from the navicular tuberosity distally to the insertion of the anterior tibial tendon on the medial cuneiform bone. An osteoperiosteal flap, $\frac{1}{2}$ inch wide, is raised extending from the navicular tuberosity to the cuneiform, thus exposing the naviculocuneiform joint. The flap is sectioned near the anterior tibial tendon insertion and reflected proximally. In the process, the tuberosity of the navicular is excised and saved in order to serve as a graft for the cuneiform osteotomy. The articular cartilages and subchondral bone are then removed from the surfaces of the naviculocuneiform joint.

Next, the naviculocuneiform joint is transfixed with a threaded wire or small-fragment cancellous screw. The osteotomy in the medial cuneiform is opened up dorsally in an effort to elevate the longitudinal arch, and the bone taken from the tuberosity is impacted into the opening. The osteoperiosteal flap is then advanced distal to the anterior tibial tendon and in a more plantar location and is sutured to the surrounding ligaments and remaining portion of the intact posterior tibial tendon insertion. The hindfoot should be held in supination, and the forefoot should be slightly plantarflexed (pronated) in order to elevate the longitudinal arch.

The plantar calcaneonavicular (spring) ligament and the plantar insertion of the posterior tibial tendon are then sutured into the osteoperiosteal flap in order to strengthen the support of the talar head. If necessary, Lovell has suggested that the heelcord may be lengthened cautiously. Clinical judgment is necessary for this determination. The wound is closed and a below-knee cast applied, with the hindfoot held in slight varus and equinus and the forefoot mildly plantarflexed. This position is just the opposite of that employed to correct the cavovarus foot (see Chapter 4). The initial cast is a nonwalking cast and is kept on for 6 weeks. It is then changed to a walking cast, which remains for an additional 6 weeks, for a total period of 12 weeks of cast immobilization. An example of the results of this procedure is seen in Figure 6-7.

*The Durham Flatfoot Operation.* Of the procedures described previously, those that have been performed most commonly to correct symptomatic flexible flatfoot at the Intermountain Unit of the Shriners Hospital are the Durham and the Miller flatfoot plasties. The Durham procedure was reported initially by Caldwell in 1953.[9] In our maximum, 26-year follow-up study of 17 children in whom 33 feet were operated on, 95% had good to excellent results. It must be emphasized that all of these children were selected for the operation because they continued to have painful symptoms despite all nonoperative and conservative efforts or because their deformity was so great that normal, everyday weight bearing caused excessive shoe wear and breakdown.

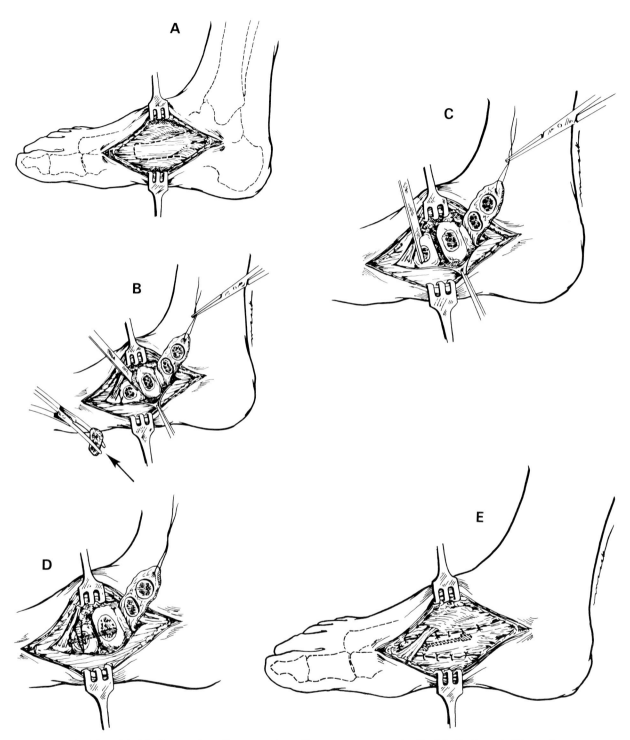

FIG. 6-6. The "Scottish Rite" procedure for correction of severe, symptomatic, flexible flatfoot. **A,** Through a generous curvilinear incision that parallels the course of the posterior tibial tendon, an osteoperiosteal flap of the insertion of that tendon is outlined. **B,** Utilizing a curved flat osteotome, this osteoperiosteal flap is elevated in distal-to-proximal fashion, with the base of the flap being attached to the distal end of the talus. In the process, a generous portion of the medial tuberosity of the navicular is excised (arrow). The articular cartilages are removed from the naviculocuneiform joint. **C,** An opening-wedge osteotomy of the medial cuneiform is then accomplished. **D,** The fragment of bone removed from the navicular is fashioned so as to fit into the opening osteotomy of the cuneiform, and a compression screw is placed across the osteotomy and into the navicular bone. **E,** The osteoperiosteal flap is then advanced distally beneath the insertion of the anterior tibial tendon, and the plantar calcaneonavicular ligament is advanced and tightly secured to the advanced tendon.

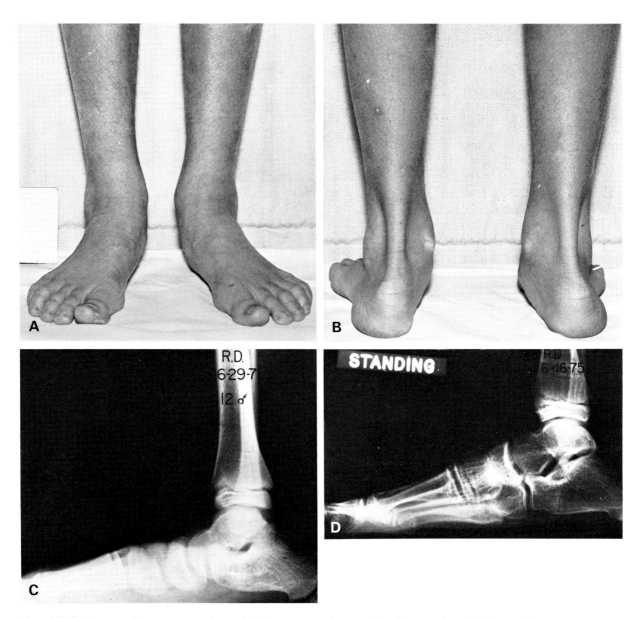

FIG. 6-7. **A,** Preoperative anteroposterior and (**B**) posteroanterior standing photographs and (**C**) standing roentgenogram. Note the impressive sag of both the talonavicular and naviculocuneiform joints. **D,** The postoperative lateral standing film demonstrates full correction of the foot and a solid naviculocuneiform fusion following a "Scottish Rite" flatfoot plasty. (Courtesy of Dr. Wood W. Lovell, Atlanta, Georgia.)

In 1935, Durham devised this procedure to correct the symptomatic "severe, third-degree" flatfoot. He cautioned that the operation was *not* designed to correct the rigid or spastic flatfoot. Caldwell also emphasized that the foot must be flexible and that muscle power must be normal for this procedure to succeed. He further felt that the ideal age for the procedure was between 10 and 14 years of age. Caldwell further proposed that the heelcord be lengthened between 4 and 6 weeks prior to performing the flatfoot operation if the ankle could not be dorsiflexed "with ease" to 95° with the foot held inverted. This flatfoot procedure is described as follows and illustrated in Figure 6-8.

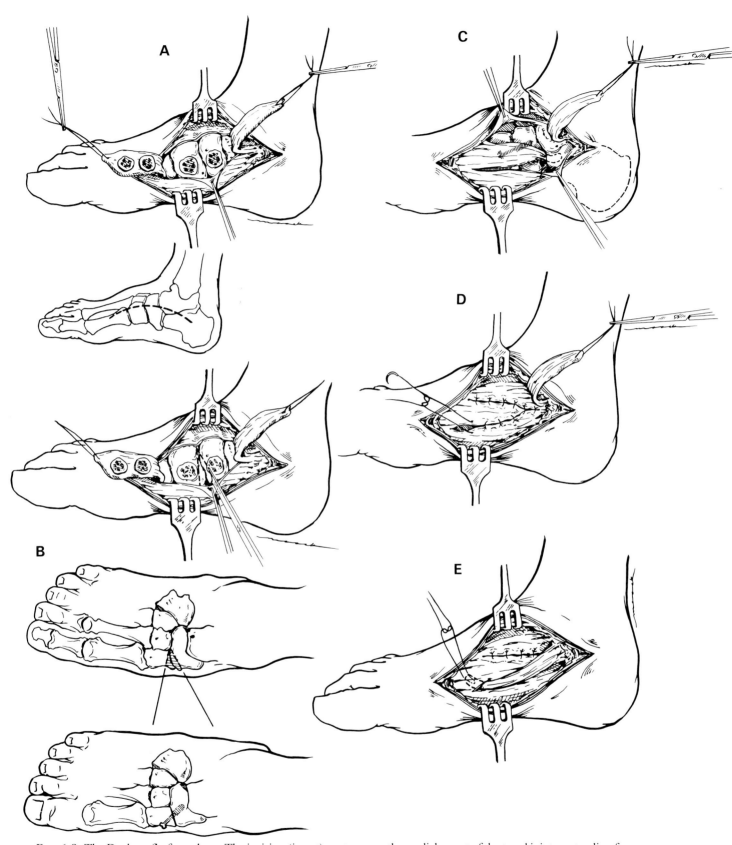

FIG. 6-8. The Durham flatfoot plasty. The incision (insert) centers over the medial aspect of the tarsal joints, extending from the region of the sustentaculum tali to the base of the first metatarsal. **A**, The incision is deepened, exposing the posterior tibial insertion. This tendon is detached from its distal insertion and reflected proximally. An osteoperiosteal flap, with its base attached distally, is developed over the navicular and cuneiform bones. **B**, The articular surfaces of the naviculo-cuneiform joint are excised with appropriate wedges of underlying bone, and the raw bone surfaces of this joint are firmly opposed and held by a compression lag screw or similar device. **C**, The osteoperiosteal flap is then sutured proximally under the plantar surface of the sustentaculum tali. **D**, The remaining deep fascia is sutured to this flap, and (**E**) the posterior tibial tendon is advanced and sutured under tension into the plantar surface of the navicular.

The incision is the same as for the Scottish-Rite or Miller procedure. Thereafter, five essential steps are followed. First, the posterior tibial tendon is sectioned at its insertion into the navicular. Second, a ligamentous flap is raised from the medial and plantar aspects of the foot, beginning at the navicular and with the base of the flap located distally at the base of the first metatarsal. Third, a naviculocuneiform arthrodesis is accomplished. Fourth, the ligamentous flap is inserted into the sustentaculum tali, and finally, the posterior tibial tendon is reattached to its insertion on the navicular bone.

Although all features of the operation are important, Caldwell feels that the most difficult and critical step is the insertion of the ligamentous flap into the sustentaculum tali. This flap, when pulled taut into this location, re-establishes the longitudinal arch and reinforces the plantar calcaneonavicular (spring) ligament. The surrounding ligamentous structures are firmly sutured to this flap, and the posterior tibial tendon is advanced into a prepared bed on the plantar aspect of the navicular.

The naviculocuneiform fusion done previously is stabilized either by an inlay graft or by a transfixion-threaded pin or small-fragment screw (my preference). After wound closure, a below-knee cast is applied. The position of the foot and the postoperative care are the same as for the Miller and Scottish-Rite procedures. Figure 6-9 shows a patient who has undergone this procedure.

*The Kidner Procedure.* Some young, preadolescent children have a flexible flatfoot with an accessory navicular bone. This ossicle is located within the substance of the posterior tibial tendon where the tendon usually inserts into the navicular bone. Kidner proposed that the attachment of the posterior tibial tendon to the abnormal accessory bone interfered with the normal insertion of the tendon on the plantar aspect of the navicular and thus vitiated the strength of the posterior tibial tendon in its support of the longitudinal arch.[35] In addition, the accessory navicular (called prehallux) creates an abnormal prominence over the medial side of the foot, often resulting in tenderness due to pressure, and in the development of a bursa over the prominence.

In some instances, weight bearing causes pain owing to the traction effect exerted upon the mobile, accessory bone. The combination of a sagging longitudinal arch, tenderness, and pain upon weight bearing led Kidner to devise an operation that could solve all three problems. Thus, the accessory ossicle is removed and the posterior tibial tendon is rerouted into a more plantar position, as described in the following. It should be emphasized that this operation should be reserved only for those young patients under 10 to 12 years who have flexible flatfeet and whose symptoms justify the procedure.

The incision is made over the medial aspect of the joint, centering over the prominence created by the accessory navicular. It should extend from the medial malleolus as far distally as the first metatarsal so as to expose the entire plantar and medial course of the posterior tibial tendon (Fig. 6-10). The tendon is freed up from its attachments to the

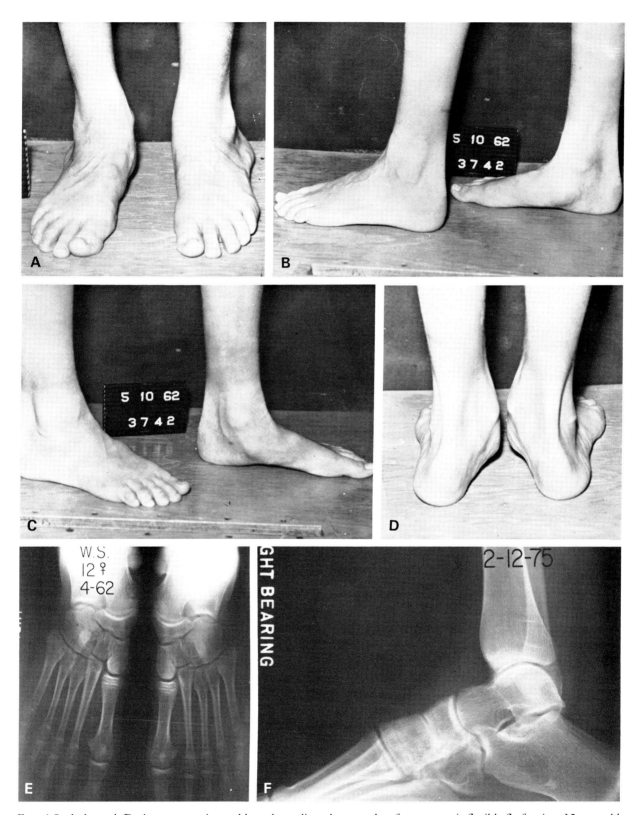

Fig. 6-9. **A** through **D**, Anteroposterior and lateral standing photographs of symptomatic flexible flatfeet in a 12-year-old girl. **E**, Note the widely divergent talocalcaneal angle and the abducted midfoot and forefoot seen in the anteroposterior roentgenogram. Because of painful symptoms and unsightly shoe wear, she underwent a Durham flatfoot operation. **F** through **K**, The photographic and radiographic appearances of the feet 13 and 18 years later.

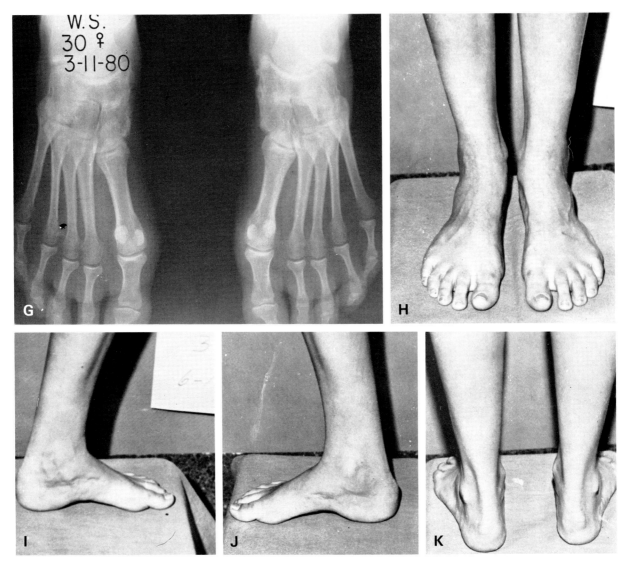

FIG. 6-9. *continued*

accessory navicular, the navicular, and the first cuneiform, but its attachment to the proximal aspect of the first metatarsal must be carefully preserved. This is necessary so that the freed-up portion of the posterior tibial tendon can be translocated underneath the navicular and sutured to the capsule and soft tissues of the plantar aspect of the navicular.

A groove in the undersurface of the navicular can be created in order to retain the translocated tendon in a more stable position. The medial, projecting portion of the navicular should also be excised so that it is flush with the head of the talus and the medial cuneiform. As the sutures are tied, the tendon is placed under slight tension, the hindfoot is held in mild varus, and the forefoot is held in slight *pronation* in order to elevate the longitudinal arch. The translocated tendon then not only reinforces the plantar calcaneonavicular (spring) ligament, but also provides dynamic support to the arch. A below-knee cast is applied with the foot held *as described previously*.

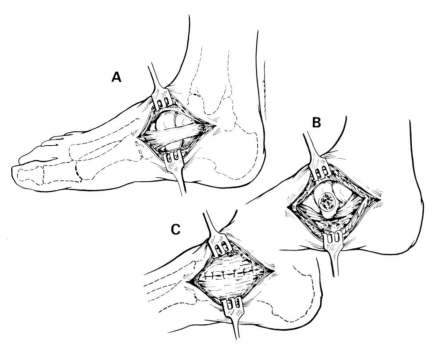

Fig. 6-10. Kidner method of treating flexible flatfoot. Usually there is an accessory navicular bone that must be excised in the process of translocating the posterior tibial tendon beneath the head of the talus and the talonavicular joint. **A,** Through a generous incision, centering over the posterior tibial tendon as it inserts into the navicular bone and also into the metatarsocuneiform joint, this tendon is identified and freed up from its soft-tissue attachments. **B,** Leaving its distal insertion undisturbed, the tendon is translocated beneath the head of the talus and talonavicular joint. It is sutured to the plantar surface by means of several well placed nonabsorbable sutures. **C,** The deep fascia is then closed over the tendon translocation, and a below-knee cast is applied.

## Rigid Planovalgus Foot

Not all severe flatfeet are flexible. A small number of flatfeet, occurring predominantly in adolescents, are substantially rigid and in many instances symptomatic. The patients either have symptoms of pain or fatigue or complain of great difficulty in shoe fitting and rapid shoe wear. These feet, although relatively rigid, have no tarsal coalition (see Chapter 9); no other obvious cause for their lack of flexibility is present except for a longstanding planovalgus deformity that has resulted in adaptive bone, joint, and soft-tissue changes sufficient to produce a rigid deformity (Fig. 6-11). Because these feet are rigid and not passively correctable, they do not qualify for any of the nonoperative or operative types of treatment described so far in this chapter.

The operative treatment of the rigid, symptomatic flatfoot in this adolescent age group can only consist of one procedure, namely, a corrective triple arthrodesis. This foot deformity is not easy to correct, and the triple arthrodesis requires a special kind of technique. In my experience, it is not technically feasible to correct this rigid deformity satisfactorily through one incision. In order to correct the *planovalgus* component of the forefoot and midfoot, two incisions are necessary. My preferred technique is described as follows and demonstrated in Figure 6-12.

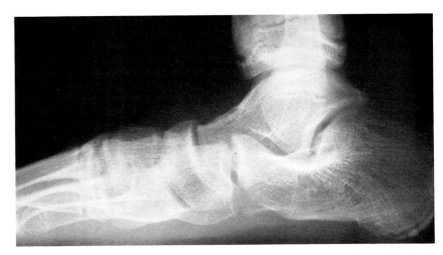

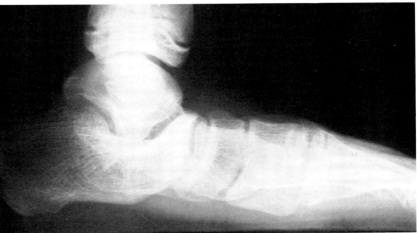

FIG. 6-11. Lateral standing roentgenograms of a 14-year-old male with rigid, painful flatfeet that, because of their lack of flexibility, are not candidates for flatfoot plasties as described in Figures 6-4, 6-7, and 6-9. The only predictable procedure for this kind of foot is triple arthrodesis (see Figure 6-12).

## TRIPLE ARTHRODESIS FOR RIGID FLATFOOT

In order to properly correct the abduction of the midfoot and forefoot and the talonavicular sag in the longitudinal arch, a medial incision is necessary, in addition to the conventional lateral incision made over the sinus tarsus in routine triple arthrodeses. The first incision is made over the sinus tarsus, and the calcaneocuboid, subtalar, and talonavicular joints are appropriately exposed. In this rigid foot deformity, the talonavicular joint is encountered much more medially than usual. The articular surfaces and appropriate bony wedges are removed from the calcaneocuboid and subtalar joints.

A medial incision is then made over the talonavicular joint, extending from the medial malleolus to the naviculocuneiform joint. The talonavicular joint is exposed, and a generous, wedge-shaped excision of this joint is made. The segment of bone and cartilage must be appropriately excised so as to correct the abduction of the forefoot and midfoot as well as the flattened longitudinal arch; it is therefore somewhat of a biplane wedge. Thus, the forefoot and midfoot must be

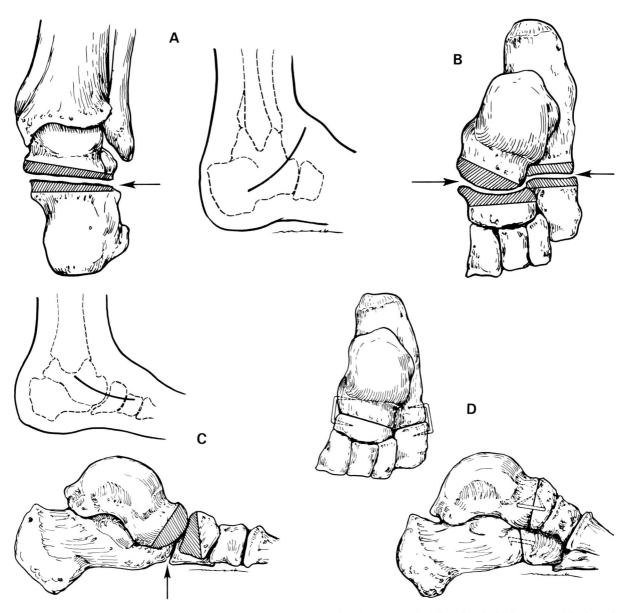

FIG. 6-12. Two incisions are required to correct a severe, rigid flatfoot by means of triple arthrodesis. **A** (Insert), The lateral incision permits evacuation of the sinus tarsus and exposure of the calcaneocuboid and subtalar joints. The talonavicular joint is difficult to expose properly through this incision in a rigid flatfoot. **A** and **B** show the configurations of the wedges removed from the calcaneocuboid and subtalar joints through the lateral exposure. **C** (Insert), The medial incision exposes the posterior tibial tendon, which overlies the talonavicular joint. The posterior tibial tendon is split, and the talonavicular joint can be easily exposed. The biplane wedges of the joint that are removed are depicted in **B** and **C**. **D**, The raw bone surfaces exposed by the arthrectomies just described are then firmly opposed and held in the corrected position by some form of internal fixation (staples) or transfixion.

adducted, plantarflexed, and pronated at the talonavicular joint in order to achieve correction. A staple or some other internal fixation device is then inserted across the talonavicular joint to maintain correction.

Attention is then turned to the lateral incision, where the raw bony surfaces of the calcaneocuboid joint must be properly opposed and similarly transfixed. Usually, the denuded surfaces of the subtalar joint will fall into contact with each other once the talonavicular and calcaneocuboid joints are properly reduced and internally fixed. Once the denuded joint surfaces have been apposed satisfactorily and fixed properly, and the foot has been adequately corrected, the wounds are closed, and an above-knee cast is applied. The routine postoperative care for triple arthrodesis consists of an above-knee cast for 3 to 6 weeks, followed by a below-knee walking cast for an additional 6 weeks. An example of a case of a rigid flatfoot treated in this manner is seen in Figure 6-13.

In summary, a defensible approach to the care of the child or adolescent with flexible flatfoot requires that one answer and place into proper perspective the following questions: (a) Is it possible to accurately quantitate what constitutes a flexible flatfoot? (b) Can any type of device alter the growth, development, or final adult configuration of a flexible flatfoot? (c) How much pain or shoe deformation can or should be tolerated? (d) Which surgical procedure can correct the flexible flatfoot most appropriately? (e) Are the results of such surgical correction so uniformly successful that the flatfoot can be predictably improved? (f) Does the mere presence of a flexible flatfoot require treatment of any sort?

I have found it difficult to answer any of these questions convincingly, and I therefore find it almost impossible to adopt any program of treatment except one that is based on a highly individualized analysis of each factor as it relates to each patient. In so doing, I have found that surgical treatment of a nonparalytic, *asymptomatic,* flexible, idiopathic flatfoot is rarely indicated.

On the other hand, a small number of adolescent patients have severe planovalgus foot deformities that are not flexible. Such feet are usually symptomatic, and these patients nearly always require or desire surgical correction. These feet must be distinguished from rigid foot deformities due to tarsal coalition and other causes of symptomatic, rigid flatfoot (discussed in Chapter 9). These rigid feet nearly always are treated surgically through a corrective triple arthrodesis.

*References*

1. Armstrong, G.: Evans elongation of lateral column of the foot for valgus deformity. J. Bone Joint Surg., *57B*:530, 1975.
2. Basmajian, J. V., and Bentzon, J. W.: An electromyographic study of certain muscles of the leg and foot in the standing position. Surg. Gynecol. Obstet., *98*:662, 1954.
3. Basmajian, J. V., and Stecko, G.: The role of muscles in arch support of the foot. J. Bone Joint Surg., *45A*:1184, 1963.
4. Bettman, E.: The treatment of flatfoot by means of exercise. J. Bone Joint Surg., *19*:821, 1937.
5. Bleck, E. E.: The shoeing of children: Sham or science? Dev. Med. Child Neurol., *13*:188, 1971.
6. Bleck, E. E., and Berzins, U. J.: Conservative management of pes valgus with plantar flexed talus flexible. Clin. Orthop., *122*:85, 1977.
7. Blount, W. P.: *Fractures in Children.* Huntington, N.Y., Krieger, 1977, p. 185.
8. Butte, F. L.: Navicular-cuneiform arthrodesis for flat-foot. J. Bone Joint Surg., *19*:496, 1937.

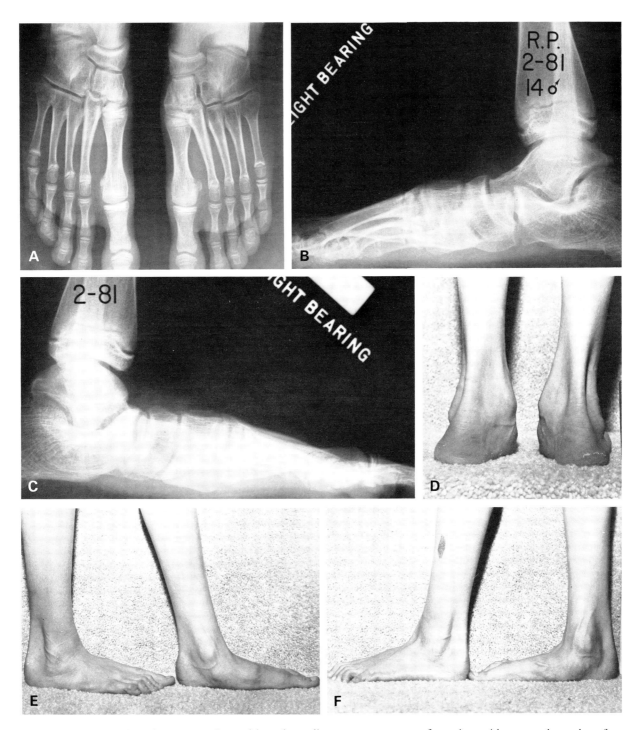

FIG. 6-13. **A**, **B**, and **C**, Anteroposterior and lateral standing roentgenograms of a patient with severe planovalgus foot deformity. **D**, **E**, and **F**, Standing preoperative photographs. These feet were painful and had undergone such extensive adaptive change that they were not flexible enough to qualify for flatfoot plasty. Thus (**G** and **H**), a corrective triple arthrodesis was done.

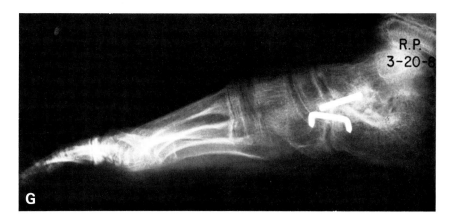

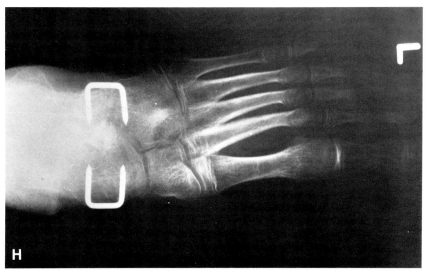

FIG. 6-13. *continued*

9. Caldwell, G. D.: Surgical correction of relaxed flatfoot by the Durham flatfoot plasty. Clin. Orthop., *2:*221, 1953.

10. Chambers, E. F. S.: An operation for the correction of flexible flatfeet of adolescents. West. J. Surg., *54:*77, 1946.

11. Chandler, F. A.: Children's feet, normal and presenting common abnormalities. Am. J. Dis. Child., *63:*1136, 1942.

12. Clark, W. A.: A rebalancing operation for pronated feet. J. Bone Joint Surg., *13:*867, 1931.

13. Crego, C. H., and Ford, L. T.: An end-result study of various operative procedures for correcting flat feet in children. J. Bone Joint Surg., *34A:*183, 1952.

14. Davy, R.: On excision of the scaphoid bone for the relief of confirmed flatfoot. Lancet, *1:*675, 1889.

15. Duchenne, G. B.: *Physiology of Motion.* Philadelphia, W. B. Saunders, 1959, p. 337.

16. Durham, H. A., cited by Caldwell, G. D.: Surgical correction of relaxed flatfoot by the Durham flatfoot plasty. Clin. Orthop., *2:*221, 1953.

17. Dwyer, F. C. (1960): Osteotomy of the calcaneum in the treatment of grossly everted feet with special reference to cerebral palsy. In "Huitieme Congres Internationale de Chirurgie Orthopedique," New York, 4–9 Septembre, 1960. Société Internationale de Chirurgie Orthopedique et de Traumatologie, p. 892. Bruxelles.

18. Evans, D.: Calcaneo-valgus deformity. J. Bone Joint Surg., *57B:*270, 1975.

19. Fisher, F. R.: Paralytic deformity of the foot. Lancet, *1:*112, 124, 214, 1889.

20. Giannestras, N. J.: *Foot Disorders—Medical and Surgical Management.* 2nd Edition. Philadelphia, Lea & Febiger, 1973, p. 139.

21. Gleich, A.: Beitrag Zur Operativen Plattfussbehandlung. Arch. Klin. Chir., *46:*358, 1893.

22. Gocht, H.: Schenenoperation beim Pes plano-valgus. Z. Orthop. Chir., *14:*693, 1905.

23. Golding-Bird, C. H.: Operations on the tarsus in confirmed flatfoot. Lancet, *1:*677, 1889.

24. Grice, D. S.: An extra-articular arthrodesis of the subastragalar joint for correction of paralytic flat feet in children. J. Bone Joint Surg., *34A:*927, 1952.

25. Haraldsson, S.: Pes plano-valgus staticus juvenilis and its operative treatment. Acta Orthop. Scand., *35:*234, 1964–65.

26. Harris, R. I., and Beath, T.: Hypermobile flatfoot with short tendon Achilles. J. Bone Joint Surg., *30A:*116, 1948.

27. Helfet, A.: A new way of treating flatfeet in children. Lancet, *1:*262, 1956.

28. Hicks, J. H.: The function of the plantar aponeurosis. J. Anat., *85:*414, 1951.

29. Hoke, M.: An operation for the correction of extremely relaxed flatfeet. J. Bone Joint Surg., *13:*773, 1931.

30. Inman, V. T.: The human foot. Manitoba Med. Rev., *46:*513, 1966.

31. Jack, E. A.: Naviculo-cuneiform fusion in the treatment of flat foot. J. Bone Joint Surg., *35B:*75, 1953.

32. Jones, B. S.: Flatfoot—a preliminary report of an operation for severe cases. J. Bone Joint Surg., *57B:*279, 1975.

33. Jones, R. L.: The human foot. An experimental study of its mechanics and the role of its muscles and ligaments in support of the arch. Am. J. Anat., *68:*1, 1941.

34. Keith, A.: The history of the human foot and its bearing on orthopaedic practice. J. Bone Joint Surg., *11:*10, 1929.

35. Kidner, F. C.: The prehallux (accessory scaphoid) and its relation to flatfoot. J. Bone Joint Surg., *11:*831, 1929.

36. Kite, J. H.: The treatment of flatfeet in small children. Postgrad. Med., *15:*75, 1954.

37. Koutsogiannis, E.: Treatment of mobile flat foot by displacement osteotomy of the calcaneus. J. Bone Joint Surg., *53B:*96, 1971.

38. Legg, A. T.: The treatment of congenital flatfoot by tendon transplantation. Am. J. Orthop. Surg., *10:*584, 1912–13.

39. Lichtblau, S.: A medial and lateral release operation for club foot. A preliminary report. J. Bone Joint Surg., *55A:*1377, 1973.

40. Lord, J. P.: Correction of extreme flatfoot. JAMA, *81:*1502, 1923.

41. Lovell, W. W., Price, C. T., and Meehan, P. L.: The foot. In *Pediatric Orthopaedics,* Edited by W. W. Lovell and R. B. Winter. Philadelphia, J. B. Lippincott, 1978.

42. Lowman, C. L.: An operative method for correction of certain forms of flatfoot. JAMA, *81:*1500, 1923.

43. Meary, R.: On the measurement of the angle between the talus and the first metatarsal. Symposium: Le Pied Creux Essentiel. Rev. Chir. Orthop., *53:*389, 1967.

44. Milch, H.: Reinforcement of the deltoid ligament for pronated flatfoot. Surg. Gynecol. Obstet., *74:*876, 1942.

45. Miller, O. L.: A plastic flat foot operation. J. Bone Joint Surg., *9:*84, 1927.

46. Morton, D. J.: *The Human Foot.* New York, Columbia University Press, 1935, p. 119.

47. Muller, E.: Ueber die Resultate der Ernst Muller'schen Plattfussoperation. Beitr. Klin. Chir., LXXXV, 424, 1913.

48. Niederecker, K.: Operationsverfahren zur Behandlung des Plattfusses. Chir., 182–183, 1932.

49. Ogilvy, C.: An operation for the permanent correction of weak feet in children. J. Orthop. Surg., I, 343, 1919.

50. Ogston, A.: On flatfoot and its cure by operation. Br. Med. J., *9:*110, 1884.

51. Ozonoff, M. B.: *Pediatric Orthopedic Radiology.* Philadelphia, W. B. Saunders, 1979, p. 300.

52. Perthes: Über modellierende Osteotomie bei Plattfussen mit schwerer Knockendeformitat. Zentralbl. Chir., XL, 548, 1913.

53. Phelps, A. M.: The etiology, pathology, and treatment of flat-foot. Post-Graduate, VII, 104, 1892.

54. Roberts, P. W.: An operation for valgus feet. JAMA, LXXVII, 1571, Nov. 12, 1921.

55. Rose, G. K.: Correction of the pronated foot. J. Bone Joint Surg., *44B:*642, 1962.

56. Ryerson, Ed. W.: Tendon transplantation in flatfoot. Am. J. Orthop. Surg., *7:*505, 1909–10.

57. Schede, Fr.: Die Operation des Plattfusses. Z. Orthop. Chir., L, 528, 1928.

58. Soule, R. E.: Value of bone pin arthrodesis in the treatment of flat-foot. JAMA, LXXVII, 1871, 1921.

59. Staheli, L. T.: Corrective shoes for children. Pediatr. Digest, *20*(5):22, 1978.

60. Staheli, L. T., and Giffin, L.: Corrective shoes for children: A survey of current practice. Pediatrics, *65*(1):13, 1980.

61. Stokes, W.: Astragaloid osteotomy in the treatment of flatfoot. Trans. Acad. Med. Ireland, III, 141, 1885 (Ann. Surg., II, 279, 1885).

62. Tachdjian, M. O.: *Pediatric Orthopedics.* Philadelphia, W. B. Saunders, 1972, p. 1397.

63. Trendelenburg, F.: Ueber Plattsfussoperationen. Arch. Klin. Chir., *39:*751, 1889.

64. Weinlechner, cited by Zadek, I.: Transverse-wedge arthrodesis for the relief of pain in rigid flat-foot. J. Bone Joint Surg., *17:*455, 1935.

65. Wilms, M.: Operative Behandlung des Plattfusses und Klumpfusses. Dtsch. Med. Wochenschr., XXXIX, 1032, 1913.

66. Zadek, I.: Transverse-wedge arthrodesis for the relief of pain in rigid flat-foot. J. Bone Joint Surg., *17:*453, 1935.

# 7

# Paralytic Equinovarus and Paralytic Planovalgus

The paralytic forms of equinovarus and planovalgus present such unusual and singular problems that I feel a separate chapter to be justified for their discussion. The etiology is implied in the title; that is, these special manifestations of equinovarus and planovalgus are clearly the result of some neuromuscular abnormality or neurologic deficit. Nearly always, in both deformities, muscle imbalance is involved, and correction of the deformity and restoration of muscle balance are the prime goals of treatment. These two foot deformities are discussed separately because each presents a different set of diagnostic and therapeutic problems.

It is important to emphasize that the outward manifestations of paralytic equinovarus are the same as those of congenital equinovarus (Fig. 7-1): the ankle is in equinus, the hindfoot in varus, and the forefoot adducted and often supinated. In paralytic equinovarus, the program of treatment is governed largely by whether the neurologic disturbance is the result of an upper-motor-neuron lesion (spastic paralysis) or a lower-motor-neuron lesion (flaccid paralysis). Further, the duration of the muscle imbalance has a substantial bearing upon the degree of rigidity, flexibility, soft-tissue contractures, and resulting adaptive bony changes. Both of these factors have enormous bearing upon any treatment program. As a further, major difference between the paralytic and congenital deformities, however, it should be established at the outset that, in paralytic deformities, no basic *intrinsic* abnormalities in the size, shape, or degree of osseous development are present.

The most frequent neuromuscular or neurologic conditions that produce an equinovarus foot deformity are cerebral palsy (upper-motor-neuron) and a variety of peripheral nerve lesions (lower-

*Paralytic Equinovarus*

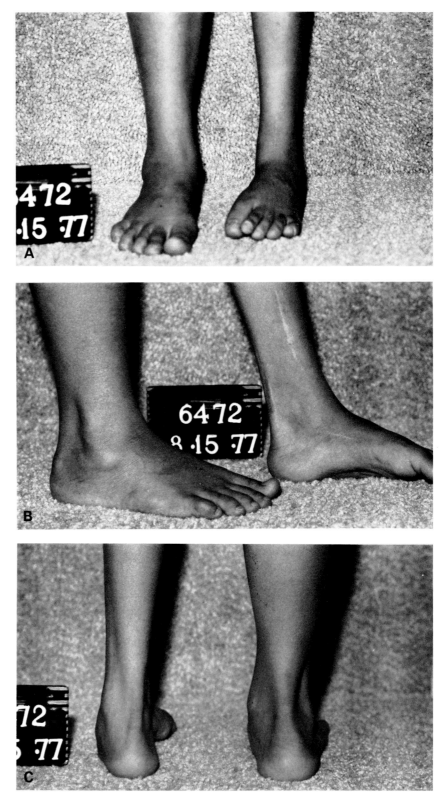

FIG. 7-1. An example of a paralytic equinovarus foot deformity in a 9-year-old male with left spastic hemiparesis. All components of the equinovarus are plainly evident, as seen in the adducted and supinated forefoot (**A** and **B**) and the varus heel (**C**). This patient had undergone previous tendon transfers of unknown type, as evidenced by the scars.

motor-neuron). Other clinical neuromuscular disorders can produce this deformity; a specific example is that seen in dystonia musculorum deformans. The basic issue, however, usually resolves itself into whether the equinovarus is caused by muscle imbalance due to *spastic* or *flaccid* paralysis. In this regard, it is important to distinguish the conditions referred to in this chapter from those encountered in the cavovarus foot deformity, even though they may clearly overlap (see Chapter 3). In fact, a pure distinction between a paralytic equinovarus foot and a paralytic cavovarus foot may be only one of degree. It is important to emphasize and reinforce the principles involved in the treatment of the paralytic foot deformities that result from neuromuscular lesions.

Tachdjian points out that, in instances in which only the triceps surae is spastic and contracted, the deformity often produced is equinovalgus,[51] whereas spasticity that also involves the posterior tibial and the toe flexor muscles more often results in equinovarus. In these instances, the varus of the forefoot is often more prominent than the equinus, and the child therefore toes-in when walking.

During motor testing, it is necessary to test anterior tibial function with the knee both extended and flexed (gastrocnemius relaxed). Voluntary anterior tibial function may not be demonstrable unless the patient flexes the hip and knee simultaneously. This Strumpell or "mass reflex" maneuver will often elicit voluntary anterior tibial function by means of synkinesia, which has also been termed the "confusion" or automatic reflex.

NONOPERATIVE TREATMENT. The conservative treatment of spastic paralytic equinovarus in the young child without fixed deformity revolves around passive stretching of all contracted and spastic muscle units and efforts at active rehabilitation of the ankle dorsiflexors and evertors. Night splints or, preferably, bivalved casts are used at night. These are designed to *maintain* passive correction and must be above-knee devices in order to keep the gastrocnemius stretched out to length.

SURGICAL TREATMENT: CONCEPTS AND PRINCIPLES. Fundamentally, the ideal solution to any deformity produced by paralytic muscle imbalance is to correct the deformity by whatever means necessary and then to balance the musculature as well as possible. In other words, the fact that the deformity has resulted from muscle imbalance ultimately *mandates* muscle-balancing procedures. Considering the problem as it relates to spastic paralysis, many well established, fundamental principles dictate the appropriate form of treatment. It is essential to understand these principles of muscle and tendon surgery in spastic paralysis of the foot and ankle.

First, and extremely important, the heelcord should never be overlengthened; thus, ankle dorsiflexion of only 5 or 10° is all that should be attempted or achieved when surgically correcting equinus in spastic paralysis. Second, no tendon should be completely transferred

## EQUINOVARUS DUE TO SPASTIC PARALYSIS

beyond the midline of the foot. Thus, if transfer of anterior tibial function is desired, a split anterior tibial tendon transfer is much preferred.

Finally, if the posterior tibial tendon is considered to be a deforming force, it should simply be lengthened in situ just above the medial malleolus, and it should be transferred anteriorly (nonphasic transfer) *only* when no other means exists of providing dorsiflexion of the foot and ankle. The reason for this precaution is that a substantial possibility exists of creating a calcaneus foot deformity, which may be more difficult to treat than the original equinovarus deformity. With these guidelines in mind, the appropriate treatment for the equinovarus foot due to spastic paralysis can be synthesized more effectively. These basic principles are applied as follows.

First, the equinovarus deformity of the foot must be corrected. In the case of spastic equinovarus, this usually can be achieved passively. On the other hand, in instances of longstanding deformity, passive correction may not be possible; surgical correction (medial release and/or lateral-column shortening) therefore may be required. In adolescents with a longstanding deformity, sufficient adaptive change may have occurred in the bones and joints such that triple arthrodesis is required.

Secondly, the muscle imbalance must be corrected as completely as possible. This demands an accurate appraisal of all muscle function about the foot and ankle. Because muscle function and spastic paralysis are often the result of "reflex action," one must be familiar with the techniques of physical examination that permit appropriate assessment of muscle function in the foot of a child with cerebral palsy. I have found that a careful physical examination may be a sufficient basis for the decision governing muscle-balancing procedures; however, Perry has effectively used electromyographic gait analysis in synthesizing a surgical plan to correct muscle imbalance resulting from spastic paralysis.[40]

SURGICAL TECHNIQUES. As noted previously, *surgical* correction of the foot deformity is not commonly required because the foot is usually flexible, especially when examined under anesthesia. If surgical correction *is* found to be necessary, however, the approach is based upon the same principles used in treating congenital equinovarus. Usually, however, paralytic deformities can be corrected more easily and readily than the congenital form, because paralytic deformities rarely exhibit the rigid soft-tissue changes in the joint capsules and tendinous retinacula commonly found in congenital or developmental foot deformities. Nonetheless, to some degree, the same type of surgical release of contracted tendinous and ligamentous structures may be necessary to correct the foot satisfactorily, especially in older children with longstanding paralytic deformities.

*The Equinus Deformity.* Overactivity of the triceps surae may contribute to the equinovarus deformity during gait, despite the examiner's ability to dorsiflex the hindfoot passively to neutral. This often requires heelcord lengthening, which can be done either percutaneously or by the open technique. I personally prefer the percutaneous method (Fig. 7-2). Tachdjian, on the other hand, prefers the White procedure of open sliding lengthening of the heelcord, as described by Banks and Green.[5] He appropriately emphasizes, however, that the ultimate result depends less upon the technique of triceps surae lengthening than upon the postoperative care. I am in complete agreement with this concept.

In cases in which the gastrocnemius is shown to be the muscle principally responsible for equinus, it can be selectively lengthened (weakened) while preserving normal soleus function. Three procedures have been devised that elongate the conjoined aponeurotic tendon of the gastrocnemius and soleus at midleg level while leaving intact the underlying muscle fibers. The first of these includes that described by Vulpius and Stoffel (transverse or V-shaped tendon incisions) and a modification by Baker (tongue-in-groove type incision).[2,55] The second is that described by Silverskiold, which consists of a proximal gastrocnemius recession in which the two heads of origin are transferred distal to the knee.[48] His procedure also includes partial neurectomy of the tibial motor nerves to the gastrocnemius.[36] Silver and Simon, in most instances, had excellent results with this procedure, with the few failures (recurrent equinus) related principally to improper preoperative evaluation of dorsiflexor muscle power rather than to the procedure itself.[46] The third procedure, originated by Strayer, consists of distal gastrocnemius recession, in which the gastrocnemius muscle is completely separated from the conjoined tendon in order to sever all afferent reflex pathways from the Achilles tendon to the gastrocnemius.[49] The ankle is then passively dorsiflexed, and the gastrocnemius tendon is sutured to the underlying soleus muscle.[53]

Tachdjian points out that although each of these procedures has the advantage of preserving soleus function for pushoff, they also have disadvantages. Because the dynamic support to the knee is removed posteriorly, recurvatum is a potential complication. He therefore believes that the Silverskiold procedure is contraindicated in those cases in which the hamstrings may require lengthening at a later date, or when the knee hyperextends to some degree during stance or gait. I agree with this and have rarely seen the need for the Silverskiold procedure. Because of the potential problem of retraction of the gastrocnemius muscle after it is completely freed up from the soleus, Tachdjian also does *not* advocate the Strayer procedure. I prefer the Vulpius procedure (Fig. 7-3), although in recent years I have lengthened the Achilles tendon percutaneously in the great majority of instances of equinus contracture, irrespective of whether the problem appears to reside in the gastrocnemius alone, or in both soleus and gastrocnemius.

Pierrot and Murphy devised a novel procedure in which they advanced the insertion of the Achilles tendon anteriorly to the dorsum of the os calcis just posterior to the subtalar joint.[41] This operation does

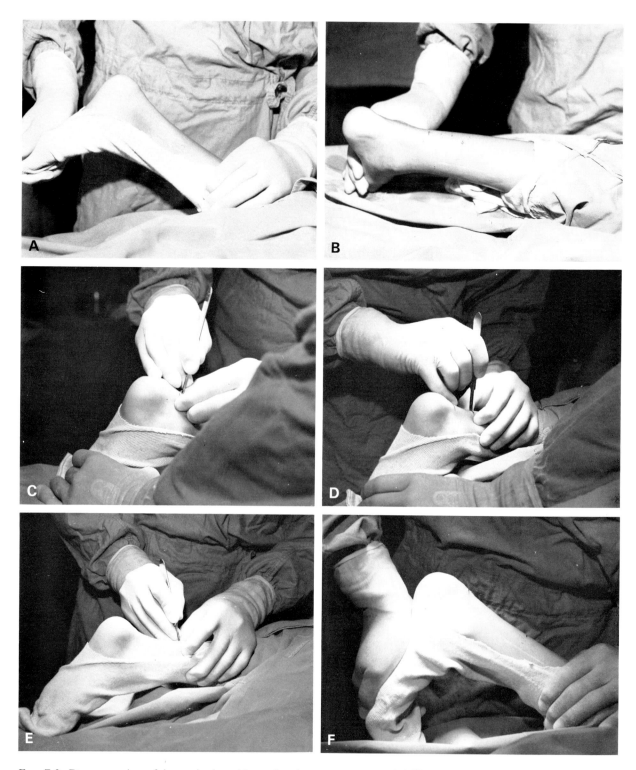

FIG. 7-2. Demonstration of the method used in performing a percutaneous Achilles tendon lengthening. This can be (and usually is) done with the patient in the supine position. For demonstration purposes, however, the patient is prone in this series of photographs. **A**, Tightness of the tendon preventing full dorsiflexion can be seen. **B**, Three small, transverse puncture wounds are made over the heelcord. **C, D,** and **E,** The distal and proximal cuts in the tendon are made laterally, and the center one is made medially. This offers greatest protection to the neurovascular bundle. **F,** Finally, the foot and ankle are carefully dorsiflexed to the appropriate degree.

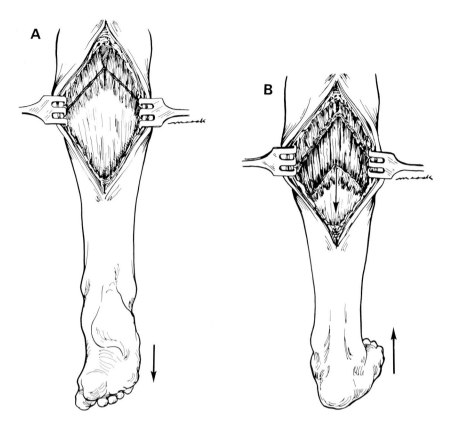

FIG. 7-3. My preferred method of performing a selective lengthening of the gastrocnemius is that originally described by Vulpius. **A,** Through a 2- or 3-inch vertical incision centering over the musculotendinous junction, the aponeurosis of the gastrocnemius is exposed. **B,** A vertically directed, chevron-shaped incision is made in the gastrocnemius aponeurosis, and with the knee held extended, the foot and ankle are gently but firmly dorsiflexed. This elongates the gastrocnemius, leaving the underlying soleus intact. This procedure is best done with the patient in the prone position.

not change the resting length of the triceps surae, but does substantially diminish the lever arm upon which it acts. They found that this transfer weakens the muscle by 48% when the limb is at rest and when the fulcrum for the triceps surae is at the ankle joint. At pushoff, however, in which the fulcrum is closer to the metatarsal heads, the plantar flexion effect of the triceps surae is weakened by only 15%. Pierrot and Murphy reported 75% good to excellent results; Throop, DeRosa, Reeck, and Waterman reported 90% good and excellent results in their series.[41,52] I have had no personal experience with this procedure, having been satisfied with the simpler procedure of lengthening the Achilles tendon.

Once the deformity has been corrected and muscle-balancing procedures have been deemed essential, a variety of operations can be considered. In most cases, varus-valgus deformities are caused by an imbalance in the muscles of inversion (posterior and anterior tibial) and eversion (peroneals). The long toe flexors may also contribute to varus deformity, and it has been noted that spasticity of the abductor hallucis longus may contribute to the deformity.

To correct equinovarus secondary to posterior tibial spasticity, Tachdjian recommends lengthening the posterior tibial tendon in the distal third of the leg. If the Achilles tendon is lengthened, it is done through the same incision. The technique involves making two incisions 5 cm apart through the tendon, well above the point at which the muscle fibers terminate on the tendon. The foot is then forced into valgus in order to effect the fractional lengthening. Care is taken to avoid total release of the posterior tibial tendon so as to prevent progressive valgus that may occur. Majestro, Ruda, and Frost described a modification of the frequently performed stepcut or Z-plasty lengthening of a hyperactive or contracted posterior tibial tendon, in which an intramuscular lengthening is performed.[33]

Baker and Hill described rerouting of the posterior tibial and peroneal tendons anterior to the malleoli in varus and valgus deformities, respectively.[4] Bisla, Louis, and Albano reported mediocre results at best with this technique;[7] because of similar poor results, I stopped using this procedure years ago.

Hoffer, Reiswig, Garrett, and Perry, after analyzing electromyographic data on anterior tibial function in patients with spastic varus hindfoot deformities, elucidated two basic patterns of muscle activity.[24] One occurs when the anterior tibial tendon is inappropriately hyperactive during gait. For these patients, excellent results were obtained using the split anterior tibial tendon transfer, often in conjunction with some of the procedures mentioned earlier that are designed to correct equinovarus deformity.

For the paralytic spastic equinovarus foot, Tohen, Cameron, and Barrera described a procedure consisting of transfer of the extensor tendons of the toes and the anterior tibial tendon to the central or lateral aspect of the dorsum of the foot.[53] In so doing, they were able not only to eliminate a dynamic deforming force, but also to use the new extensor as a dorsiflexor of the ankle, primarily because of its function in response to the abnormal Babinski reflex and to the triple flexion response.

My experience has demonstrated that the most satisfying and effective technical procedure designed to provide the needed muscle balance in the equinovarus foot is the "Rancho" operation described by Hoffer, Reiswig, Garrett, and Perry.[24] It was initially designed for use in adult hemiplegics, but we have found it equally effective in balancing the muscles of the foot and ankle in children with this deformity. It produces a substantial degree of lasting correction without necessitating any type of bone and joint stabilization.

*The "Rancho" Procedure.* In the typical patient with spastic equinovarus, this operation involves three procedures: (1) open elongation (weakening) of the posterior tibial tendon, (2) percutaneous lengthening (weakening) of the Achilles tendon, and (3) transfer of the lateral half of the anterior tibial tendon into the cuboid bone. This combination of procedures embodies the fundamentals of tendon transfer surgery in the patient who has a muscle imbalance of the foot due to spastic paralysis as outlined previously, namely, the overpowering muscles (posterior tibial and triceps surae) are weakened by lengthening, and the hemitransfer of the anterior tibial tendon adheres to the principle of not transferring tendons beyond the midline. The operation therefore prevents any overpull that lateral transfer of the entire anterior tibial tendon might cause. The technical details of the procedure are outlined as follows and illustrated in Figure 7-4.

Four open incisions usually are necessary. The first, 1 inch long, is made over the course of the posterior tibial tendon just above the medial malleolus. Through this incision, the tendon of the posterior tibial muscle is lengthened by a "Z" cut and is then repaired in the lengthened position with the foot held in maximum eversion. This wound is closed and a percutaneous heelcord lengthening performed. In my experience, this technique (previously mentioned) of percutaneous Achilles tendon lengthening has proven eminently satisfactory in all instances of heelcord contracture resulting from neuromuscular causes. In 25 years of experience, I have not found an open heelcord lengthening to be necessary in a *child* or young *adolescent* with equinus deformity due to heelcord contracture resulting from any form of *neuromuscular* disease.

Clearly, care must be exercised during this procedure, because injudicious overlengthening of the Achilles tendon is a distinct hazard since it may produce a calcaneus deformity. The percutaneous incisions necessary to lengthen the heelcord do not require formal skin closure.

The next incision centers over the insertion of the anterior tibial tendon. It is 1½ inches long and parallels the most distal extension of the tendon into its insertion on the medial (first) cuneiform bone. The tendon is isolated and split in half longitudinally; the lateral half is then detached from its insertion and dissected free from its soft-tissue, synovial, and retinacular attachments as far proximally as possible.

A third incision, 1½ inches long, is then made anteriorly in the midline of the lower leg just above the extensor retinaculum. The lateral half of the anterior tibial tendon is extracted through this incision, and the incision over the normal anterior tibial tendon insertion is closed. A fourth incision, 1½ inches long, is then made over the cuboid bone, which is exposed subperiosteally over its dorsal and lateral aspects. A drill hole directed in a dorsoplantar direction is made in this bone; it should be large enough in caliber to accommodate the lateral half of the anterior tibial tendon. This tendon is then transferred under the extensor retinaculum and over the short extensor muscle belly to the lateral incision and is then placed into the hole prepared in the cuboid bone. This transferred portion of the anterior tibial tendon is then sutured into the soft tissues and periosteum, with the distal end of the tendon having been placed into the prepared osseous bed of the cuboid. During the suture process, the foot is held in mild eversion, with the ankle neutral or placed in 5° of dorsiflexion.

The next step requires clinical judgment in deciding whether to suture together the two halves of the split anterior tibial tendon in the proximal (pretibial) incision in order to provide equal tautness to the

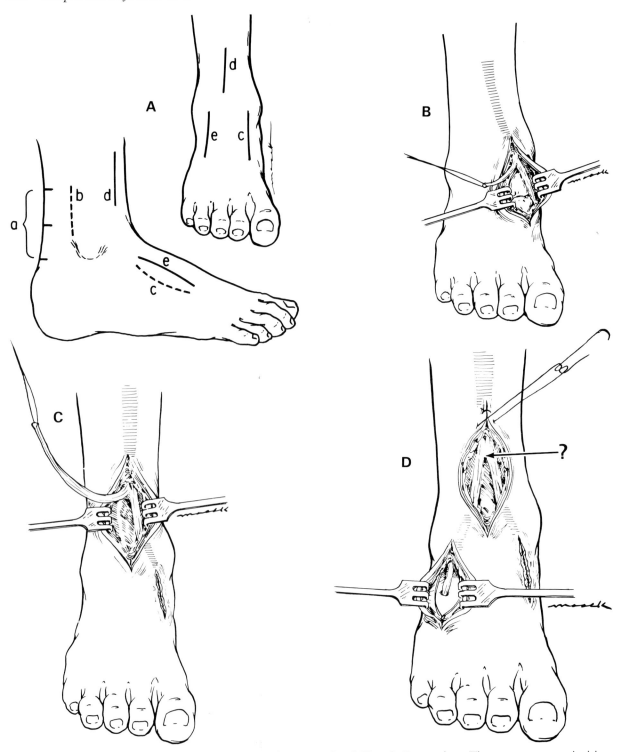

FIG. 7-4. **A**, Five incisions are necessary to perform the conventional "Rancho" procedure. Three percutaneous incisions (a), approximately 1 inch apart, are made over the lower 2 inches of the Achilles tendon (see Figure 7-2). Through a 1½-inch incision (b) just above the medial malleolus, the posterior tibial tendon is lengthened by the fractional or "Z" technique. **B**, Following this, a 2-inch oblique incision (c) is made over the distal course of the anterior tibial tendon, which is exposed and split into two equal halves. The lateral half is severed from its insertion and freed from all soft-tissue and synovial attachments. **C**, A second vertical incision, 2 inches long (d), is made just above the extensor retinaculum, and the lateral half of the tendon is split further proximally and delivered into the wound. **D**, A third incision, 2 inches long (e), exposes the cuboid bone, and the lateral half of the anterior tibial tendon is passed under the extensor retinaculum and inserted into a hole in the cuboid. The surgeon's judgment governs whether or not the split halves of the tendon should be sutured under equal tautness.

lateral (transferred) and medial halves of the tendon. Intuitively, I prefer to suture the two halves under approximately equal tension as long as the foot is held in mild eversion. The fourth wound is then closed and a below-knee cast applied, with the foot and ankle held in slight dorsiflexion and the foot in mild eversion.

The cast is removed in 6 weeks, and a below-knee, double-upright brace is prescribed, which must have a plantar flexion stop and free dorsiflexion. I have found it important to avoid spring-loaded dorsiflexion braces in patients with spastic paralysis. The postoperative care involving gradual elimination of the brace must be highly individualized. Figure 7-5 gives an example of a patient who has had this surgical program for spastic paralytic equinovarus deformity.

In some cases in which the anterior tibial muscle is not strong enough to justify the operation just described, anterior transfer of the posterior tibial tendon is justified. Bisla, Gritzka, Turner, and their respective co-workers all reported good to excellent results in treating this deformity by transferring the posterior tibial tendon through the interosseous membrane.[7,19,54] The tendon must be rated at least good, and the tendon should be transferred *to the midline,* that is, to the second or third cuneiform bone. As a matter of principle, it is clear that the ankle must be in slight dorsiflexion at the time of transfer and that the tendons should not be implanted under too much tension. Hoffer agrees that in the case of an equinovarus deformity in which the posterior tibial muscle is strong and the anterior tibial muscle is weak, anterior transfer of the posterior tibial tendon is indicated and justified. I share Hoffer's approach to this muscle-balancing program; namely, that if the anterior tibial muscle is strong, then the split transfer is indicated, in addition to lengthening the posterior tibial tendon. An advantage of this approach is that the transfer is phasic rather than nonphasic. In the *absence* of a good or better anterior tibial muscle, however, anterior transfer of the posterior tibial tendon is indicated as illustrated in Figure 7-6.

## EQUINOVARUS DUE TO FLACCID PARALYSIS

The same basic principles employed in the treatment of spastic (upper-motor-neuron) paralysis apply to the flaccid (low-motor-neuron) paralysis; specifically, that the deformity is corrected first by whatever means necessary, and then a muscle-balancing operation is performed to maintain correction and prevent recurrence.

In most cases of equinovarus due to lower-motor-neuron (anterior horn cell or peripheral nerve) paralysis, the strength and voluntary control of the functioning musculature can be accurately assessed. Furthermore, in flaccid paralytic equinovarus, if tendons must be transferred, it is possible to predict with substantial accuracy their post-transfer function. This is in contrast to spastic equinovarus deformities, in which muscle response is largely the result of involuntary reflex action.

In most cases of equinovarus due to flaccid paralysis, the major problem is weak and ineffective evertors and dorsiflexors rather than

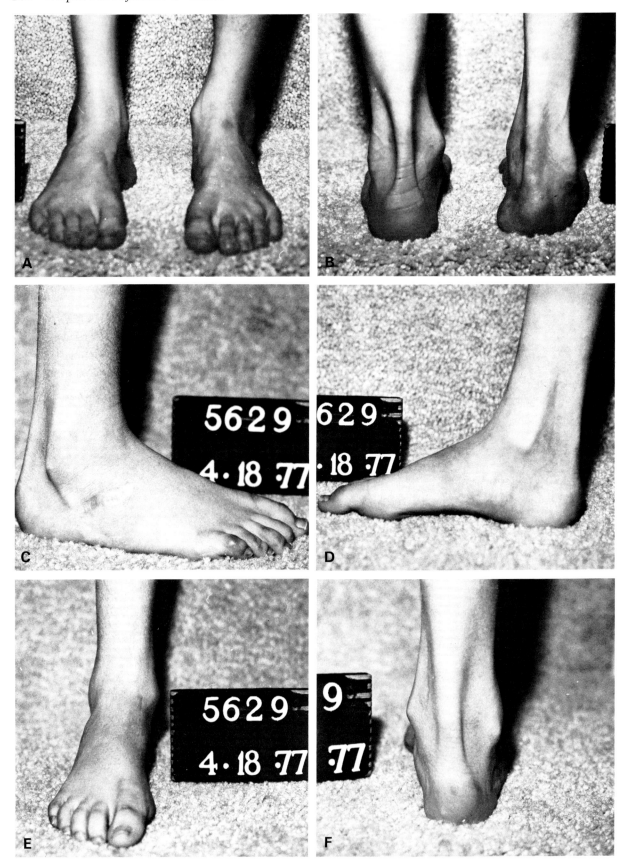

FIG. 7-5. **A** and **B**, Preoperative standing photographs of the right foot in a 9-year-old boy with spastic hemiplegia, showing spastic equinovarus deformity. Strong anterior tibial and posterior tibial tendon strength was elicited by both active and reflex functional testing, and the heelcord was contracted. Thus, the heelcord was lengthened percutaneously and the posterior tibial tendons were lengthened through an open procedure, and a split anterior tibial tendon transfer was accomplished. **C** through **F**, The result 2 years later.

overpowering or spastic invertors and plantar flexors. Thus, although in both types, the overall effort is directed towards correcting the deformity and balancing muscle function, the flaccid paralytic deformity differs substantially from spastic equinovarus in the methods by which correction is achieved.

In equinovarus deformity due to lower-motor-neuron disease, just as in treating the same deformity in upper-motor-neuron lesions, the surgeon must direct his initial efforts at correction of the deformity, either nonoperatively (through manipulation and cast applications) or operatively. In rare cases, this decision can be made only after examination under general anesthesia, when the true flexibility or correctability of the foot can be established.

Following correction, appropriate muscle-balancing procedures must be accomplished. This must clearly be governed by the availability of transferable motor units. In most instances the tendon transfers will result in anterior transfer of the posterior tibial tendon through the interosseous membrane into the dorsum of the foot so that it will serve as a dorsiflexor and evertor of the foot.

In this deformity, posterior tibial function is strong, and unless this influence is removed, the equinovarus deformity will persist. In a report that encompassed a thorough review of the orthopedic literature, Watkins, Jones, Ryder, and Brown attempted to put into proper perspective the technique of anterior transfer of the posterior tibial tendon.[56] They found that transfer of this tendon anteriorly to serve as the dorsiflexor of the foot and ankle was not well established and had received little attention. These authors gave Ober credit for describing transplantation of the posterior tibial tendon about the medial malleolus into the dorsum of the foot in order to serve as the dorsiflexor.[37] Mayer, however, believed that the procedure was not biomechanically sound because the method of transfer resulted in an indirect pull of the transferred tendon upon the foot and ankle.[35] Lipscomb and Sanchez, however, reported excellent results with this technique.[32] Watkins, Jones, Ryder, and Brown, on the other hand, preferred to transfer the posterior tibial tendon anteriorly through the interosseous membrane into the dorsum of the foot. In reviewing the literature, they found that Putti and Durham successfully transferred this tendon by this technique in a number of patients.[13,42]

My personal experience reflects poor success with translocation of the posterior tibial tendon anterior to the medial malleolus; and, therefore, I agree completely that for most effective transfer function, the tendon should be transferred anteriorly through the interosseous membrane so that the resulting function of the transferred tendon will accomplish dorsiflexion of the foot and ankle more directly.

If the posterior tibial muscle does not have sufficient strength for transfer, Tachdjian and others have recommended lateral transfer of the anterior tibial tendon to the base of the second or third metatarsal. It should not be placed more laterally because a valgus deformity may result. In selected situations, I have employed the split transfer of the anterior tibial tendon, as reported by Hoffer, in correcting the muscle imbalance in flaccid paralytic equinovarus.

If the toe extensors are strong enough (Grade IV), these tendons may also be transferred to the midfoot (extensor shift) to strengthen the dorsiflexion power of the foot and ankle. Clearly, a major gray area may surface in these deliberations, in which a combination of clinical judgment and the availability of muscle and tendon transfers will ultimately provide the best possible solution to the muscle-balancing problem.

In the *older child* and adolescent with an equinovarus deformity due to flaccid paralysis, just as in comparable deformities due to spastic paralysis, the therapeutic problem usually encompasses some degree of bone and joint deformity as well as a substantial degree of hindfoot instability. Therefore, in many instances, these pathologic changes require a correcting and stabilizing triple arthrodesis as a preliminary step to any effort at tendon transfers. The procedure consists of removal of appropriate wedges of bone and cartilage in order to correct as well as stabilize the foot. The operative procedure is similar, if not identical, to that used to correct an advanced deformity in congenital equinovarus.

The tendon transfer program must be based upon the two factors mentioned earlier:(1) evaluation and quantitation of the functional musculotendinous units that are available and that qualify for transfer, and (2) determination of the most appropriate place to transfer these available motor units. A "cookbook" answer to this complex issue is not possible; clearly, each case must be evaluated and treated according to its own singular set of circumstances. In the majority of instances, however, a transferable posterior tibial tendon will be available and is best transferred through the interosseous membrane (Fig. 7-6). Figure 7-7 gives an example of the surgical methods of approaching the treatment of this deformity.

## Paralytic Planovalgus

The deformity opposite to equinovarus is planovalgus (flatfoot). As with equinovarus, planovalgus is frequently seen in paralytic conditions, both spastic and flaccid, and manifests itself as a moderately severe flatfoot. The heel is in valgus, and the longitudinal arch is flattened in the weight-bearing position (Fig. 7-8). As with the equinovarus deformity, it is due either to almost complete lack of muscle power or to a muscle imbalance that exists about the foot and ankle. In the case of planovalgus, however, the type or pattern of the imbalance is quite different from that encountered in equinovarus. For example, in the planovalgus foot, posterior tibial tendon function is usually weak or absent, and peroneal muscle strength is good or strong (spastic or normal). On the other hand, both often have a common denominator, namely, a tight, contracted or strong triceps surae muscle-tendon group. In this regard and this regard only, there is some similarity to the muscle imbalance problem discussed in the earlier section dealing with paralytic equinovarus foot deformities.

The same basic considerations apply to paralytic planovalgus foot deformity as to the paralytic causes of equinovarus. Thus, these deformities can be produced by either upper- (spastic) or lower-motor-

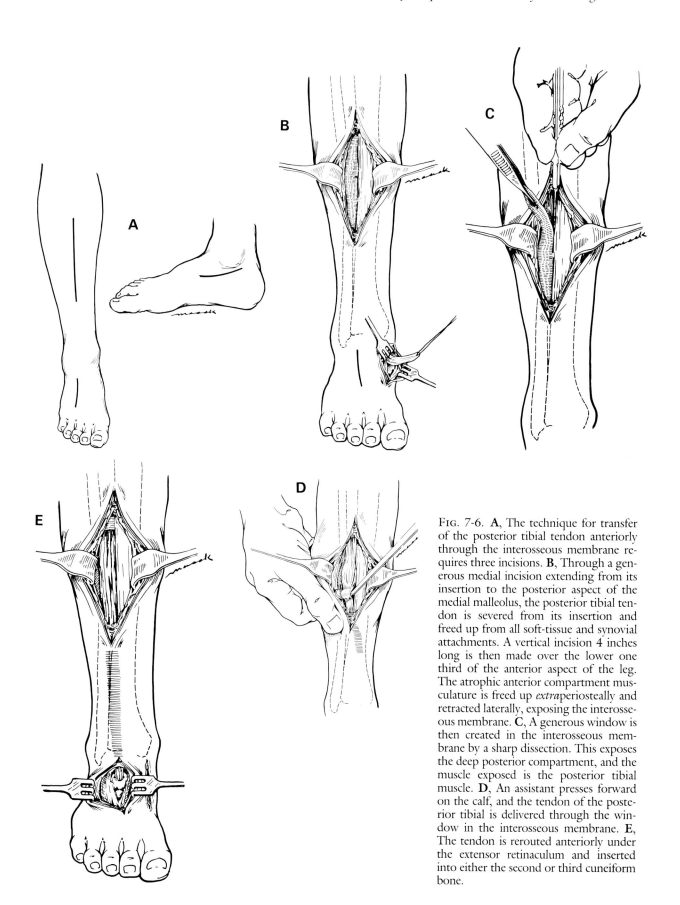

Fig. 7-6. **A**, The technique for transfer of the posterior tibial tendon anteriorly through the interosseous membrane requires three incisions. **B**, Through a generous medial incision extending from its insertion to the posterior aspect of the medial malleolus, the posterior tibial tendon is severed from its insertion and freed up from all soft-tissue and synovial attachments. A vertical incision 4 inches long is then made over the lower one third of the anterior aspect of the leg. The atrophic anterior compartment musculature is freed up *extra*periosteally and retracted laterally, exposing the interosseous membrane. **C**, A generous window is then created in the interosseous membrane by a sharp dissection. This exposes the deep posterior compartment, and the muscle exposed is the posterior tibial muscle. **D**, An assistant presses forward on the calf, and the tendon of the posterior tibial is delivered through the window in the interosseous membrane. **E**, The tendon is rerouted anteriorly under the extensor retinaculum and inserted into either the second or third cuneiform bone.

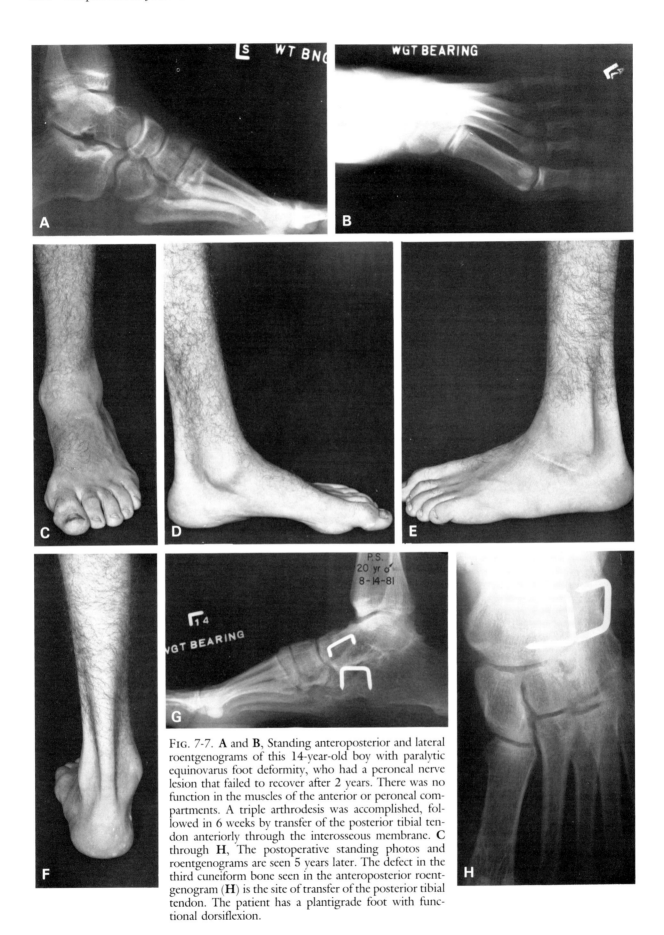

FIG. 7-7. **A** and **B**, Standing anteroposterior and lateral roentgenograms of this 14-year-old boy with paralytic equinovarus foot deformity, who had a peroneal nerve lesion that failed to recover after 2 years. There was no function in the muscles of the anterior or peroneal compartments. A triple arthrodesis was accomplished, followed in 6 weeks by transfer of the posterior tibial tendon anteriorly through the interosseous membrane. **C** through **H**, The postoperative standing photos and roentgenograms are seen 5 years later. The defect in the third cuneiform bone seen in the anteroposterior roentgenogram (**H**) is the site of transfer of the posterior tibial tendon. The patient has a plantigrade foot with functional dorsiflexion.

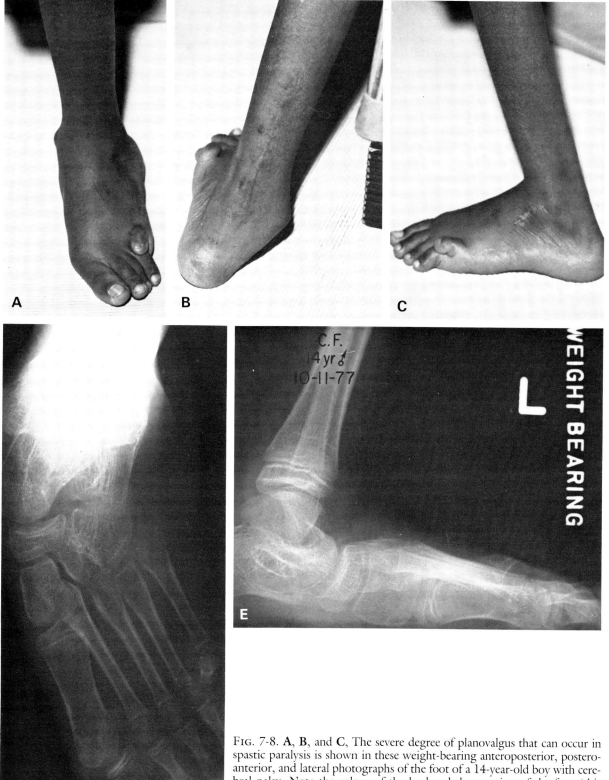

FIG. 7-8. **A**, **B**, and **C**, The severe degree of planovalgus that can occur in spastic paralysis is shown in these weight-bearing anteroposterior, postero-anterior, and lateral photographs of the foot of a 14-year-old boy with cerebral palsy. Note the valgus of the heel and the eversion of the foot (this patient had undergone a prior open heelcord lengthening). **D** and **E**, Weight-bearing anteroposterior and lateral roentgenograms showing the abduction of the midfoot and forefoot and the sagging longitudinal arch due to a severe break in the talonavicular articulation.

neuron lesions (flaccid). Also, the same basic principles should be observed with respect to treatment of either of these deformities. In most instances of paralytic flatfoot, the deformity is passively correctable, and only in older children and adolescents who have developed adaptive bony change will it ever be necessary to correct the foot deformity by means of major bone or joint operations. In these instances, the corrective procedure nearly always will consist of a stabilizing corrective triple arthrodesis (see p. 247). In younger children, passive, nonoperative correction can most often be achieved, and the major program of surgical treatment will consist of simpler stabilization operations (subtalar arthrodesis) and muscle-balancing procedures. As in the case of deformities due to *upper*-motor-neuron lesions and those due to *lower*-motor-neuron lesions, each must be considered separately.

PLANOVALGUS DUE TO SPASTIC PARALYSIS

Planovalgus is a common problem in patients with spastic paralysis, irrespective of the cause of the spasticity. The heelcord is usually tight or contracted, the forefoot is in a variable degree of abduction, the midfoot shows a flattened longitudinal arch, and the heel is in valgus (Fig. 7-8). Upon weight bearing, the heel may not even touch the floor. Under heavy sedation or general anesthesia, the foot deformity is nearly always passively correctable in children and young adolescents. The heelcord is nearly always contracted in these patients, however, and passive dorsiflexion at the ankle may be impossible to demonstrate. Upon muscle testing, the peroneal muscles are usually strong or spastic and usually overpower the weaker or less active posterior tibial and anterior tibial musculature. Weight bearing in the presence of a tight heelcord contributes to the development and perpetuation of the problem.

Tachdjian describes the pathomechanics as follows: The bowstring effect of the contracted triceps surae forces the hindfoot into valgus because the os calcis rotates and displaces posterolaterally under the talus. Consequently, the support of the sustentaculum tali beneath the head of the talus is lost, and the talus therefore drops into a more vertical position than normal. Because the hindfoot cannot be dorsiflexed, dorsiflexion occurs principally at the midfoot, and this combination produces a rocker-bottom deformity of the foot. Weight bearing is then abnormal, being concentrated over the head of the talus rather than the heel. Valgus of the hindfoot then can be increased even further if the peroneals are at all spastic.

THERAPEUTIC CONCEPTS. I find this particular foot deformity much more difficult to treat than the opposite deformity, namely, paralytic spastic *equinovarus*. Certain fundamental principles, however, may help in developing an effective therapeutic plan for this challenging deformity. First, it is essential to establish that the foot is passively correctable. If it is rigid, then a totally different problem surfaces, because *simple* bone stabilization or muscle-balancing procedures are not considered until the deformity has been corrected. Second, the cause of the heelcord contracture or spasticity must be accurately determined, i.e., whether it lies in the soleus, the gastrocnemius, or both. This will determine to some extent the kind of triceps surae lengthening operation that will be required (see p. 227). Third, the age of the patient must be considered. In young children, hindfoot bony stabilization procedures may be contraindicated or totally inappropriate, whereas in older children, such procedures may be essential to achieve or maintain a satisfactory correction. Finally, the degree of functional disability that the planovalgus deformity produces must be assessed. In this regard, it is extremely important to emphasize that the simple presence of a spastic planovalgus foot does *not* mandate surgical correction. Finally, the functional capacity of the patient must be considered. Treatment may not be indicated for a patient who has a low demand for ambulation or who does not walk at all.

Once all of these determinants have been fully considered, a logical and defensible program of treatment can be synthesized. One often must assume that the patient will become ambulatory and therefore will need treatment, especially the young child, whose ambulatory potential has not yet been realized.

METHODS OF TREATMENT. Tachdjian recommends conservative management of these deformities in early childhood (i.e., Thomas heel, medial heel wedge, longitudinal arch support, and a valgus "T" strap if an ankle-foot orthosis is worn), but he emphasizes the need for early surgical correction in some cases to prevent the development of a rigid valgus deformity. Tachdjian also recommends an Achilles tendon lengthening and, if the peroneal tendons are contributing to the deformity, he performs fractional lengthenings of these peroneal tendons. Postoperatively, active rehabilitation of the anterior tibial is emphasized by means of physical therapy. If *disabling* heel valgus persists by age 6 or 7 years, an extra-articular subtalar arthrodesis (Grice procedure) is recommended.

Baker and Dodelin claimed that the indications for and goals of the Grice procedure in cerebral palsy patients with planovalgus are no different than in those patients with poliomyelitis.[3,18] They conceded, however, that one might expect less consistent results because of the unpredictable nature of an upper- as compared to a lower-motor-neuron lesion. Nevertheless, they reported good to excellent results in 29 cases involving 17 patients who underwent the Grice procedure. Of the 29 procedures, 15 were done on feet with spasticity only, 10 on feet with combined spasticity and athetosis, and 4 on feet with athetosis only. The Grice procedure was combined with gastrocnemius lengthening in all cases and with peroneal tendon transfer in 2 cases. Varus deformities developed in 5 patients, attributed in most cases to an overactive posterior tibial. In 3 cases severe enough to warrant treatment, the varus was successfully corrected by posterior tibial tenotomy.

Grice himself agreed with Baker and Dodelin that the extra-articular subtalar fusion is useful in cerebral palsy patients with planovalgus deformity. As with the poliomyelitis patients, the os calcis must be placed into its corrected position under the talus *before* fusion. Grice felt that stabilization of the corrected hindfoot may restore balance to the foot since the overactivity of the peroneals and triceps surae *may* be diminished. Grice erroneously felt that tendon transfers seldom will be needed in these cerebral palsy patients, but he correctly pointed out that the necessity for tendon transfers should be determined only after the fusion is accomplished, to avoid the problem of overcorrection. It has been shown, however, that if some degree of muscle balance is not achieved, with continued growth, a rigid planovalgus deformity will develop, because of the fused subtalar joint. This deformity may be more difficult to treat than the original, more flexible deformity (see p. 215).

Ingram felt that the extra-articular subtalar fusion is the procedure of choice for the treatment of severe planovalgus in cerebral palsy, especially in the age group from 4 to 9 years.[27] He emphasized the need to correct deformities of the soft tissues prior to the procedure, but in contrast to Grice, he believed that the arthrodesis should be *preceded* by attempts to balance the muscles. Several authors have reported generally excellent results with this procedure in cerebral palsy patients with severe planovalgus deformity, and their conclusions parallel those just listed.[4,29]

Silver and Baker and their respective co-workers described calcaneal osteotomies that produced good results in treating the spastic planovalgus deformity.[4,47] Silver's approach is basically a modification of that described by Dwyer, in which either a closing medial-wedge or an opening lateral-wedge osteotomy is performed, augmented by the insertion of a bone graft in the latter instance.[14] He recommends a minimum age of 3 years and a maximum age of 9 years to qualify for this procedure, after which a triple arthrodesis should be performed in order to achieve correction. Baker's technique consists of a horizontal osteotomy made from the lateral side, just beneath the posterior articular surface. The osteotomy site is opened up and held with bone graft, and in this fashion, valgus can be corrected. In a few cases, this procedure was combined with a subtalar bone block.

It is evident from the foregoing review of pertinent literature that a substantial degree of latitude exists with respect to the concepts and the methods of executing the techniques available in managing this problem. Over the years, after having attempted all of the foregoing procedures, I have adopted the following approach to treatment of this challenging problem.

The major goal of treatment, as with all paralytic foot deformities, is to correct the deformity and then to balance the musculature of the foot. As indicated earlier, this is not an easy task in instances of spastic planovalgus, but by using the principles outlined earlier, I have had greatest success with the following program. In the young child with a flexible flatfoot due to spastic paralysis, and in whom the heelcord is contracted, the most appropriate treatment mandates simple lengthening of some component of the triceps surae. If the contracture is principally in the gastrocnemius musculotendinous unit, a selective gastro-cnemius lengthening, such as the Strayer or the Vulpius (Fig. 7-3) operation, is most appropriate. If the contracture involves *both* components of the triceps surae, percutaneous elongation of the entire Achilles tendon is essential in order to correct the equinus contracture. Following either of these procedures, an above-knee cast is worn for 4 weeks, and then a well molded ankle-foot orthosis is fabricated that supports the patient's longitudinal arch and also prevents plantar flexion of the foot and ankle (see Fig. 5-16). This rather simple operative and orthotic approach is usually all that is necessary in the child under 6 or 7 years of age.

Older children may require a more complicated therapeutic program that may include a stabilizing procedure such as a subtalar bone block. In addition, not only must the triceps surae be lengthened, but also, the need for tendon transfers or tendon lengthenings (weakening) must be carefully considered in an effort to balance the musculature. This latter issue is not easy to determine in the case of spastic paralysis. In most situations, simple lengthening (weakening) of the peroneals, if they are spastic, is all that can be done safely.[51]

The indications for a subtalar bone block (extra-articular subtalar arthrodesis) are *not* well established in foot deformities due to spastic paralysis. For this reason, it is essential to clearly understand the expected goal of the subtalar bone block, as it applies not only to flatfoot resulting from spastic paralysis, but also to planovalgus feet resulting from flaccid paralysis. This operation is *not* a *corrective* procedure, but rather simply a *stabilizing* operation. One of the most important prerequisites for it is a flexible and/or passively correctable hindfoot. As emphasized by Grice, *passive* restoration of the normal talocalcaneal relationship is an essential prerequisite, and the bone block is then employed simply to *maintain* this correction.[18] Furthermore, the extent to which this hindfoot correction will be maintained is directly related to the amount of growing the foot still has to do and to the presence of acceptable muscle balance that exists after successful fusion. In other words, if a successful subtalar bone block is accomplished for planovalgus in a growing child in whom substantial spastic overpull of the peroneal muscle groups persists, then not only will the valgus deformity recur with growth, but also the hindfoot will assume a rigid valgus position because of the now fused subtalar joint. Thus it is essential to carefully weigh the stabilizing value of the subtalar bone block against its possible disadvantages in the presence of spastic muscle imbalance. My great concern over this issue has led me to substantially reduce the number of subtalar bone block procedures I have done in recent years for this condition. It has been my experience that, in this particular foot deformity, soft-tissue and tendon releases are usually all that are necessary, followed by the rather continuous use of a well constructed ankle-foot orthosis.

In adolescent spastic planovalgus feet, the same considerations must be taken into account as have been discussed earlier. These deformities may *not* be passively correctable, however, and the patient may be too old (over age 10 years) for a successful subtalar bone block. Thus, in these instances, a triple arthrodesis may be necessary to stabilize as well as to correct the deformity. Also, the same considerations obtain with respect to muscle-balancing procedures as outlined previously. A triple arthrodesis done in an older child or adolescent is an excellent corrective and stabilizing operation, but in the presence of a substantial muscle imbalance, and with the passage of time (even after active growth has ceased), the initial planovalgus deformity will recur gradually to some degree, and the hindfoot will then be rigid because of the triple arthrodesis.

In summary, therefore, the treatment of the planovalgus foot due to spastic paralysis is complicated, and the therapeutic guidelines are not well established. If any substantial doubt exists about the need for a stabilizing operation, it probably should *not* be done. The difficulty and unpredictability of balancing the foot musculature in the spastic planovalgus foot may compromise the value of any stabilizing effect of either a subtalar bone block (in children and young adolescents) or a corrective triple arthrodesis (in older adolescents).

Maintaining flexibility of the foot in spastic paralytic deformities is important, and the use of modern ankle-foot orthoses, accompanied by appropriate soft-tissue releases, has radically reduced the need for stabilizing procedures in my current treatment of these problems.

One of the frequently coexisting and causally related deformities in the spastic planovalgus foot is hallux valgus. Holstein has appropriately emphasized this relationship,[26] and it is an important consideration because any efforts to correct the hallux valgus will predictably fail as long as the planovalgus deformity persists. Conversely, a spastic equinovarus deformity (in which hallux valgus is almost never seen) that is converted to a planovalgus deformity nearly always will gradually develop a hallux valgus deformity within a short period of time with weight bearing.

## PLANOVALGUS DUE TO FLACCID PARALYSIS

As discussed earlier, the foot deformities produced by lower-motor-neuron lesions (flaccid paralysis) can be evaluated more accurately and respond quite differently to a treatment program than do similar deformities resulting from upper-motor-neuron lesions (spastic paralysis). The explanation lies in the same basic principles as they apply to any deformity resulting from paralysis that produces muscle absence or imbalance; that is, the residual muscle function in lower-motor-neuron paralysis can be accurately assessed, the behavior of any needed tendon transfer procedures can be rather accurately predicted, and the indications for bony stabilization or corrective operations therefore are more easily established.

According to Ingram,[27] paralysis of the posterior tibial muscle alone can cause planovalgus. The principal action of the posterior tibial muscle is to invert the foot at the talonavicular joint during plantar flexion. When this is paralyzed, a substantial degree of the support to the head of the talus is lost, and abduction of the midfoot and forefoot develops, in addition to valgus of the heel. The toe flexors, now laterally positioned, are unable to substitute for this inverting function and therefore cannot prevent this deformity from occurring. Most functions of the foot, such as gait and pushoff, are carried out by plantar flexion, and paralysis of the posterior tibial tendon therefore becomes a severe impairment.

My observations indicate that the planovalgus deformity resulting from lower-motor-neuron lesions is usually the result of weak anterior and posterior tibial muscle function, accompanied by good or normal peroneal muscle strength. In most instances, also, the heelcord is contracted because its action is relatively unopposed by the weak anterior tibial muscle. The weakness or absence of posterior tibial muscle function further contributes to the flattening of the longitudinal arch, because the *pronating* or plantarflexing action of this muscle on the midfoot and forefoot is vitiated. As noted in earlier chapters (1, 5, 6), the integrity of normal muscle balance and function is essential in order to maintain normal development and configuration of the bones and joints of the foot and ankle. When the muscle imbalance just noted occurs, a planovalgus deformity is almost certain to occur.

THERAPEUTIC CONCEPTS. Historically, tendon transfers and stabilizing procedures have been the main issues emphasized. In contrast to the problems encountered in spastic planovalgus, the management of this deformity in flaccid paralysis is much more consistent. Tachdjian recommends that one peroneal muscle at most be transferred, and it should rarely, if ever, be transferred past the midline, i.e., the second ray. The balance between the anterior tibial, posterior tibial, and peroneus longus tendons as they act upon the first metatarsal should always be considered. It is important to emphasize that transfer of the peroneus longus to the dorsum of the foot in the presence of normal anterior tibial muscle function will often result in a dorsal bunion of the first metatarsal head if the posterior tibial tendon is paralyzed.

Fried and Hendel devised a procedure in which the peroneus longus is routed posterior to the ankle and inserted through the sheath of the posterior tibial tendon and then into the plantar aspect of the navicular in order to substitute for the paralyzed posterior tibial tendon.[16] Alternatively, they recommended transfer of the toe flexors in the same fashion, or even transfer of the great toe extensor posteriorly through the interosseous membrane into the plantar aspect of the navicular.

I have attempted these transfers in a limited number of patients with only fair success. On the other hand, Fried and Moyseyev used the transfers in 20 patients with severe planovalgus and reported full correction in 7 and slight to moderate deformity, either varus or valgus, in 13; none of these, however, required further tendon operations. The need for hindfoot stabilization was to be determined when the patients reached skeletal maturity. Only 1 of these 20 patients had recurrent planovalgus severe enough to be considered a failure.[17]

Often associated with equinovalgus or planovalgus is clawing of the toes. This deformity results from a substitution pattern in which the toe extensors attempt to assist the weak anterior tibial muscle in dorsiflexing the ankle. The clawtoe deformity usually disappears if the extensors are effectively transferred prior to the development of fixed deformities. The Jones and Hibbs procedure, however, i.e., proximal interphalangeal joint fusion and transfer of the extensor tendons to the cuneiforms or to the metatarsal necks, may be necessary if rigid deformities of the toes have developed.[22,28]

As with all deformities that result from paralytic muscle imbalance, the goals of treatment remain the same, namely, the deformity must first be corrected and stabilized, and then attempts to correct the muscle imbalance must be made. These fundamental principles cannot be violated; however, the implementation of the available solutions to the problem may be quite variable, simply because the degree of severity of the problem can vary widely from one instance to another. It is, therefore, difficult to propose a "cookbook" solution to a specific case, except as it can be synthesized through the application of these principles.

Few children with paralytic planovalgus under the age of 5 years require any treatment except for a plastic foot orthosis such as the UCB splint (Fig. 3-15), whose purpose is to support the longitudinal arch during the child's growth. It should not be considered a corrective device. After age 5 years, it usually becomes necessary to determine whether or not surgical stabilization of the hindfoot (subtalar joint) by means of an extra-articular arthrodesis is indicated and/or justified. This is the type of foot for which Grice originally intended the subtalar bone block. It is especially valuable when tendons are available for transfer. In these instances, the bone block serves to stabilize the hindfoot, and this enables one or more of the peroneal muscles to be transferred in an effort to achieve muscle balance. In the case of a flail foot (no transferable muscle), the value of the subtalar bone block is greatly vitiated, because in these instances and at this age, the foot and ankle cannot be rendered free of an orthosis by any combination of surgical procedures.

Therefore, in this young age group, the following program of treatment is suggested. In those children under age 5 years, the paralytic flexible flatfoot is best treated by a simple foot or foot-and-ankle orthosis designed to support the foot and ankle. It is essential, however, to correct any heelcord tightness, either nonoperatively or operatively. After age 5, a subtalar bone block is justified if muscles are available for transfer. This stabilization procedure (bone block) should be considered the first part of a two-stage operation. Any program of tendon transfer clearly must be governed by the functioning muscle units that qualify for transfer; i.e., they must rate at least Grade IV in strength, because most muscles lose about one functional grade after transfer. Also, the transfers are preferably phasic in nature, so that they will convert to their new function more easily and effectively. This latter issue, however, is not nearly as critical in treatment of the flatfoot due to lower-motor-neuron lesions (flaccid paralysis) as it is in instances of upper-motor-neuron paralysis, because conversion of a nonphasic transfer is usually much more successful in lower-motor-neuron paralysis.

Since the major motor loss in these kinds of deformities involves the posterior tibial muscle, it is most appropriate that the surgeon attempt to substitute for that motor unit. The means of accomplishing this involve highly individualized issues in which the surgeon's experience and intuition must play a major role.

After age 12 or 13 years, the paralytic flatfoot is subject to the same principles of treatment as in the younger years, but the child is now in the triple arthrodesis age group. Thus, instead of performing a subtalar bone block, the need for a stabilizing (and if necessary, corrective) triple arthrodesis is the first consideration, *provided* that muscles are available for transfer. The triple arthrodesis is then followed by the most appropriate tendon transfer procedures, as outlined previously. In the event of a flail flatfoot, in which the foot and ankle are totally paralyzed (but *not* in the case of an *insensitive* flail foot), a pantalar arthrodesis may be indicated.

Because arthrodeses of the joints of the hindfoot and ankle are so commonly necessary in the treatment of paralytic deformities, it seems reasonable to deal with these important operations in a separate section. Depending upon the techniques employed, these procedures are designed to accomplish three main goals: (1) hindfoot and/or ankle stabilization, (2) correction of foot deformity, and (3) improvement in function of the lower limbs. The purpose of stabilization for paralysis or weakness about the foot and ankle is to reduce the number of joints that the paretic or paralyzed muscles must be called upon to control. Four major categories of arthrodesis about the foot and ankle exist: (1) subtalar extra-articular arthrodesis, (2) triple arthrodesis, (3) ankle arthrodesis, and (4) pantalar arthrodesis, which includes both ankle and triple arthrodesis. Other bone stabilization procedures that do not involve arthrodesis include anterior or posterior bone blocks at the ankle. These are now outmoded because of past failures and will not be discussed further.

Grice, in 1959, first reported an extra-articular method of fusion of the subtalar joint using the insertion of autogenous tibial bone grafts between the talus and calcaneus in the sinus tarsus.[18] It was designed to stabilize the paralytic valgus foot and to maintain the height of the longitudinal arch. This procedure interferes minimally with longitudinal growth of the foot, but if a solid fusion is accomplished, growth in height is arrested *at the talocalcaneal joint*. The procedure was developed principally to stabilize the hindfoot in the treatment of flaccid paralytic planovalgus, as described earlier in this chapter.

Preoperatively, it is imperative to determine that the os calcis can be restored passively to its normal position beneath the talus. Failure to ensure normal talocalcaneal relationships will result in a foot that has a valgus heel in fixed equinus and an abducted forefoot. With weight bearing, the talus may then be tilted into valgus within the mortise. Thus, the Grice procedure should not be performed if the os

*Stabilizing (Arthrodesing) Procedures in Paralytic Equinovarus and Paralytic Planovalgus*

calcis cannot be placed in its normal position under the talus. Also, it is essential to correct ankle equinus either operatively or nonoperatively prior to or at the time of the subtalar arthrodesis.

Valgus of the *ankle* can be a late complication of the subtalar arthrodesis. In paralyzed lower limbs, the distal fibular epiphysis frequently is seen proximal to its normal location. Sometimes it can be found proximal to the distal tibia (see p. 191). If the bone graft for the subtalar arthrodesis is removed from the ipsilateral tibia, as Grice described, then stimulation of the distal tibial epiphysis potentially can accentuate the ankle valgus. To reduce the likelihood of this complication, Chigot and Sananes recommended taking the graft from the ipsilateral fibula well above the level of the ankle.[9] This not only avoids the problem of creating significant cortical weakness in the tibia, but also potentially can stimulate growth in the shortened fibula. For these same reasons, since 1962, I have used the fibula exclusively as the graft source in performing subtalar extra-articular arthrodesis (Fig. 5-7).

Tachdjian points out that if one uses the fibula, the segment removed should not be too long and that periosteal closure should be meticulous in order to promote osseous continuity of the fibula. It is well known that a fibular nonunion may cause valgus of the ankle owing to failure of the distal fibula to grow normally. Thus, I agree with Tachdjian that when bilateral Grice procedures are performed, short grafts from each fibula, rather than a large graft from a single fibula, should be removed. I also strongly recommend that autogenous bone be used rather than bone from a bank.

Brown, Seymour, and Evans described a modification of the bone block procedure initially described by Batchelor.[6,8,45] The extra-articular subtalar fusion is accomplished by placing a fibular graft through the neck of the talus into the calcaneus in a dorsal-plantar direction without exposing the sinus tarsus. Because of a high rate of pseudoarthrosis (41%) and generally unsatisfactory results (53%) in his series of 34 patients, Gross reported that the conventional technique described by Grice was much more reliable than the Batchelor procedure.[20] I completely agree with this conclusion.

Dennyson and Fulford described a modification of the Batchelor procedure in which the talus is transfixed to the os calcis by a screw placed through the talar neck, followed by packing of cancellous bone chips around the screw.[11] They reported solid union in 45 of 48 patients. In my opinion, however, the technique of extra-articular subtalar arthrodesis as originally described by Grice, but using the fibular graft, is substantially superior to any currently known modification.

It is not clear who originally described the triple arthrodesis of the hindfoot, largely because of the definition of what constitutes a triple arthrodesis. In a thorough historical review of the literature, Hart analyzed the evolution of arthrodesing procedures of the hindfoot joints.[21] The interested reader should refer to this study for more detailed data dealing with the issue of tarsal arthrodesis. Schwartz accomplished a similar review.[44]

Ryerson placed the triple arthrodesis into proper perspective in 1923 by emphasizing that it is designed not only to provide hindfoot stability, but also to correct any bone or joint deformity of the hindfoot.[43] As a prerequisite to triple arthrodesis, the talus must be stable within the ankle mortise. If it is not, pantalar arthrodesis may be indicated. Flint and MacKenzie have shown that in nearly half of those feet with flaccid paralytic equinovarus, the talus may be subluxated anteriorly within the mortise.[15] If not recognized, this may lead to persistent subluxation and later degenerative changes in the ankle joint after successful triple arthrodesis. In cases in which anterior talar subluxation is detected on preoperative plantar flexion views, Flint and MacKenzie suggest that ankle arthrodesis be considered. I have not seen the high incidence of anterior subluxation they describe; I agree, however, that it should be looked for in all patients undergoing triple arthrodesis. Several variations of Ryerson's triple arthrodesis have been developed, including those designed by Hoke and Dunn to correct the calcaneocavus deformity (Fig. 5-1).[12,25] In this procedure, as described in Chapter 5, posterior displacement of the foot on the talus indirectly transfers the ankle to a more central position on the foot, and the posterior lever arm is lengthened, which then provides mechanical advantage to a weak or paralyzed triceps surae muscle or to muscles transferred to the calcaneus.

Another variation of the triple arthrodesis, described by Lambrinudi in 1927, was designed for use in the foot that has no dorsiflexor function.[30] In order to keep the foot from dropping into plantar flexion, appropriate wedges of bone are excised from the subtalar joint. The talus is then locked in its equinus position, and the remainder of the foot can be dorsiflexed on the talus, resulting in a spurious but effective correction of ankle equinus (see Fig. 2-40).

Minor variations of the Ryerson triple arthrodesis are also employed to correct deformities in equinovarus and planovalgus. Thus, the triple arthrodesis is an extremely versatile and useful procedure that, when properly done, gives effective long-term results.[1,31]

## COMPLICATIONS AND PROBLEMS WITH TRIPLE ARTHRODESIS

Marek and Schein found avascular necrosis of the talus to be a complication of either triple or pantalar arthrodesis.[34] As one would expect, they found that it is more likely to occur after wide excision of the head and neck of the talus, and also that it is somewhat age related, occurring more frequently in adolescents and adults than in younger children. On the other hand, Struckman, in a long-term review of 38 cases, found that necrosis of the talus was much more common when triple arthrodesis was done under age 7 years.[50] Thus, it appears that the incidence of talar necrosis is most likely to occur in either those young children (in whom the operation should *not* be done) or in older adolescents and adults.

Hill, Wilson, Chevres, and Sweterlisch reported the results of over 40 triple arthrodeses performed on children age 5 to 8 years and followed for an average of 9 years.[23] Although they performed these procedures at a much earlier age than is customary, they waited until the navicular ossification was large enough to allow fusion with the talus. The incidence of pseudoarthrosis was approximately 20%, and approximately 12% required revision to correct residual deformity. The foot was ultimately shortened by an average of 2 cm. Recognizing this situation, Tachdjian emphasizes the well accepted concept that to avoid disturbing growth of the tarsal bones, which occurs concentrically at their periphery, triple arthrodesis should be deferred until age 10 to 12 years in girls and 12 to 14 years in boys, at which time the foot has essentially reached skeletal maturity.

Other problems associated with foot stabilization have been reported. Following triple arthrodesis, the ankle is subjected to many forces that otherwise would be dissipated or cushioned by the intertarsal joints. As a consequence, degenerative arthritis of the ankle can be a long-term sequela of triple arthrodesis. In a long-term follow-up study, however, Adelaar and associates showed that this untoward change following triple arthrodesis is not common.[1]

According to Crego and McCarroll, residual foot deformity has been reported in as high as 20% of feet following triple arthrodesis.[10] They attributed most of these failures to residual muscle imbalance following the triple arthrodesis. In keeping with this observation, Ingram and Peabody both agreed that correction of dynamic deformities cannot be maintained by arthrodesis alone in a growing child. With growth, the deformities will gradually recur.[27,39]

Patterson, Parrish, and Hathaway reported an 18% failure rate in triple arthrodesis, most of which they attributed to residual deformities.[38] Most were related to inadequate initial correction, but others resulted from such factors as insufficient immobilization, failure to align the foot properly, loss of position at the time of cast change, pseudoarthrosis, persistent muscle imbalance, and the fact that the operation was performed at too early an age when the bones were not sufficiently mature.

Pseudoarthrosis of one or more joints has been a common problem with triple arthrodesis, and its incidence ranges from 9 to 23% in the reported series. Most of the pseudoarthroses, up to 89%, have involved the talonavicular joint. By using internal fixation (staples) or transfixion, I have rarely had failure of fusion of any joint in performing the triple arthrodesis. My observations dictate that fusion fails most often because of technical errors, especially when no internal fixation or transfixion is used.

The pantalar arthrodesis (tibiotalar, talocalcaneal, talonavicular, and calcaneocuboid) is most often indicated in instances of totally paralyzed (flail) foot and ankle (see Fig. 5-18). In my opinion, the only virtual, absolute contraindication to this operation is the flail, insensitive foot and ankle seen most commonly in paralysis due to myelodysplasia. The same concepts and techniques apply to pantalar arthrodesis as to triple arthrodesis.

*References*

1. Adelaar, R. S., et al.: Long term study of triple arthrodesis in children. J. Bone Joint Surg., *58A:724*, 1976.
2. Baker, L. D.: Triceps surae syndrome in cerebral palsy. Surgery, *68:*216, 1954.
3. Baker, L. D., and Dodelin, R. A.: Extra-articular arthrodesis of the subtalar joint (Grice procedure). JAMA, *168:*1005, 1958.
4. Baker, L. D., and Hill, L. M.: Foot alignment in the cerebral palsy patient. J. Bone Joint Surg., *46A:*1, 1974.
5. Banks, H. H., and Green, W. T.: Correction of equinus deformity in cerebral palsy. J. Bone Joint Surg., *40A:*1359, 1958.
6. Batchelor, J. S., cited as personal communication to Seymour, N., and Evans, D. K., A modification of the Grice subtalar arthrodesis. J. Bone Joint Surg., *50B:*372, 1968.
7. Bisla, R. S., Louis, H. J., and Albano, P.: Transfer of the tibialis posterior tendon in cerebral palsy. J. Bone Joint Surg., *58A:*497, 1959.
8. Brown, A.: A simple method of fusion of the subtalar joint in children. J. Bone Joint Surg., *50B:*369, 1968.
9. Chigot, P. L., and Sananes, P.: Arthrodese de Grice, Variente technique. Rev. Chir. Orthop., *51:*53, 1965.
10. Crego, C. H., and McCarroll, H. R.: Recurrent deformities in stabilized paralytic feet. J. Bone Joint Surg., *20:*609, 1938.
11. Dennyson, W. G., and Fulford, G. E.: Subtalar arthrodesis by cancellous grafts and metallic internal fixation in children. J. Bone Joint Surg., *54A:*585, 1972.
12. Dunn, N.: Stabilizing operations in the treatment of paralytic deformities of the foot. Proc. R. Soc. Med., *15:*17, 1921.
13. Durham, H. A., cited as personal communication by Caldwell, G. D., in Watkins, M. B., Jones, J. B., Ryder, C. T., Jr., and Brown, T. H., Jr.: Transplantation of the posterior tibial tendon. J. Bone Joint Surg., *36A:*1181, 1954.
14. Dwyer, F. C.: Osteotomy of the calcaneum for pes cavus. J. Bone Joint Surg., *41B:*80, 1959.
15. Flint, M. H., and MacKenzie, I. G.: Anterior laxity of the ankle, a cause of recurrent paralytic dropfoot deformity. J. Bone Joint Surg., *44B:*377, 1962.
16. Fried, A., and Hendel, C.: Paralytic valgus deformity of the ankle; replacement of the paralyzed tibialis by the peroneus longus. J. Bone Joint Surg., *39A:*921, 1957.
17. Fried, A., and Moyseyev, S.: Paralytic valgus deformity of the foot: treatment by replacement of the paralyzed tibialis posterior muscle; a long-term follow-up study. J. Bone Joint Surg., *52A:*1674, 1970.
18. Grice, D. S.: The role of subtalar fusion in the treatment of valgus deformities of the feet. In *AAOS Instructional Course Lectures.* Vol. 16. St. Louis, C. V. Mosby, 1959, p. 127.
19. Gritzka, T. L., Staheli, L. T., and Duncan, W. R.: Posterior tibial tendon transfer through the interosseous membrane to correct equinovarus deformity in cerebral palsy: An initial experience. Clin. Orthop., *89:*201, 1972.
20. Gross, R. H.: A clinical study of the Batchelor subtalar arthrodesis. J. Bone Joint Surg., *58A:*343, 1976.
21. Hart, V. L.: Arthrodesis of the foot in infantile paralysis. Surg. Gynecol. Obstet., *64:*794, 1937.
22. Hibbs, R. A.: An operation for "claw-foot." JAMA, *73:*1583, 1919.
23. Hill, N. A., Wilson, H. J., Chevres, R., and Sweterlisch, P. R.: Triple arthrodesis in the young child. Clin. Orthop., *70:*187, 1970.
24. Hoffer, M. M., Reiswig, J. A., Garrett, A. M., and Perry, J.: The split anterior tibial tendon transfer in the treatment of spastic varus hindfoot of childhood. Orthop. Clin. North Am., *5:*31, 1974.
25. Hoke, M.: An operation for stabilizing paralytic feet. J. Orthop. Surg., *19:*494, 1921.
26. Holstein, A.: Hallux valgus—an acquired deformity of the foot in cerebral palsy. Orthop. Trans., *2:*246, 1978.

27. Ingram, A. J.: Anterior poliomyelitis. In *Campbell's Operative Orthopaedics*. 6th Edition. Edited by A. S. Edmondson and H. A. Crenshaw. St. Louis, C. V. Mosby, 1980, p. 1418.

28. Jones, R.: The soldier's foot and the treatment of common deformities of the foot. Part II, Claw foot, Br. Med. J., *1*:749, 1916.

29. Keats, S.: Operative orthopedics. In *Cerebral Palsy*. Springfield, Illinois, Charles C Thomas, 1970, p. 218.

30. Lambrinudi, C.: New operation on dropfoot. Br. J. Surg., *15*:193, 1927.

31. Lee, G., and Coleman, S. S.: Calcaneal cavus foot. Read at Shriners Annual Alumni Scientific Meeting, Salt Lake City, 1965.

32. Lipscomb, P. R., and Sanchez, J. J.: Anterior transplantation of the posterior tibialis tendon for persistent palsy of the common peroneal nerve. J. Bone Joint Surg., *43A*:60, 1961.

33. Majestro, T. C., Ruda, R., and Frost, H. M.: Intramuscular lengthening of the posterior tibialis muscle. Clin. Orthop., *79*:59, 1971.

34. Marek, F. M., and Schein, A. J.: Aseptic necrosis of the astragalus following arthrodesing procedures of the tarsus. J. Bone Joint Surg., *27*:587, 1945.

35. Mayer, L.: Tendon transplantations on the lower extremity. In *AAOS Instructional Course Lectures*. Vol. 6. Ann Arbor, J. W. Edwards, 1949, p. 189.

36. Mooney, V., and Goodman, F.: Surgical approaches to lower extremity disability secondary to strokes. Clin. Orthop., *63*:142, 1969.

37. Ober, F. R.: Tendon transplantation in the lower extremity. N. Engl. J. Med., *209*:52, 1933.

38. Patterson, R. L., Parrish, F. F., and Hathaway, E. N.: Stabilizing operations on the foot. J. Bone Joint Surg., *32A*:1, 1950.

39. Peabody, C. W.: Tendon transposition: An end-result study. J. Bone Joint Surg., *20*:193, 1938.

40. Perry, J.: Personal communication, 1981.

41. Pierrot, A. H., and Murphy, O. B.: Heel cord advancement: A new approach to the spastic equinus deformity. Orthop. Clin. North Am., *5*:117, 1974.

42. Putti, V., cited by Mayer, L.: The physiological method of tendon transplantation in the treatment of paralytic drop-foot. J. Bone Joint Surg., *19*:389, 1937.

43. Ryerson, E.: Arthrodesing operations of the feet. J. Bone Joint Surg., *5*:453, 1923.

44. Schwartz, R. P.: Arthrodesis of subtalus and midtarsal joints of the foot. Historical review, pre-operative determinations, and operative procedure. Surgery, *20*:619, 1946.

45. Seymour, N., and Evans, D. K.: A modification of the Grice subtalar arthrodesis. J. Bone Joint Surg., *50B*:372, 1968.

46. Silver, C. M., and Simon, S. D.: Gastrocnemius muscle resection (Silverskiold operation) for spastic equinus deformity in cerebral palsy. J. Bone Joint Surg., *41A*:1021, 1959.

47. Silver, C. M., Simon, S. D., and Litchman, H. M.: Calcaneal osteotomy for valgus and varus deformities of the foot in cerebral palsy: Preliminary report, presentation, American Academy for Cerebral Palsy Meeting, New York City, 1964.

48. Silverskiold, N.: Reduction of the uncrossed two joint muscles of the leg to one joint muscle in spastic conditions. Acta. Chir. Scand., *56*:315, 1923–24.

49. Strayer, L. M., Jr.: Recession of the gastrocnemius, an operation to relieve spastic contracture of the calf muscles. J. Bone Joint Surg., *32A*:671, 1950.

50. Struckman, J. S.: Triple arthrodesis in young children. Presented at the Western Orthopedic Association, 1970. J. Bone Joint Surg., *53A*:396, 1971.

51. Tachdjian, M. O.: *Pediatric Orthopedics*. Philadelphia, W. B. Saunders, 1972.

52. Throop, F. B., DeRosa, G. P., Reeck, C., and Waterman, S.: Correction of equinus in cerebral palsy by the Murphy procedure of tendocalcaneus advancement: A preliminary communication. Dev. Med. Child Neurol., *17*:182, 1975.

53. Tohen, F. A., Cameron, P. J., and Barrera, J. R.: The utilization of abnormal reflexes in the treatment of spastic foot deformities. A preliminary report. Clin. Orthop., *47:77*, 1966.

54. Turner, J. W., and Cooper, R. R.: Anterior transfer of the tibialis posterior through the interosseous membrane. Clin. Orthop., *83:241*, 1972.

55. Vulpius, O., and Stoffel, A.: *Orthopaedische operationstebre*. 2nd Edition. Stuttgart, Ferdinard Enke, 1920.

56. Watkins, M. B., Jones J. B., Ryder, C. T., Jr., and Brown, T. H., Jr.: Transplantation of the posterior tibial tendon. J. Bone Joint Surg., *36A:1181*, 1954.

# Teratologic Equinovarus Congenita

The major purpose for including a separate chapter on this unusual foot problem is that it represents the most difficult challenge of all equinovarus deformities. This foot always requires surgical correction, usually through radical, complete releases most often accomplished relatively early in infancy. This deformity resists *any* form of treatment, tends to recur, and nearly always requires day-and-night postoperative bracing through the first several years of life. This particular type of equinovarus is most frequently associated with arthrogryposis multiplex congenita or occurs in conjunction with other multiple congenital skeletal deformities.

According to Middleton, the condition now known as arthrogryposis multiplex congenita was described by Otto as early as 1841.[8,9] The term itself, however, was introduced by Stern in 1923.[11] Sheldon, in 1932, believed that the disorder was primarily a deficiency of muscle or muscle fibers due to an unknown cause.[10] Subsequently, Adams and associates subdivided the condition into two distinct clinical syndromes, "neuropathic" and "myopathic," based upon their conception of the pathologic process.[1] Some controversy still remains concerning the possibility that these are one and the same conditions, the differences simply representing variations in the manifestation of the process.

    The etiologic factors have been explored from several standpoints. These include mechanical (positional), "neurogenic," and myopathic causes. The mechanical concept has not been well accepted, despite the fact that Wynne-Davies noted arthrogryposis in instances of oligohydramnios, reduced fetal movements, and breech deliveries. These factors, however, had rather uncommon relationships in the patients reviewed in several British centers by both Wynne-Davies and Lloyd-Roberts and Lettin.[7,13]

*Arthrogryposis: Etiology and Pathogenesis*

The "neurogenic" cause of arthrogryposis has been more well accepted because of the rather strong evidence found by Drachman and Banker who identified histologic findings of denervation atrophy.[2] Equally common is the concept of amyoplasia as the cause of arthrogryposis. Several authors have identified absence of muscle function or even dystrophic muscle changes in postmortem studies.

At present, no proven cause appears to account for all of the manifestations of this unique and unusual condition. The important thing to remember is that these children often have severely restricted joint motion and do not respond to surgical procedures in the usual way. Excessive scarring tends to occur despite well performed operations, and these children have especially resistant congenital equinovarus foot deformities.

Arthrogryposis is uncommon, but the incidence varies considerably from one community to another. Williams reported that 120 cases were seen in The Royal Children's Hospital in Melbourne in 20 years, an average of only 6 patients per year.[12] He also cited a study in Helsinki in which the incidence was found to be 3 per 10,000 live births.

The absence of normal function and the rigidity of the joints are further complicated by the fact that the arthrogrypotic joints have a distinct tendency to develop stiffness and fibrosis following any type of open surgical procedure. One must keep these observations in perspective whenever operating on teratologic joints in general and arthrogrypotic joints in particular. Despite these overwhelming problems, many of these patients become gainful, contributing citizens later in adult life; a substantial number, however, become totally disabled as the result of the immense disability caused by the lack of effective muscle and joint function. Many patients with arthrogryposis multiplex congenita just disappear, ultimately leaving no trace of their whereabouts, at least for purposes of routine follow-up studies. At the Intermountain Unit of the Shriners Hospital, Salt Lake City, Utah, we conducted a search of all patients with a diagnosis of arthrogryposis multiplex congenita and were able to find only 2 patients over the age of 21.[4] Surprisingly, no record could be found of the deaths of the remaining patients.

To what extent these factors enter into a decision to implement treatment of the teratologic foot is clearly a highly individualized problem. Each case must be considered on the basis of its own merits; ultimately a decision *in favor* of treatment is usually reached.

## Clinical Features

The foot has a rather typical equinovarus appearance, but it is extremely rigid and possesses all of the features of arthrogryposis. Williams describes the limbs in arthrogryposis as being "featureless." Not only are the normal skin creases absent, but dimples are often seen in the extensor surfaces of the affected joints. The subcutaneous fat is also increased, usually at the expense of the mass or volume of musculature. Such a situation often makes vein puncture difficult, an important consideration when general anesthesia is contemplated (see p.

259). Substantially reduced motor power is demonstrable in essentially all the muscles of the leg and the foot. The skin creases are usually poorly defined, and the soft tissues of the leg are grossly atrophic (Fig. 8-1). Cutaneous sensory modalities are preserved, but the deep tendon reflexes are absent or weak. The rigidity of the deformity and the reduced muscle strength of the leg and foot are the factors largely responsible for the difficulty encountered in treating this particular deformity. The rigidity in some cases proves to be a tarsal coalition that is encountered in the course of surgical correction.

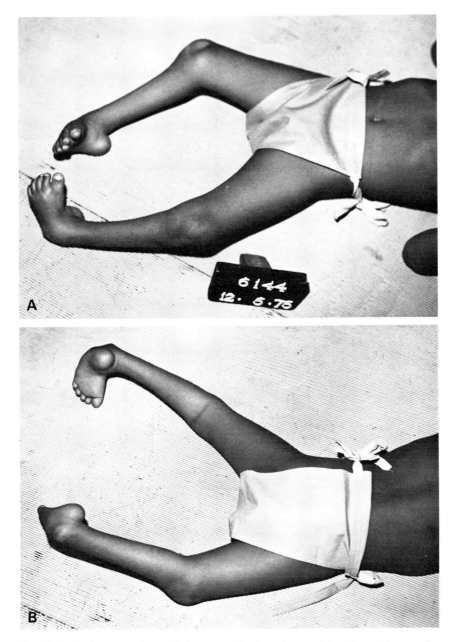

FIG. 8-1. Arthrogryposis multiplex congenita in a 2-year-old patient. Observe the "featureless" thighs and legs and the obviously severe and rigid congenital equinovarus, in addition to the knee flexion contractures.

### Radiographic and Pathologic Features

The roentgenographic findings are often indistinguishable from those seen in the conventional congenital equinovarus. In some instances, however, the findings are grossly abnormal. Commonly, an ossification center is missing in the talus or calcaneus, and in many cases the ossification centers are smaller than normal and are abnormally shaped (Fig. 8-2). These aberrations undoubtedly reflect the effect of poor muscle and joint function.

Pathologically, the joints about the talus (the peritalar joint) may be poorly formed, and intra-articular adhesions may be found. Thus, the rigidity is due both to intra- and extra-articular causes. These factors account for the difficulty in achieving correction either nonoperatively or operatively and explain why astragalectomy may be the only possible method of correction in young children. As noted earlier, it is not rare to encounter a tarsal coalition, especially in the talocalcaneal joint.

### Concepts of Treatment

The decision to treat skeletal deformities of such severity and magnitude is based upon several important factors: (1) the probability of survival, (2) the likelihood of ambulation, and (3) the character and degree of abnormality of the foot. Thus, it is important to identify all associated or accompanying visceral and skeletal abnormalities in order to place the foot problem into perspective. Clearly, a major foot

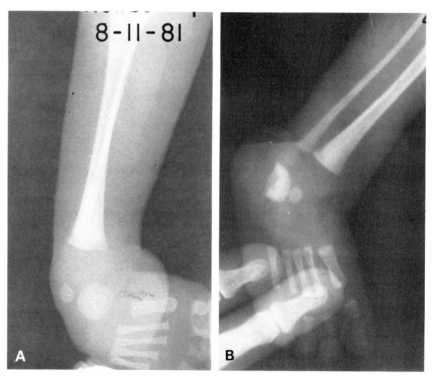

FIG. 8-2. Examples of the abnormal ossification centers occurring in teratologic (arthrogrypotic) clubfeet. **A**, The talus is unusually small, and the calcaneus is essentially spherical. **B**, The calcaneus has a rectangular shape, and the talus is similarly small.

operation should be delayed until any life-threatening visceral abnormalities are corrected or stabilized. Also, it is helpful to determine, as well as possible, whether a foot operation is likely to assist ambulation. This obviously necessitates accurate appraisal of the configuration and function of the remainder of the lower limbs, as well as the functional capabilities of the upper limbs. In many instances, however, this determination cannot be made with sufficient confidence in the first few months of life and thus does not represent a major factor in the decision to implement treatment. Also, in nearly all cases, the parents will want the feet corrected whether or not ambulation will be possible. To what extent the degree of severity of the foot abnormality enters into the decision is a highly variable judgmental issue, and guidelines are difficult to develop. Again, in most, if not all instances, the decision to carry out a treatment program will be overwhelmingly affirmative and will counter or over-ride any factors except for life-threatening, coexisting visceral abnormalities. This is especially so because these children are invariably bright and intelligent, and the parents will strongly desire correction of these deformed feet.

When the decision is made to treat such feet, the initial program should consist of the application of corrective casts in the same manner as described in Chapter 2. If the patient has a true arthrogrypotic teratologic clubfoot, however, substantial nonoperative correction of the disturbed bony relationships should *not* be expected because of the unusually rigid and recalcitrant character of these feet. The principal reasons for even attempting to correct these particular feet nonoperatively are to stretch out the skin and subcutaneous tissues and to help determine accurately whether nonoperative correction can be achieved (usually never).

Also, it is prudent to wait a few weeks or months until the child is more mature and will therefore be a better candidate for general anesthesia. As a matter of fact, the risks of general anesthesia are reported to be substantially higher during the first few months of life in these children than in normal children.[5] Also, it is not unusual that "cut down" vein punctures will be required to provide appropriate intravenous fluid replacement if necessary.

Weekly manipulations and cast changes should be monitored by careful physical and strategic radiographic examinations. In nearly all instances, the hindfoot will rarely show any substantial evidence of correction even after 12 to 16 weeks of conscientious efforts. By this time, however, the medial aspect of the foot should have become somewhat elongated, and the foot will be big enough and the child old enough that operative correction can be carried out more safely. Surgical release, however, is rarely done on a selective basis, because, in nearly *all* instances, all of the soft tissues will require radical and complete severance or elongation.

## Surgical Technique

It is not necessary to repeat the technical details of the operations that are described in Chapter 2 because, in principle, the same procedures are employed. Because of the great difficulty encountered in correcting these feet, however, and because of the gross motor weakness that so often exists, simple tenotomy, with or without repair of the tendons on the medial and posterior aspects of the foot and ankle, is usually the most practical method of elongating the tendons.

Williams actually removes a segment of the Achilles tendon when correcting the equinus. I sometimes have found it necessary also to resect the posterior tibial tendon in the medial release procedure. The ligamentous structures must be sectioned completely about the talus as well as the ankle joints, except for the deep tibiotalar portion of the deltoid ligament. This can be called a peritalar capsulotomy or capsulectomy. At the same time, correction will often necessitate *excision* of the laciniate ligament and its retinacula. A pin is always placed across the talonavicular joint, and a well padded cast is applied. Care must be taken not to achieve too much correction at the time of the operation. The danger to wound healing and the skin and soft tissues is considerable and must be carefully observed.

Postoperatively, it is important to change casts frequently, and the cast application must be preceded by the usual gentle manipulation of the foot into greater degrees of correction. The sequential cast change must be continued until maximum or optimum correction has been achieved. Usually at 6 weeks postoperatively, the talonavicular pin may be removed, but the corrective cast applications should continue. In some situations, these maneuvers may require 8 or 10 weeks for satisfactory correction. Then a holding cast is applied, which remains for an additional 4 to 6 weeks.

Following removal of the holding cast, the feet are placed into toe-out clubfoot shoes attached to a dorsiflexion-assist brace that has a right-angle plantar flexion stop. As long as the child is nonambulatory, an outward-rotation bar is placed on the soles of the shoes with the feet outwardly rotated about 30 to 45° (Fig. 8-3). This is designed

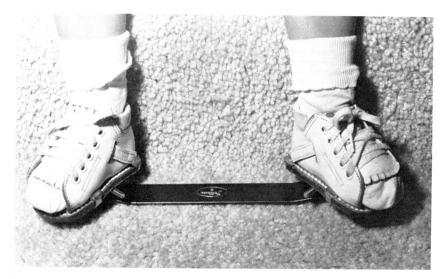

FIG. 8-3. A crossbar attached to outwardly rotated shoes is appropriate to maintain correction postoperatively after the postoperative casts have been removed in the nonambulatory child (see also Figure 2-14).

to maintain eversion and outward rotation in conjunction with the dorsiflexion effect of the brace on the foot and ankle. This position may have to be achieved gradually, and care is necessary to ascertain that the foot is held snugly in this position within the shoes. Special care must be taken to see that the heel of the foot is held properly in the shoes. These retaining devices must remain on day and night, but it is important to take the feet out of the shoes and braces two or three times a day to check any possible pressure areas and so that the feet can be carried through a passive range of motion, especially dorsiflexion and eversion. With proper instructions, the parents can usually do this effectively.

This method of postoperative care must be followed for several years. Depending upon the child's ambulatory capacity and whether he has any functional muscles, this program can be modified as the child grows and develops. The important principles to observe are that (1) this deformity has a notorious tendency to recur, (2) tendon transfers usually are not practical, (3) each time the foot is operated upon, correction becomes more difficult and finally, (4) salvage procedures are frequently necessary, even when the most conscientious efforts have been exerted.

The four most frequently employed salvage procedures used for these feet include (1) lateral-column shortening, (2) astragalectomy, (3) distal tibial anterior closing-wedge osteotomy, and (4) triple arthrodesis. Although these procedures all have been discussed in detail in Chapter 2, each will be briefly discussed and illustrated here as it applies specifically to this type of clubfoot, because certain special considerations obtain in these instances of teratologic equinovarus.

*Salvage Procedures in Teratologic Equinovarus*

Lateral-column shortening is much more likely to be required in this deformity because of its recalcitrant and longstanding nature and inexorable tendency to recur. The lateral column of these feet is best shortened by calcaneocuboid resection, either through complete joint resection or by the Lichtblau technique, in which only the distal end of the calcaneus is resected.[3,6] Often, however, this joint fuses spontaneously, irrespective of the method of lateral-column shortening (Fig. 8-4).

Astragalectomy is the ultimate salvage procedure (except for ankle disarticulation) in teratologic clubfeet. This procedure is usually reserved for children in the 3- to 5-year age group, but it may be equally effective in older children (Fig. 8-5). Williams has observed spontaneous fusion occurring between the tibia and the navicular and the calcaneus. This often is accompanied by the development of equinus, which will then require corrective osteotomy.

Anterior closing-wedge osteotomy of the tibia is a salvage procedure in which correction usually lasts only a year or two because the growth of the tibia causes the equinus deformity to recur. Nevertheless, it is a convenient and rather rapid method of correcting equinus in children too young for triple arthrodesis. It is frequently necessary even after astragalectomy (Fig. 8-6).

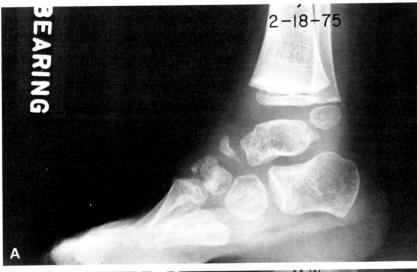

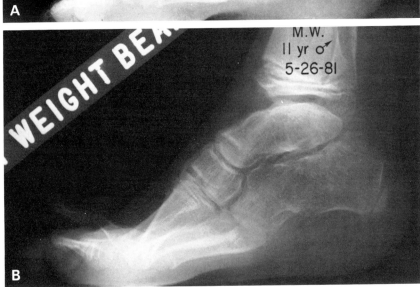

FIG. 8-4. **A,** Lateral standing roentgenogram of an 11-year-old boy who underwent a calcaneus resection for severe arthrogrypotic clubfoot at 5 years of age. **B,** The spontaneous fusion of the calcaneocuboid joint, as well as of the talonavicular joint, is seen 6 years later.

Triple arthrodesis is reserved for children in whom correction has been maintained well enough through their growth period that they have avoided astragalectomy but whose deformities are persistent enough to justify surgical correction. Towards the age of skeletal maturity, this is best achieved by triple arthrodesis. One must remember, however, that the ankle joint in these feet is usually not totally normal, and a substantial degree of foot and ankle rigidity is thus inevitable. Realizing the rather low demands that are usually made on these feet, however, the acceptance of increased rigidity in exchange for a plantigrade foot seems justified.

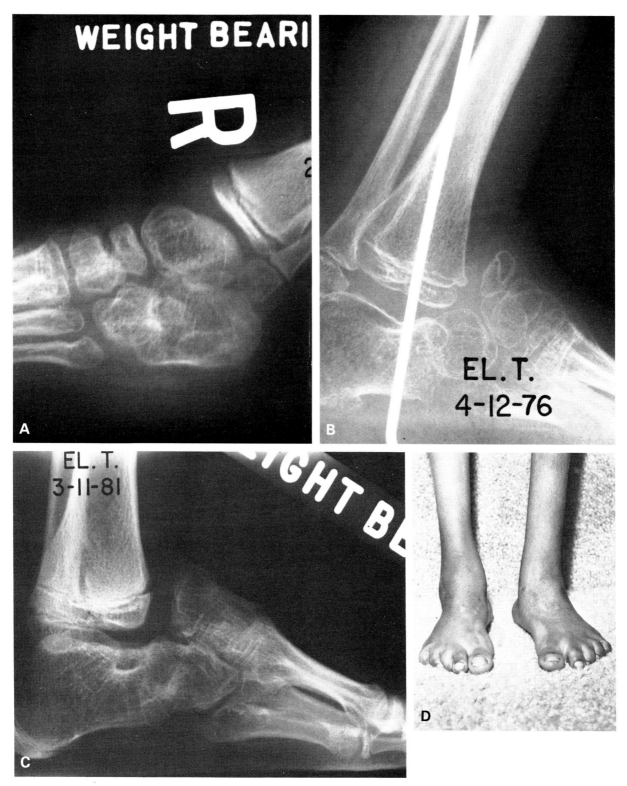

FIG. 8-5. **A**, Attempted weight-bearing lateral film of a foot with residual stigmata of severe congenital equinovarus deformity due to arthrogryposis multiplex congenita. This patient had undergone three previous posterior release procedures, and the region of the ankle and Achilles tendon were extensively scarred. **B**, Six weeks following astragalectomy, the improved plantigrade appearance of the foot is evident. **C**, Correction maintained 5 years later. **D**, **E**, and **F**, Clinical photographs also showing results of correction.

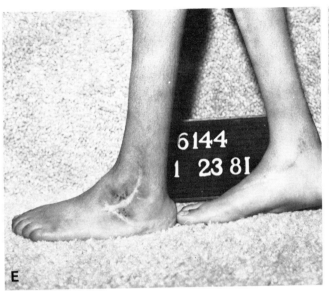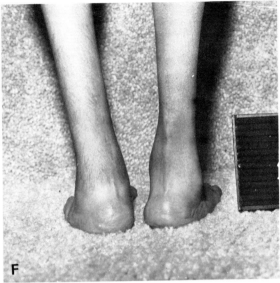

Fᴵɢ.. 8-5. *continued*

*References*

1. Adams, R. D., Denis-Browne, D. and Pearson, C. M.: *Diseases of Muscle, a Study in Pathology.* New York, Harper & Row, 1967, p. 310.
2. Drachman, D. B., and Banker, B. Q.: Arthrogryposis multiplex congenita: Case due to disease of anterior horn cells. Arch. Neurol., *5:*77, 1961.
3. Evans, D.: Relapsed clubfoot. J. Bone Joint Surg., *43B:*722, 1961.
4. Jacobs, L., and Coleman, S. S.: Unpublished data.
5. Jordan, W. R.: Personal communication, 1981.
6. Lichtblau, S.: A medial and lateral release operation for club foot. A preliminary report. J. Bone Joint Surg., *55A:*1377, 1973.
7. Lloyd-Roberts, G. C., and Lettin, A. W. F.: Arthrogryposis multiplex congenita. J. Bone Joint Surg., *52B:*494, 1970.
8. Middleton, D. S.: Studies on prenatal lesions of striated muscle as a cause of congenital deformity. Edinburgh Med. J., *41:*401, 1934.
9. Otto, A. G.: Monstrorum sec centorum descriptio anatomica in vratislaviae museum. Anatomico-Pathologicum Vratislaviense, 1841.
10. Sheldon, W.: Amyoplasia congenita. Arch. Dis. Child., *7:*117, 1932.
11. Stern, W. G.: Arthrogryposis multiplex congenita. JAMA, *81:*1507, 1923.
12. Williams, P.: The management of arthrogryposis. Orthop. Clin. North Am., *9:*67, 1978.
13. Wynne-Davies, R.: Family studies and the cause of congenital clubfoot—talipes equinovarus, talipes calcaneovalgus and metatarsus varus. J. Bone Joint Surg., *46B:*445, 1964.

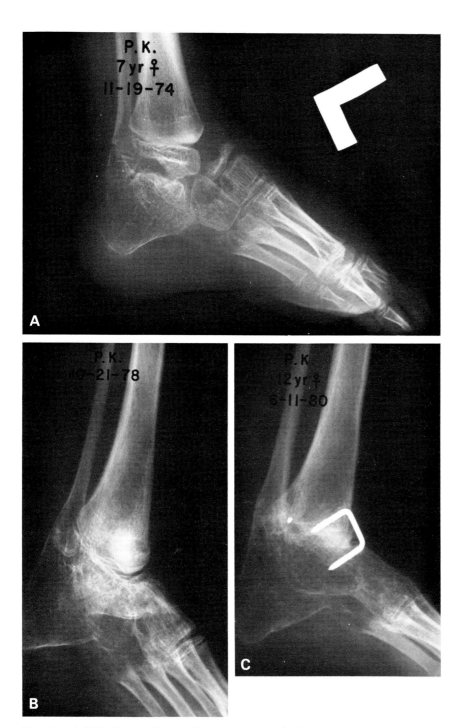

FIG. 8-6. **A**, This 7-year-old girl with arthrogryposis had undergone astragalectomy 1 year previously as salvage treatment for a severe clubfoot deformity. **B**, Four years later, the equinus deformity had recurred. In addition, spontaneous fusion of the ankle and triple joint had taken place. **C**, An anterior closing-wedge osteotomy of the distal tibia (through the physis) was accomplished to correct the equinus.

# Miscellaneous Disorders

This chapter attempts to complete the discussion of complex foot deformities in children as they were defined and classified in Chapter 1. Clearly, it is impossible to claim that this text has appropriately dealt with *all* complicated foot problems in children. This is because a substantial number of rare and atypical abnormalities of the foot cannot be classified in a meaningful way. Many foot abnormalities occur as a manifestation of terminal limb deficiencies or as the result of rare and unusual developmental defects. Examples include the "lobster foot," gigantism, absence of digital rays, and the bizarre foot resulting from failure of segmentation as seen in Apert's syndrome. Because of their rare and unusual nature, these will not be discussed, since each must be approached in such a highly individualized manner. Thus, this section deals with the following conditions: metatarsus adductus (serpentine foot), tarsal coalition, peroneal spastic foot, and disorders of the foot following peripheral nerve injuries due to intramuscular injections.

*Metatarsus Adductus (Serpentine Foot)*

This rather uncommon disorder demands special attention because it often requires surgical correction. It must be carefully separated from the much more common and usually self-correcting condition known as metatarus varus. In this regard, it is essential that the deformity be clearly described and that terminology be agreed upon. Much confusion surrounds this latter issue, because metatarsus adductus is often confused with metatarsus varus, and frequently the same term is used interchangeably for both. This unfortunate and disconcerting situation has often led to misunderstanding regarding treatment. In order for this particular discussion to be valid and effective, therefore, the name metatarsus adductus will be used for the complex condition discussed in the following sections.

CLINICAL APPEARANCE    Characteristically, the hindfoot is in valgus (pronation), the midfoot has a substantial loss of the normal longitudinal arch, and the forefoot is adducted and supinated. Thus, the foot assumes a "Z" or serpentine appearance both clinically and radiographically (Fig. 9-1). Usually, this abnormality is not manifested until early childhood after the patient has been walking for a year or two. This somewhat paradoxic deformity is difficult to treat with any type of ankle-foot orthoses, and it often creates shoe-fitting and shoe-wear problems that, when sufficiently great, justify surgical correction.

The alternate foot deformity, called here metatarsus varus, is commonly seen in infants and differs substantially from the foot just described. The hindfoot is nearly always normal and there is no loss of the longitudinal arch, yet the forefoot is adducted. The deformity thus produces a C-shaped foot that is most often positional and nearly always responds to conservative measures such as passive stretching, splintage, or, in unusual circumstances, a short period of manipulation and cast applications. By way of comparison, this foot is illustrated in Figure 9-2.

Whether or not this particular nomenclature is accepted is not important; what is important is to agree that these deformed feet represent two distinctly different foot abnormalities. In metatarsus adductus, the rarer situation, the problem is complex and not uncommonly requires surgical correction. In metatarsus varus, surgical correction is virtually never required. The definitions employed are proposed simply to avoid confusion in the discussion that follows.

TREATMENT    As with all complex foot deformities, the degree of severity in manifestation of the serpentine foot varies widely. Only those feet that demonstrate substantial cosmetic or shoe-fitting problems should be considered candidates for surgical correction. Clearly, the decision to operate on this type of foot must be predicated upon the observations that the foot is not improving during growth and development and is sufficiently deformed to justify correction. The answers to these two important issues are highly individual. Clinical judgment on the part of the physician, combined with the needs of the patient and parents, will ultimately result in an acceptable decision regarding treatment. Usually such a decision will not be reached, nor will it be necessary, before the patient is 5 to 7 years old. Also, the type of surgical procedure required is more effectively accomplished, and the results more predictable, after the tarsal bones have become more mature. This is because appropriate correction often will require some type of operation on the tarsal bones.

The basic approach to correction of this unusual deformity is based upon the premise that the hindfoot is flexible and that correction of the adducted and supinated forefoot will adequately correct all components of the deformity. In order to do this, a soft-tissue (plantar) release is essential, in addition to some method of elongating the medial column of the midfoot and forefoot, in some instances accompanied by lateral-column shortening. An operative procedure to solve

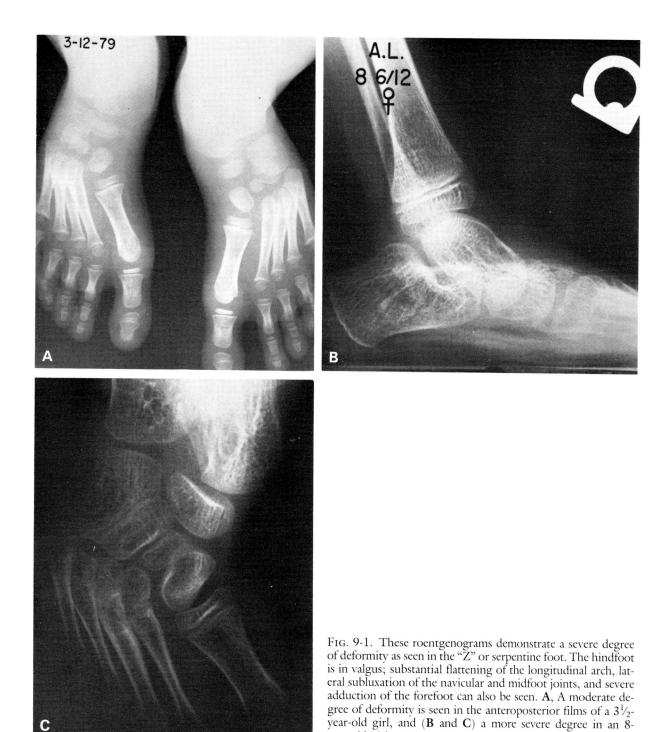

FIG. 9-1. These roentgenograms demonstrate a severe degree of deformity as seen in the "Z" or serpentine foot. The hindfoot is in valgus; substantial flattening of the longitudinal arch, lateral subluxation of the navicular and midfoot joints, and severe adduction of the forefoot can also be seen. **A**, A moderate degree of deformity is seen in the anteroposterior films of a 3½-year-old girl, and (**B** and **C**) a more severe degree in an 8-year-old girl.

this problem in younger children has been described by Goldner.[17] For older children (over 6 years), I prefer the opening-wedge osteotomy of the medial cuneiform, as described in Chapter 2 (Fig. 9-3).

*Metatarsus Varus*

As noted previously, metatarsus varus is a common foot disorder, most often encountered at birth and in early infancy. Also, as outlined earlier, several clinical features distinguish it from metatarsus adductus.

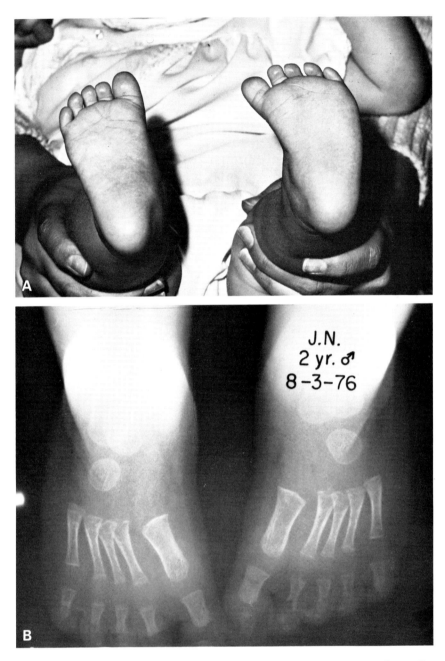

FIG. 9-2. Plantar photographs of a metatarsus varus foot (right). Compare its configuration to that on the viewer's left. **A**, The reason for the term "C" foot is readily apparent. **B**, Anteroposterior roentgenograms of a 2-year-old male with metatarsus varus. The right foot (viewer's left) shows more metatarsus varus than the left.

These cases of metatarsus varus nearly all are corrected during the first or second year, either spontaneously or by simple, nonoperative means. A rare patient may enter childhood with a persistent deformity that is usually dynamic; that is, the varus configuration usually can be corrected passively, but upon stance and when walking, the forefoot is decidedly adducted. Whether or not this dynamic deformity is serious enough to justify surgical correction is highly controversial, because it

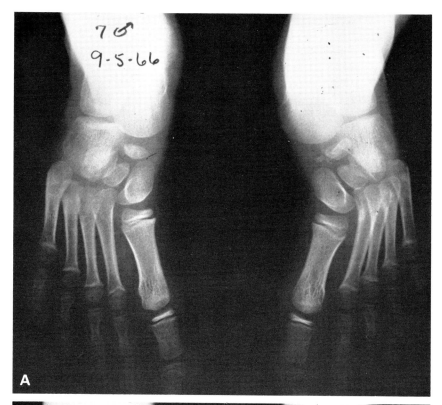

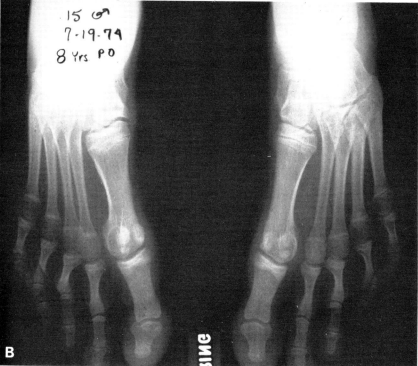

FIG. 9-3. **A**, Anteroposterior weight-bearing roentgenogram showing a "serpentine" or metatarsus adductus foot in a 7-year-old boy. Because of the degree of deformity and the failure of the feet to improve, an opening-wedge osteotomy of the medial cuneiform (Fowler procedure) was accomplished. **B**, The satisfactory radiographic result is seen in the anteroposterior weight-bearing film taken 8 years later at nearly complete skeletal maturity.

rarely persists through adulthood. In some rare instances of severe deformity, however, operative correction *may* be indicated.

The basic reason proposed for the persistent, dynamic forefoot adduction is an abnormal insertion of the posterior tibial tendon. Browne and Paton demonstrated that in these persistent cases the posterior tibial tendon inserts predominantly on the medial cuneiform, essentially bypassing the navicular bone.[7] Although the tendon provides a token "slip" to the navicular, its primary attachment is more distal, and it therefore performs a different function than normally. Instead of plantarflexing and inverting the foot at the talonavicular joint, it adducts the forefoot at the naviculocuneiform and cuneiform metatarsal joints.

The treatment Browne and Paton propose consists of transferring the tendon from the abnormal insertion just described to its normal insertion on the navicular bone. They reported satisfactory results in 10 children, 5 of whom had bilateral deformities (hence a total of 15 feet). It is important to emphasize that the average age at which the children were being operated upon was only 20 months.

I have had no personal experience with this operation, and as yet I have not seen a case of metatarsus varus for which I felt it to be justified. I do not mean to criticize the procedure, but rather to emphasize the fact that it is rarely necessary.

## Tarsal Coalition

Failure of the tarsal bones to segment represents one of the most interesting of all the complex foot deformities. By definition, a tarsal coalition involves fibrous, cartilaginous, or bony union between two or more tarsal bones, thus forming a single bone that exhibits the combined characteristics of both or all bones involved. A variety of radiographic and pathologic manifestations is associated with the condition, but all exhibit a variable degree of hindfoot rigidity on physical examination. Some are completely or relatively asymptomatic and thus never require any treatment. Indeed, individuals may pass through life never fully aware that they had a tarsal coalition. On the other hand, many require treatment of one sort or another, and surgical correction is not uncommonly necessary. Cowell has written extensively about this curious problem, and the reader is referred to his contributions, from which much of this section has been derived.[13]

This condition was known before the discovery of the x-ray in 1895. According to Conway and Cowell, the earliest allusion to this skeletal defect was made by Buffon in 1750.[8,11] Cruveilhier illustrated an example of a calcaneonavicular coalition in 1829.[14] Conway and Cowell credit Kermission, in 1898, as being the first to demonstrate a tarsal coalition by roentgenographic examination.[11,27] Slomann believed that tarsal coalition was related to the condition known as "peroneal spastic flatfoot," a disorder described later in this chapter.[39] Conway and Cowell reviewed the world's literature on the subject of tarsal coalition, and all who desire a thorough and exhaustive discussion of the radiologic aspects of this subject should read their classic contribution to our knowledge of this subject. They found that certain special radiographic techniques are often required for diagnosis and accurate depiction of the problem. They also identified some secondary radiographic changes and described a heretofore unrecognized variant of talocalcaneal coalition involving the anterior facet, a lesion that cannot be seen on routine roentgenograms. Furthermore, in reviewing the family histories, a distinct mode of genetic transmission was identified in the developmental forms of the condition.

The causes of tarsal coalition are both developmental and acquired. In the former, there is a strong genetic influence, an observation studied in depth by Cowell and others.[45] In addition to Cowell's studies, Wray and Herndon have written most extensively on this issue. They prefaced their analysis by concluding that the asymptomatic nature of many tarsal coalitions and the difficulty in making the radiographic diagnosis of some of these tarsal anomalies, especially talocalcaneal coalition, are the major factors that have contributed to our relative lack of meaningful genetic studies in these conditions.[45] They reported three cases of calcaneonavicular bar in three successive generations of one family and concluded that this heritable pattern was most consistent with a single gene mutation, autosomal dominant, with *reduced penetrance,* being responsible for the anomaly.

ETIOLOGY AND
GENETIC CHARACTERISTICS

Leonard came to a slightly different conclusion in his study of 31 patients with tarsal coalition.[30] He studied 98 of their first-degree relatives (parents and siblings) and found that 33% of the parents and 56% of the siblings, or a total of 39%, had tarsal coalition. Slightly more than one third of these were of a different type from that affecting the index patient. The 39% figure is substantial when compared to the overall incidence in the general population of less than 1%. Also of interest is that none of these relatives ever complained of painful feet. Leonard concluded that tarsal coalitions are inherited as a unifactorial disorder, autosomal-dominant in type, with nearly *full penetrance.*

Several cases reported in the literature seem to corroborate a genetic cause for several types of tarsal coalition. These include calcaneonavicular coalition,[16,30,45] talocalcaneal coalition,[12,44] talonavicular coalition,[6,23,28,36] and massive tarsal coalition.[4]

The association of talonavicular synostosis with symphalangism is well known.[3,10] Both types of symphalangism (involvement of the proximal interphalangeal joints of the hand versus the distal interphalangeal joints) are caused by an autosomal dominant gene. Talonavicular synostosis has been reported only with the proximal interphalangeal variety of symphalangism.

Wray and Herndon felt that the strongest evidence points to distinct genetic mutations, for each type of abnormal fusion rather than to a single gene that predisposes to the various clinical types of coalition. They support this idea with the observation that two separate genes appear to be responsible for the two types of symphalangism. On the other hand, the work of Leonard seems to challenge this concept. Leonard showed that different types of coalitions were present in several first-degree relatives of index patients with a given type of tarsal coalition. Thus, we can conclude that tarsal coalition is genetically determined, although the exact mode of inheritance currently remains somewhat controversial.

PATHOGENESIS

It was long believed that tarsal coalitions could be attributed to the fusion of accessory ossicles to adjacent tarsal bones. Pfitzner deserves much of the credit for this concept. The German anatomist, in 1896, published an article describing two small accessory bones occasionally found coexisting with tarsal coalitions,[35] namely, the os sustentaculum (middle facet talocalcaneal coalition) and the os calcaneum secondarium (calcaneonavicular coalition).

Jack, in 1954, was one of the first to disagree with this concept.[24] He felt that radiographic evidence showed only a small portion of the anomalies to be derived from an accessory ossicle that had fused with adjacent tarsal bones. He believed that the origin of the abnormality was related to the early differentiation of the mesenchyme that was destined to become the specialized tissues of the hindfoot. His hypothesis was basically that primitive mesenchyme failed to differentiate and segment. Harris supported this hypothesis when she showed, in 1955, that such anomalies can occur in the fetus, a fact that has since become well known and accepted.[19] These scientific findings thus refute the concept of fusion of accessory ossicles to adjacent tarsals.

Tarsal coalitions resulting from acquired causes include those following operations (subtalar arthrodesis and triple arthrodesis) and those due to inflammatory disorders such as rheumatoid arthritis (with resultant subtalar arthrodesis), to trauma (fracture with spontaneous arthrodesis), and degenerative changes in the tarsal joints producing arthrodesis. In these instances of acquired coalition, genetic factors obviously have little, if any, causative role.

CLINICAL
MANIFESTATIONS

The four most common examples of tarsal coalition, in order of frequency, are those involving the calcaneonavicular, the talocalcaneal, the talonavicular, and the calcaneocuboid joints. If the coalition is fibrous, it is possible to have nearly normal tarsal motion. If the coalition is cartilaginous, the motion will be substantially reduced, and if the coalition is osseous, depending on the location of the union, most, but not all, hindfoot motion will be lost. As noted previously, because a coalition conceptually may proceed from fibrous to cartilaginous to bony union during growth, physical findings may change with skeletal maturation. The diagnosis therefore is rarely made in infancy and early childhood simply because the patient is almost invariably asymptomatic and because the motion of the tarsal bones will be normal or nearly so (no osseous coalition).

Although an unknown number of tarsal coalitions are painless, symptoms, when they do occur, usually develop during adolescence. This is not only because young children rarely complain of foot pain, irrespective of the nature of the foot deformity, but also because the tissue joining the bones does not ossify (thus increasing rigidity) until this age. Most patients complain of aching pain related to activity and usually located in the hindfoot region. Walking over irregular terrain is an especially common related factor. Several of my patients first experienced symptoms when they attempted a new and more advanced physical activity such as ballet or gymnastics.

The foot may appear completely normal on outward inspection. The configuration of the foot, longitudinal arch, and the attitude of the hindfoot and forefoot are often indistinguishable from normal. On the other hand, some will exhibit a distinctly flattened longitudinal arch with a valgus heel. It is this foot to which Slomann must have referred when he related tarsal coalition to the "peroneal spastic flatfoot."[40] Rarely, according to Conway and Cowell, a tarsal coalition may be associated with a cavus foot. Also, I have encountered cartilaginous tarsal coalitions when operating on teratologic clubfeet.

The striking physical finding in the adolescent child is the sharply limited passive motion of the tarsal bones. This is especially evident when examining the subtalar joint motion, if the coalition is in the talocalcaneal joint. A similar but lesser degree of reduction in subtalar motion is evident in calcaneonavicular coalition, but hindfoot motion will be less restricted in coalitions involving the calcaneocuboid joint.[37]

"Peroneal spasm" has been referred to frequently in these feet. It is surely possible to have some degree of spasm in any foot that is painful; in the painless coalition, however, it is difficult to demonstrate whether this is a true spasm or whether the tightness of the peroneals is simply a secondary adaptive change in the foot that has sharply restricted tarsal joint motion. Nevertheless, it is this poorly understood but commonly associated finding that has created some of the confusion about the two conditions, which in this chapter are clearly separated from each other.

Each of these conditions involving failure of segmentation poses somewhat different diagnostic problems both clinically and radiologically. Thus, each will be discussed separately from the standpoint of diagnosis and treatment.

CALCANEONAVICULAR COALITION. As noted previously, the degree of reduction of tarsal joint motion found on clinical examination reflects whether the coalition is fibrous, cartilaginous, or bony. These findings, coupled with the symptoms of either pain or rigidity, prompt the radiographic studies necessary to establish the diagnosis.

*Diagnosis.* In all suspected coalitions, more than the standard anteroposterior and lateral roentgenograms are required to demonstrate the lesion. In the case of calcaneonavicular fusion, one may suspect a bony bar in these conventional views, but an oblique projection of the foot, taken at approximately 45°, is essential to establish the diagnosis. Even then, Conway and Cowell claim that some coalitions may be missed unless additional views are taken in various degrees of obliquity.[11]

In the case of a solid bony bar, the diagnosis is usually rather easy

(Fig. 9-4). In instances in which the bar is fibrous or cartilaginous, however, one must use additional radiographic observations. In such cases, Conway and Cowell have observed interesting and irregular cortical surfaces at the site of the suspected coalition. As with all cases of tarsal coalition, any associated coalition should be excluded before contemplating treatment; however, coexistence of multiple tarsal coalitions in otherwise normal limbs is rare.

*Treatment.* If the patient has sufficient symptoms, treatment of some form is required. A variety of therapeutic methods is available, and an equally variable response to the different forms of treatment may occur from one patient to another. In the older child and adolescent, temporary restriction of physical activities, accompanied by mild analgesics, may alleviate the symptoms. In others, a below-knee cast for 6 weeks may be essential. Often these two modes of therapy provide lasting relief (Fig. 9-5). The reason for the pain is not always clear; equally enigmatic is why simple measures such as these solve the problem, often permanently.

A few patients in older childhood and early adolescence will not respond to the nonoperative measures just outlined. In these cases, if symptoms persist, operative treatment may be required. In the younger patient who is not yet skeletally mature and who has no secondary degenerative changes in the other tarsal joints, simple but radical excision of the fibrous, chondral, or osseous bar usually will solve the problem.

Mitchell and Gibson were the first to publish a report of a series in which a calcaneonavicular bar was excised in a group of young, symptomatic patients who did not have degenerative or adaptive changes in the hindfoot.[33] These authors did not recommend interposition of the extensor digitorum brevis, which was later described by Cowell in 1972.[13] The raw bone surfaces, however, were cauterized. In their series of 41 patients followed for an average of 6 years, satisfactory results were obtained in 31 feet and unsatisfactory results in 10. Their good results exhibited restoration of a significant degree ($> 25°$) of inversion and substantial or complete relief of pain. They reported that the bar recurred to a major degree in one third of the cases and to a slight degree in another third. They emphasized, however, that incomplete recurrence of the bar can be compatible with a mobile, painless foot.

The procedure Cowell favors is excision of the lesion accompanied by interposition of the muscle belly of the extensor digitorum brevis into the defect created by the excision.[13] This is done to prevent or discourage reformation of the bony bridge (Fig. 9-6). According to Cowell, tarsal joint motion was often increased and pain was relieved in 23 of his 26 patients, or approximately 90% successful results.[12] I have employed this operation only on two occasions, and in both patients the symptoms were relieved and tarsal motion was increased slightly.

Tachdjian has reported resecting the calcaneonavicular bar and then interposing a free fat graft,[41] much as done by Langenskiold

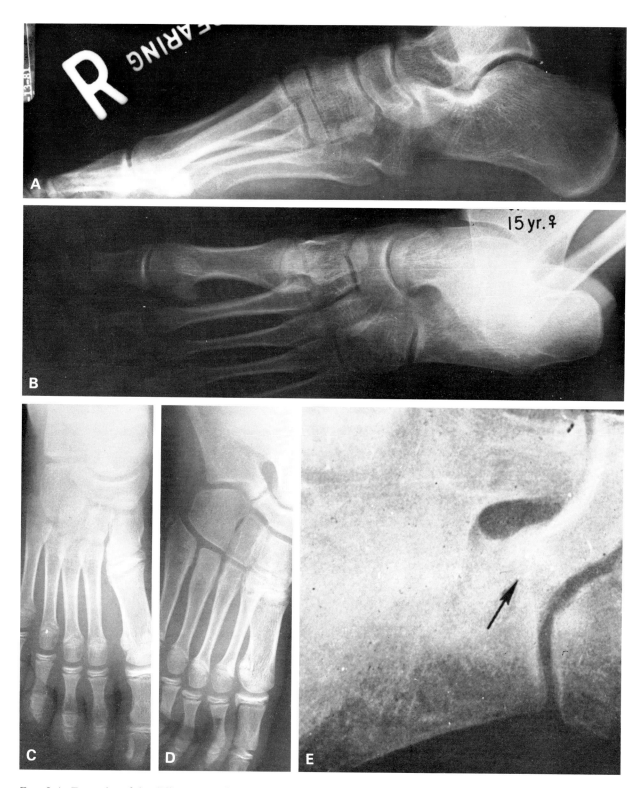

FIG. 9-4. Examples of the different manifestations of calcaneonavicular tarsal coalition. Two suggestive radiographic findings consist of (**A**) a talocalcaneal "beak" and (**B**) poor delineation of the osseous shadow in the oblique view. **C**, The anteroposterior view of a 12-year-old boy shows no obvious abnormality, but the oblique view (**D**) shows a partial calcaneonavicular coalition with sharp sclerotic margins between the two bones. **E**, A complete solid calcaneonavicular osseous union is readily seen (arrow).

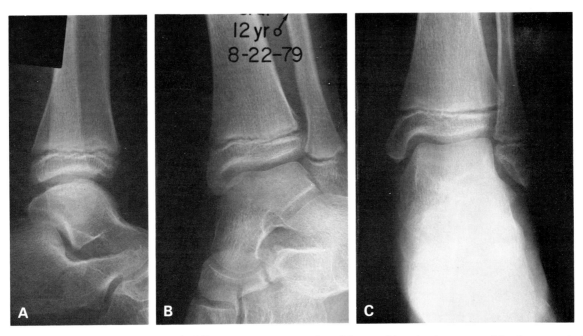

FIG. 9-5 Anteroposterior, lateral, and oblique roentgenograms in a 12-year-old male show a partial calcaneonavicular coalition. The patient had substantially restricted subtalar motion and a rather sudden onset of foot pain upon activity. A below-knee walking cast was applied for 6 weeks. One year later, he was totally asymptomatic and unrestricted in his physical activities. (Courtesy of Dr. Michael Naeve, Boise, Idaho.)

when resecting bony bridges across the physes of long bones.[29] He claims successful restoration of motion in 18 consecutive cases. All authors unanimously recommend that the procedures just described be carried out only in symptomatic patients in whom no degenerative or adaptive changes of the hindfoot have occurred. They also agree on the need for triple arthrodesis if these secondary degenerative changes exist in a patient who has sufficiently severe symptoms and is old enough to qualify for this operation.

Postoperatively, the patient wears a below-knee walking cast for 6 weeks. Thereafter the patient engages in a passive-range-of-motion exercise program in an effort to increase hindfoot motion, accompanied by a program of muscle-strengthening exercises directed towards strengthening all motor units about the foot and ankle, but especially the peroneal and posterior tibial musculotendinous units. Unrestricted activities are permitted, depending on symptoms, once the cast is removed.

In older adolescents and young adults, this more conservative program usually does not successfully relieve painful symptoms or increase motion. Secondary adaptive changes such as talonavicular "beaking" (Fig. 9-4) and/or other degenerative changes often will occur that compromise the result. In these instances, a triple arthrodesis is the only satisfactory solution when symptoms justify surgical correction and when nonoperative measures have failed. The operation consists of simply completing the triple arthrodesis, taking appropriate corrective osteocartilaginous wedges in the joints (and the bar) whenever a substantial or unattractive foot deformity might exist.

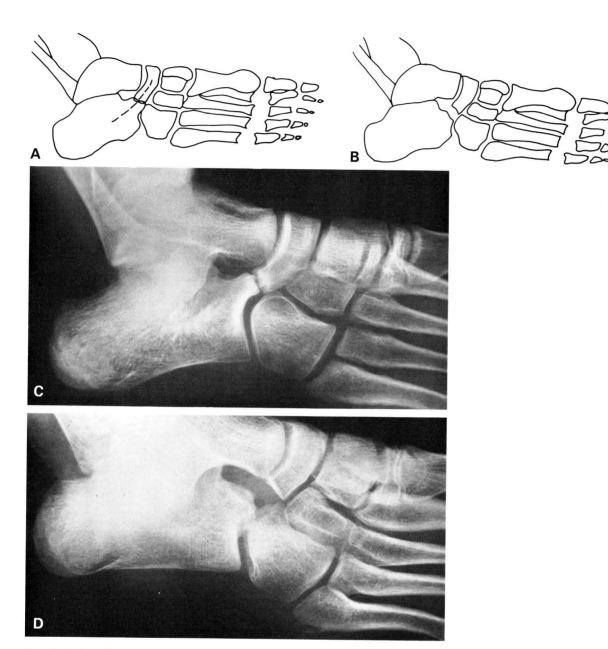

FIG. 9-6. Cowell's technique for excision of the osteochondral fusion of the calcaneus and navicular. **A,** The incision over the sinus tarsus; **B,** the amount of resection necessary to accomplish correction. **C** and **D,** Pre- and postoperative oblique roentgenograms. (Courtesy of Dr. H. R. Cowell, Wilmington, Delaware.)

TALOCALCANEAL COALITION. According to Conway and Cowell, Zuckerkandl described this particular coalition in 1877.[11,46] Later, Korvin described a special axial view that best demonstrates the lesion radiographically.[28] Others, such as Harris, Beath, Conway, and Cowell, have reaffirmed that the posteroanterior axial ("ski jump") view taken at approximately 45° from the horizontal (Fig. 9-7) is necessary to accurately identify the lesion.[11,22] It must be emphasized, however, that a single angle may not provide the view necessary to demonstrate a talocalcaneal coalition, as outlined by Harris, who suggested addi-

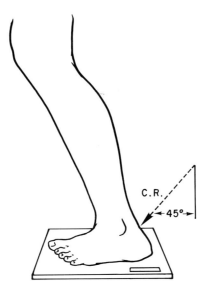

FIG. 9-7. Position of the foot and ankle on the x-ray cassette and the direction of the x-ray beam necessary for an axial view of the calcaneus or a direct view of the posterior talocalcaneal facet.

tional views taken at 30°, 35°, and 40°. The need for these extra views is well illustrated by the work of Conway and Cowell (Fig. 9-8).[11] These authors furthermore emphasized that this view of the talocalcaneal joint will not permit proper visualization of the anterior facet; therefore, if one truly suspects a subtalar coalition and the axial views do not show one, additional views are necessary.

Several "secondary signs" that can exist in one or another of the three joints of the hindfoot prompt the suspicion of a talocalcaneal coalition in one or more facets between the talus and calcaneus. As mentioned earlier, an osteophyte on the talar side of the talonavicular joint is a radiographic clue commonly encountered that suggests

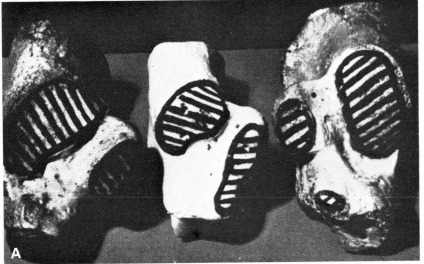
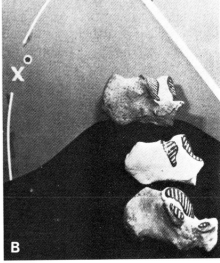

FIG. 9-8. The variations in size and configuration of the subtalar facets are well demonstrated in these specimens, shown graphically from the superior aspect of the calcaneus (**A**). **B**, The reason why different projections of the x-ray beam are essential in order to demonstrate these variations is illustrated. (Conway, J. J., and Cowell, H. R.: Tarsal coalition: Clinical significance and roentgenographic demonstration. Radiology, *92*:799, 1969.)

talocalcaneal coalition. Development of this bony spur has been attributed to increased or compensatory motion that must take place at the talonavicular joint because motion has been blocked at the talocalcaneal joint. It is a reasonable explanation because this is seen commonly several years after an extra-articular subtalar arthrodesis has been performed in children who needed a hindfoot stabilizing procedure (Fig. 9-9). In 24 cases of talocalcaneal coalition, Conway and Cowell encountered the osteophytic spur in 15 patients.[11] These authors have popularized other suggestive radiographic findings, including broadening of the lateral process of the talus and narrowing of the posterior calcaneal facet. In keeping with the concepts outlined previously, these changes have been attributed to the abnormal tarsal motions imposed by failure of the talocalcaneal segmentation.

The most common talocalcaneal coalition occurs in the region of the sustentaculum tali. A fusion of the posterior facet is much rarer. The axial views mentioned and illustrated earlier nearly always divulge a coalition of one or the other if they are present. The anterior facet cannot be seen by these views, however, and in such situations in which clinical and ancillary radiographic signs strongly suggest a talocalcaneal bar, a lateral tomogram is recommended (Fig. 9-10). The purpose of this radiographic study is to disclose a possible coalition of the anterior facet. Conway and Cowell call this the "hidden" coalition.[11] These authors have illustrated beautifully the variability of the subtalar facet joints (Fig. 9-8), and it is essential to remember these variations when attempting to interpret radiographs of this particular group of joints.

Experience with treating this more uncommon coalition has been much less extensive than with the more frequently encountered calca-

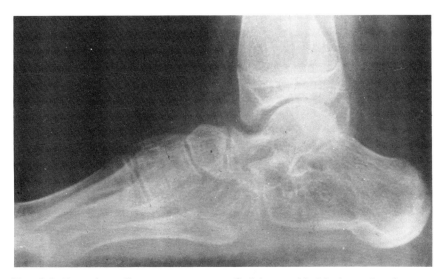

Fig. 9-9. Lateral standing roentgenogram of a 14-year-old girl who had undergone subtalar bone block 10 years earlier at 4 years of age for treatment of congenital vertical talus. The talonavicular "beak" is clearly seen, along with a solid subtalar arthrodesis. (Coleman, S. S., Stelling, F. H. III, and Jarrett, J.: Pathomechanics and treatment of congenital vertical talus. Clin. Orthop., *70*:72, 1970.)

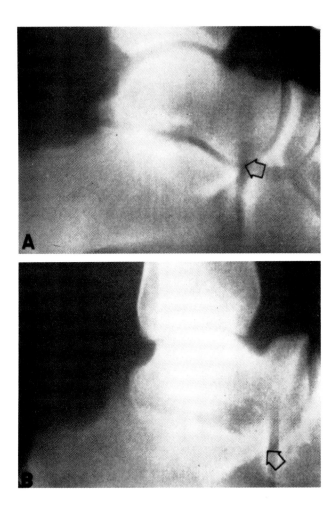

FIG. 9-10. Lateral tomograms show the difficulty in demonstrating subtalar coalition in the anterior facet. **A** shows a normal anterior facet. **B** illustrates a talonavicular "beak," suggesting a coalition, and the lack of definition of the anterior foot. (Conway, J. J. and Cowell, H. R.: Tarsal coalition: Clinical significance and roentgenographic demonstration. Radiology, *92:*799, 1969.)

neonavicular coalition. I have not attempted to excise this lesion; Conway and Cowell claim that such efforts have failed in their hands. Therefore, the treatment resolves itself into either nonoperative efforts to temporarily restrict activities, a trial of a below-knee walking cast, or a triple arthrodesis.

For surgical treatment of the symptomatic medial talocalcaneal coalition, Harris recommends a medial approach both for exposure of the subtalar and talonavicular joints and for the opportunity to recognize an incomplete, fibrous, or cartilaginous talocalcaneal bridge.[20] If the coalition is solid bone, it follows that subtalar pain cannot be a problem, and only the talonavicular joint need be fused. If the talocalcaneal bar is incomplete or is not solid bone, and/or if a valgus deformity is present that requires correction, he recommends performing a double (talonavicular and subtalar) arthrodesis. He feels that the calcaneocuboid joint need not be fused.

Dwyer, in 1976, suggested that, in those patients with excessive hindfoot valgus secondary to tarsal coalition (both calcaneonavicular and talocalcaneal), the oblique strain on the foot played an important part in propogating the symptoms.[15] He therefore suggested correcting hindfoot valgus by calcaneal osteotomy with insertion of a lateral wedge. Cain modified Dwyer's approach by performing a medial closing-wedge osteotomy of the calcaneus.[9] In both series, only those patients who had severe hindfoot valgus and did not respond to conservative measures were considered candidates for surgical correction. Both reported a consistent ability to restore the heel to normal, but residual pes planus was a frequent result. Cain, in his series of 14 patients followed for an average of approximately 8 years, reported relief of pain and improvement in motion (especially inversion) in all.

Talonavicular Coalition. Anderson is credited as being the first to describe this lesion in 1879.[1] It is seen most commonly in instances of terminal limb deficiency and is rare in otherwise normal lower limbs. Therefore, any in-depth discussion of treatment is not meaningful in this text. I have never encountered such a case; according to those who have, the radiographic diagnosis is rather uncomplicated and straightforward.

Calcaneocuboid Coalition. This lesion is not uncommon in terminal limb deficiencies such as partial or complete fibular agenesis. In otherwise normal lower limbs, however, only seven cases have been reported in the world's literature through 1969.[11] The radiographic diagnosis can be made easily by means of routine anteroposterior and lateral films of the foot. I have had no experience with treatment of this problem, but conceptually it probably should be managed in the same manner as the other tarsal coalitions described earlier.

This foot deformity can and should be separated from tarsal coalition, with which it has been associated heretofore in most publications dealing with foot abnormalities, because a peroneal spastic foot does not always have a tarsal coalition. This is an important issue and has considerable bearing upon treatment and prognosis. For example, a rigid hindfoot due to a tarsal coalition has a relatively predictable behavior depending upon the many pathologic issues outlined in the previous section. The peroneal spastic foot that does not have coalition is the result of a variety of etiologic factors, including posterior tibial tenosynovitis, subtalar joint synovitis, adhesive capsulitis of the subtalar joint, and other pathologic conditions that irritate the triple joint. One can distinguish between the rigid hindfoot in tarsal coalition and a similar finding in the condition described here, among other means, by examination under anesthesia. Thus, in the peroneal spastic foot that is *not* due to coalition, the hindfoot will often have greatly increased, if not normal, motion under anesthesia as compared to examination without anesthesia. Clearly, this is an important distinction to establish. Appropriate radiograms of the foot in older children can

*Peroneal Spastic Foot*

usually establish the presence or absence of a coalition (see previous section). Furthermore, a careful clinical examination may provide clues to some of the possible causes of irritation of the triple joint that produce the rigid hindfoot in peroneal spastic foot in which no coalition can be demonstrated radiographically.

ETIOLOGY Any condition that limits subtalar motion can produce peroneal spastic flatfoot, especially if the restricted motion is painful. At least four different major etiologic factors can be identified: those due to trauma, inflammatory disorders, and neoplasms, and a miscellaneous group. Traumatic causes of painful peroneal spastic flatfoot include lesions such as fractures of the calcaneus and talus,[13] and sprains or partial ruptures of the ligaments of the subtalar joint. Often, traumatic conditions may include osteochondral fractures of the subtalar joint and post-traumatic osteoarthritis of the tarsal joints.[12,13]

Inflammatory causes include such disorders as collagen-vascular diseases, especially rheumatoid arthritis of the tarsal joints. This may produce peroneal spasm, resulting in a painful hindfoot valgus. With arthritic destruction of the joints, the foot may acquire a fixed, painful valgus deformity.[22] Other inflammatory disorders include bacterial or mycotic osteomyelitis of the tarsal bones.[24,25] Both benign and malignant neoplasms have been reported to cause painful subtalar motion, specifically, osteoid osteoma and fibrosarcoma of the calcaneus.[12]

A small group of miscellaneous disorders have been associated with peroneal spastic flatfoot. Examples are the mucopolysaccharidoses[34] and other such conditions that distort the tarsal bones and their associated joints.

TREATMENT The treatment of peroneal spastic foot obviously depends upon the cause or causes of the problem, which must be determined before any clearcut therapeutic program can be synthesized. In most instances, the etiologic factor is one that is difficult to treat. For example, the treatment of rheumatoid arthritis of the hindfoot should be directed towards the *systemic* disease, of which the symptoms in the joints of the hindfoot are a local manifestation. This treatment can be supplemented by local measures, such as manipulation, plaster casts, and various rigid orthoses. No reports recommend local intra-articular injections for rheumatoid disease of the hindfoot. Mankin and Shepard and their respective associates found intra-articular steroids to have a deleterious effect on cartilage.[3,32] On the other hand, some rheumatologists do feel that intra-articular steroids in weight-bearing joints can be useful and safe if the joint is protected for a sufficiently long time after the injection.

For peroneal spastic flatfoot resulting from osteochondral fracture of the undersurface of the talus due to impingement by the os calcis, if no degenerative changes are present, Cowell recommended excision of that portion of the os calcis anteriorly that is responsible for the impingement, combined with interposition of the extensor digitorum brevis.[13] If degenerative changes are present at diagnosis, conservative methods such as cast immobilization are implemented; if these are ineffective, triple arthrodesis may be required.

The main purpose for including a special, brief section on these foot deformities is to emphasize the continuing problem of injury to the sciatic nerve from gluteal injections in infancy. Although the types of deformities that result from this iatrogenic factor are variable and highly singular, certain patterns emerge. This section emphasizes the potentially devastating effect of such an untoward event and illustrates the important technical means of preventing such lesions. Treatment clearly is directed towards the specific pathologic manifestations of the deformities. To a large extent, the therapeutic approaches to these problems have been thoroughly covered in previous chapters.

Over the past 15 years, I have encountered a substantial number of pediatric patients whose major problem on presentation was a severe unilateral foot deformity.[5] The fact that made many of these cases unique was that all patients had received intramuscular injections into the hip or thigh when treated for a major febrile illness in infancy. All of these children had received prior poliomyelitis immunizations. Because their clinical manifestations were so unusual and because the electromyographic studies identified the lesion in the sciatic nerve, this special category of complex foot deformities seems justified.

Concern about the possible injury to major peripheral nerves following injection is not new. As early as 1920, Turner proposed giving injections in the lateral thigh in infants and young children in order to reduce the likelihood of sciatic injury.[42] The occurrence of quadriceps fibrosis, however, as reported by Lloyd-Roberts, Thomas, and Gunn, discouraged this proposed alternative method of intramuscular injection.[18,31] This led to some sophisticated studies concerning the preferred site and method of injection. Von Hochstetter, Johnson, and Raptou developed basic concepts of intramuscular injection based on anatomic principles.[26,43] Unfortunately, these concepts occasionally either are unrecognized or ignored because the area of the sciatic nerve in the buttock continues to be violated, with the resulting tragic development of a major foot deformity.

I have identified and treated at least eight patients who fulfilled the criteria just outlined. I encountered the most recent case, representing an almost pure equinovarus deformity, in 1980. Four of these patients developed cavovarus deformities. Two exhibited calcaneocavus deformities, and one (the most recent) had an equinovarus lesion. The eighth patient had a foot palsy of nondescript nature, and was known to have had an injection into the area of the sciatic nerve in the buttocks. The paresis resolved completely, and no abnormality resulted.

The clinical case histories on these patients are reported elsewhere;[5] the important issue in this section is to bring the reader's attention to a condition whose true cause and pathogenesis often go unrecognized. The treatment in all instances was patterned on the principles enunciated in the previous chapters.

*Deformities Secondary to Sciatic Nerve Injuries in Infancy*

Unfortunately, the neurologic damage created by injecting medication into the sciatic nerve of infants is often permanent. Most of these injections damage the lateral (peroneal) division of the sciatic nerve. Anatomic reasons explain the greater susceptibility of this portion of the nerve to any kind of injury. Nevertheless, even this potential susceptibility can be obviated by attention to the precise details of intramuscular gluteal injection as described by Von Hochstetter, Johnson, and Raptou.[26,43] These authors demonstrated that a triangle is found in the gluteal area that is safe for injection of medications, especially if the needle is inserted perpendicular to the long axis of the patient's body rather than perpendicular to the skin. Three lines form this "safe" triangle. The first parallels the crest of the ilium, extending from the posterior-superior to the anterior-superior iliac spine. The other two extend from the greater trochanter to each of these iliac spines (Fig. 9-11).

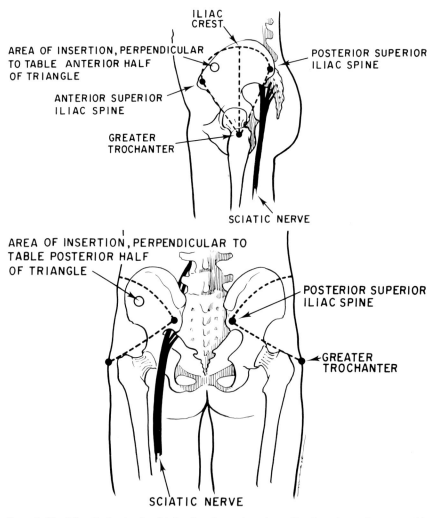

FIG. 9-11. The "safe sites" of injecting intragluteal medications in order to avoid injury to the sciatic nerve. **A,** In the side-lying technique, the preferred site is in the anterior half of the triangle. **B,** In the prone technique, the preferred area is in the posterior triangle (see text for details). (Bigos, S. J. and Coleman, S. S., unpublished data.)

The cavovarus foot was the most common deformity I encountered (Fig. 9-12). I also found two cases of calcaneocavus foot; Figure 9-13 illustrates one of them. As mentioned earlier, treatment of these foot deformities was based upon the concepts and techniques outlined in earlier chapters.

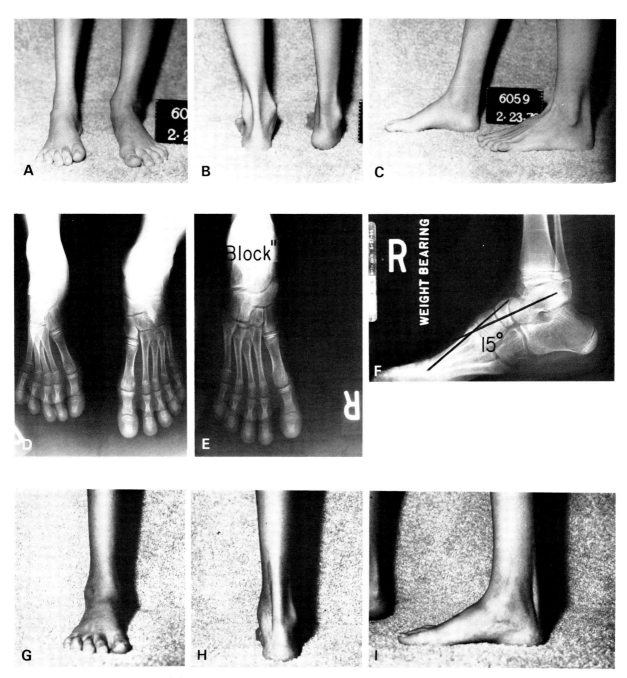

FIG. 9-12. A more common deformity encountered in sciatic nerve injuries is the cavovarus deformity, resulting from paresis of the peroneal portion of the sciatic nerve. **A**, **B**, and **C**, Preoperative standing photographs of the typical deformity. **D**, **E**, and **F**, Preoperative standing roentgenograms, including the block test. **G**, **H**, and **I**, Postoperative photos, following radical plantar release, heelcord lengthening, and tendon transfers.

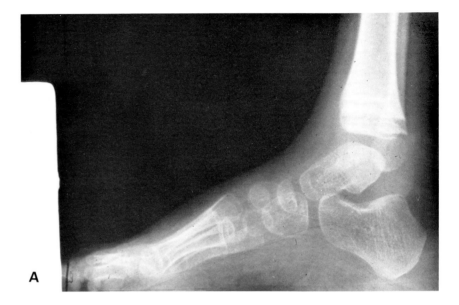

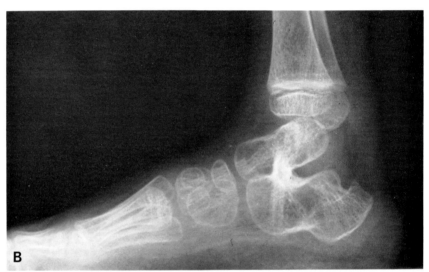

FIG. 9-13. Standing pre- (**A**) and 1-year postoperative (**B**) roentgenograms show an instance of calcaneocavus foot due to sciatic injury in infancy. (**A** and **B**). A 7-year-old boy developed a limp following a febrile illness in infancy, during which he received gluteal injections. Electromyographic studies showed denervation of the triceps surae muscle group, traceable to the sciatic nerve in the region of the buttock.

*References*

1. Anderson, R. F.: The presence of an astragalo-scaphoid bone in man. J. Anat. Physiol., *14:*452, 1879–1880.
2. Austin, F. H.: Symphalangism and related fusions of tarsal bones. Radiology, *56:*882, 1951.
3. Behrens, F., Shepard, N., and Mitchell, N.: Alteration of rabbit articular cartilage by intra-articular injections of glucocorticoids. J. Bone Joint Surg., *57A:*70, 1975.
4. Bersanti, F. A., and Samilson, R. L.: Massive familial tarsal synostosis. J. Bone Joint Surg., *39A:*1187, 1957.
5. Bigos, S. L., and Coleman, S. S.: Unpublished data reported at annual Shrine Scientific Program, Salt Lake City, Utah, April, 1980.

6. Boyd, H. B.: Congenital talonavicular synostosis. J. Bone Joint Surg., *26:*682, 1944.
7. Browne, R. S., and Paton, D. F.: Anomalous insertion of the tibialis posterior tendon in congenital metatarsus varus. J. Bone Joint Surg., *61B:*74, 1970.
8. Buffon, G. L. L.: Comte de: Histoire naturelle avec la description du cabinet du Roy. Tome, *3:*47, 1750.
9. Cain, T. J., and Hyman, S.: Peroneal spastic flatfoot, its treatment by osteotomy of the os calcis. J. Bone Joint Surg., *60B:*527, 1978.
10. Challis, J.: Hereditary transmission of talonavicular coalition in association with anomaly of the little finger. J. Bone Joint Surg., *56A:*1273, 1974.
11. Conway, J. J., and Cowell, H. R.: Tarsal coalition: Clinical significance and roentgenographic demonstration. Radiology, *92:*799, 1969.
12. Cowell, H. R.: Diagnosis and management of peroneal spastic flatfoot. In *AAOS Instructional Course Lectures.* St. Louis, C. V. Mosby, 1965, p. 94. Vol. 24.
13. Cowell, H. R.: Talocalcaneal coalition and new causes of peroneal spastic flatfoot. CORR, *85:*16, 1972.
14. Cruveilhier, J.: Anatomie pathologique du corps humain. Tome, *I:*1829–1835.
15. Dwyer, F. C.: Causes, significance and treatment of the subtaloid joint. Proc. R. Soc. Med., *69:*97, 1976.
16. Glessner, J. R., and Davis, G. L.: Bilateral calcaneonavicular coalition occurring in twin boys. CORR, *47:*173, 1966.
17. Goldner, J. L.: Personal communication, 1980.
18. Gunn, D. R.: Contractures of the quadriceps muscle. J. Bone Joint Surg., *46B:*492, 1964.
19. Harris, B. A.: Anomalous structures in the developing human foot (abstract). Anat. Res., *121:*399, 1955.
20. Harris, R. I.: Retrospect—peroneal spastic flatfoot (rigid valgus foot). J. Bone Joint Surg., *47A:*1657, 1965.
21. Harris, R. I.: Rigid valgus foot. J. Bone Joint Surg., *37A:*169, 1955.
22. Harris, R. I., and Beath, T.: Etiology of peroneal spastic flatfoot. J. Bone Joint Surg., *30B:*624, 1948.
23. Hodgson, F. G.: Talonavicular synostosis. South. Med. J., *39:*940, 1946.
24. Jack, E. A.: Bone anomalies of the tarsus in relation to peroneal spastic flatfoot. J. Bone Joint Surg., *36B:*530, 1954.
25. Johnson, J. C.: Peroneal spastic flatfoot syndrome. South. Med. J., *69:*807, 1976.
26. Johnson, E. W., and Raptou, A. D.: A study of intragluteal injections. Arch. Phys. Med. Rehabil., *46:*167, 1965.
27. Kermission, E.: Double pied bot varus par malformation osseuse primitive associe a des ankyloses congenitales des doigts et des orteils chez quatre membres d'une meme famille. Rev. Orthop., *9:*392, 1898.
28. Korvin, H.: Coalition talocalcanea. Z. Orthop. Chir., *60:*105, 1934.
29. Langenskiold, A.: An operation for partial closure of an epiphyseal plate in children and its experimental basis. J. Bone Joint Surg., *57B:*325, 1975.
30. Leonard, M. A.: The inheritance of tarsal coalition and its relationship to spastic flatfoot. J. Bone Joint Surg., *56B:*520, 1974.
31. Lloyd-Roberts, G. C., and Thomas, T. G.: The etiology of quadriceps contracture in children. J. Bone Joint Surg., *46B:*498, 1964.
32. Mankin, H. S., and Conger, K. A.: The acute effects of intra-articular hydrocortisone on articular cartilage in rabbits. J. Bone Joint Surg., *48A:*1383, 1966.
33. Mitchell, G. P., and Gibson, J. M. C.: Excision of calcaneonavicular bar for painful spasmodic flatfoot. J. Bone Joint Surg., *49B:*281, 1967.
34. Outland, T., and Murphy, I. D.: The pathomechanics of peroneal spastic flatfoot. CORR, *16:*64, 1960.
35. Pfitzner, W.: Die Variationen im Auf-bau des Fusskelets. Morphologisches Arbeiten, *6:*245, 1896.
36. Rothberg, A. S., Feldman, F. W., and Schuster, O. F.: Congenital fusion of astragalus and scaphoid: Bilateral; inherited. N.Y. J. Med., *35:*29, 1935.

37. Samuelson, K. M.: Personal communication, 1981.
38. Schreiber, R. R.: Talonavicular synostosis. J. Bone Joint Surg., *45A*:170, 1963.
39. Slomann, H. C.: On coalitio calcaneo-navicularis. J. Orthop. Surg., *3*:586, 1921.
40. Slomann, H. C.: On the demonstration and analysis of calcaneo-navicular coalition by roentgen examination. Acta. Radiol., *5*:304, 1926.
41. Tachdjian, M. D.: Personal communication, 1981.
42. Turner, G. G.: The site for intramuscular injections. Lancet, *2*:819, 1920.
43. Von Hochstetter, A.: Problems and technique of intragluteal injections. Part 2. Influence of injection technique on the development of the syringe injuries. Schweiz. Med. Wochenschr., *86*:69, 1956.
44. Webster, F. S., and Roberts, W. M.: Tarsal anomalies and peroneal spastic flatfoot. JAMA, *146*:1099, 1951.
45. Wray, J. B., and Herndon, C. N.: Hereditary transmission of congenital coalition of the calcaneus to the navicular. J. Bone Joint Surg., *45A*:365, 1963.
46. Zuckerkandl, E.: Ueber einen Fall von Synostose zwischen Talus und Calcaneus. Allg. Wein Med. Zeitung., *22*:293, 1877.

# Index

Page numbers in *italics* indicate figures; page numbers followed by "t" indicate tables.

# Cavovarusfoot

## Etiology -
a) residual clubfoot
b) neurologic
c) idiopathic - Dx. of exclusion

## Path
Varus hindfoot
Planterflexed forefoot
(windlass from FHL depressing 1st MT head indirectly)

$\left.\begin{array}{c} \\ \\ \end{array}\right\}$ ± Clawtoes

## Test hindfoot seperately -
Must eliminate the forefoot
"Block test" - tests hindfoot flexibility

If hindfoot remains in varus - Fixed deformity.
Define joint of problem -   subtalar joint = planter medial release
either                       calcaneus = osteotomy
(get skijumperview
to determine which is
at fault)

If hindfoot flexible -
Planter releases -   ± tarsal joints
                     ± metatarsal osteotomy
                     ± cuneiform osteotomy.

Tom Faciszewski, M.D

Tom Faciszewski, M.D